Women's Voices in Psychiatry

Women's Voices in Psychiatry
A collection of essays

Edited by

Gianetta Rands

Consultant Psychiatrist, Re:Cognition Health, London, UK;
Mental Capacity Act Adviser and Executive Member,
Faculty of Old Age Psychiatry, Royal College of Psychiatrists,
London, UK

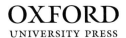
OXFORD
UNIVERSITY PRESS

OXFORD

UNIVERSITY PRESS

Great Clarendon Street, Oxford, OX2 6DP,
United Kingdom

Oxford University Press is a department of the University of Oxford.
It furthers the University's objective of excellence in research, scholarship,
and education by publishing worldwide. Oxford is a registered trade mark of
Oxford University Press in the UK and in certain other countries

Published in the United States of America by Oxford University Press
198 Madison Avenue, New York, NY 10016, United States of America

British Library Cataloguing in Publication Data

Data available

Library of Congress Control Number: 2017962124

ISBN 978–0–19–878548–4

Printed in Great Britain by
Ashford Colour Press Ltd, Gosport, Hampshire

Foreword

Gianetta Rands and I began to ruminate over dinner one evening about how faint the voices were of women in the public discourse of psychiatry, even those of the most successful in career terms, compared with men. Perhaps that is because women have often contributed in ways that have been traditionally less valued in a man's world, although the leadership and personal drive that are required to devise improved service models and change the way society regards mental disorders and disturbed families are as intellectually demanding and challenging as any research project. Gianetta suggested we needed to do more shouting about women's achievements. I agreed and this book is the fascinating result.

Women's lives have changed immeasurably in the last century but we are often still chasing an elusive cultural ideal of fulfilling many roles at the same time, negotiating the shifting priorities of love, children, ambition and financial necessity throughout our careers. Emily Wills' final marvellous poem on page 298 'The Other Women in the Wardrobe' articulates the inevitable regrets, the difficult choices, the acceptance of change and also an elegy for opportunities lost or abandoned. All these are reflected in the chapters that follow, giving women psychiatrists a chance to describe what has been important to them, not only as clinicians, scientists and professional carers but as patients, writers and prominent leaders of the profession in the United Kingdom. There are good stories here to inspire any man or woman embarking on a career in medicine today, stories which capture the essence of our recent history and provide a launchpad for the next generation of psychiatrists.

Baroness Elaine Murphy,
Member of the House of Lords
Formerly Professor of Old Age Psychiatry, University of London

Preface

To quote a companion book preface 'The provenance of this volume of essays is two-fold.'[1] First, in summer 2015, on retirement from NHS work, I presented an exit seminar entitled 'Career Reflections of a 1970s Feminist'. A colleague warned me not to be boringly nostalgic. On the contrary: I didn't feel warm nostalgia from reciting my reminiscences. Many events in my career should not be repeated. Many areas showed evidence of change for the better over the past 40 years. An aim of writing about this is to record this history so that services for people when they are mentally ill can improve. A separate aim is to describe the professional work of women psychiatrists in the twentieth century.

A version of my seminar is the first chapter in this anthology. Feedback from current psychiatry trainees made it clear how important this book is and that advances in feminism, equality, education, and our profession happen in waves, with troughs as well as peaks.

Second, I read a book review by Baroness Elaine Murphy[2] of a collection of essays called *Psychiatry: Past, Present, and Prospect*.[1] It had 3 male editors from the United States, Australia, and the United Kingdom, and 28 authors, only 3 of which were women. Where are the women's voices? Baroness Murphy's role was as reviewer; there was no reference to her ground-breaking psychiatric career as clinician, researcher, senior manager, and Cross-Bench Peer in the House of Lords.

I contacted Oxford University Press, the publisher of the book and suggested that this was a clear example of gender bias in scientific publications, adding that over 50 per cent of UK medical students and nearly 50 per cent of its psychiatrists are now women. Where were the women's voices?

For this book, I was in the right place at the right time. After years of contributing to Royal College of Psychiatrists committees I have connections with women psychiatrists and trainees throughout the United Kingdom. I had just left my National Health Service (NHS) job so had time, momentum, and energy available to dedicate to what I believe is a very important record.

This project

This book is an anthology, a collection of chapters written by women psychiatrists working in England and Wales. There is a wide age range of authors from colleagues in their 80s to colleagues in their 20s. All authors are psychiatrists, with the addition of a medical journalist and a senior NHS manager.

The range of topics covered is diverse. Women professionals seem to get themselves into niche areas for reasons that will become apparent in the chapters that follow and are largely specific to socio-political attitudes of the late twentieth century. Interspersed between the chapters are short biographical profiles of pioneering women who have contributed to psychiatry and mental health services. There is a wide range of writing styles. Some are autobiographical, some biographies, some are descriptive, and some more evidence-based analyses.

This is not meant to be a textbook. There are excellent textbooks of psychiatry that are regularly updated. This is also not a guide to mental illnesses. The Royal College of Psychiatrists has many acclaimed information leaflets about mental illnesses[3] and in 2017 published 'The Female Mind: A User's Guide' edited by Kathryn Abel and Rosalind Ramsay, both psychiatrists.

This is a collection of thoughts, opinions, and experiences of women doctors specializing in modern-day psychiatry. It is intended to be accessible to all readers interested in the mind, mental health services, and women's roles in medicine. Psychiatry and mental illnesses can be scary and mysterious, especially as portrayed in some films and literature. However, the more we understand diseases of the brain and disorders of the mind, the more fascinating they become, and the more treatable. Some emotional and personality disorders can be attributed to 'man's inhumanity to man' and that is an issue that requires research from many specialties.

I hope that the chapters in this book go some way to demystifying this fascinating specialty, to destigmatize mental illness, and to encourage young people interested in the mind to think about careers in psychiatry. Whatever the structure of health services in the future, there will always be a need for psychiatrists and other mental health professionals.

Pictures and poems

As a psychology student in the 1970s I often wondered about visual imagery and its role in memory, thinking, understanding, and problem-solving. At the time, cognitive research was predominantly about verbal skills and strategies, with little recognition of non-verbal components. In this anthology, I have encouraged authors to include pictures. This was for two main reasons: first, many of us use visual imagery to think and learn, and second because they offer stepping stones to ponder the content of these chapters. Similarly with the inclusion of poems, as they can challenge our assumptions, prompt imagery, and reframe some attitudes.

Patchworks

As I have pieced together these writings, these individual contributions from women colleagues, each carefully crafted with their own personal style and stories, I have thought about patchworks created by other groups of women and how their collective voices can still be heard. In particular, I think about the Changi quilts.

There are four Changi quilts: two in Australia, the Girl Guide quilt at the Imperial War museum, and the British quilt now in the Red Cross archive and reproduced here with their kind permission (see Figure P.1).

These quilts were embroidered by women and child prisoners of war, held in Changi jail, during the Japanese occupation of Singapore, 1942–45. Each square was embroidered by one person, telling something of herself and her family. Thread was scavenged

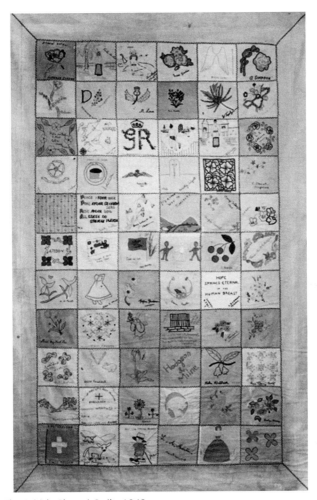

Figure P.1 The British Changi Quilt, 1942
© British Red Cross

from the seams of rotting garments and needles were precious prison trophies, sharpened on the concrete floors.

Many of the women, and men, in Changi jail in 1942 were captured during the aftermath of the Alexandra Military Hospital massacre in which hundreds of doctors, nurses and patients (including one person under anaesthetic) were killed. This hospital had been a beacon of excellence, one of the first to undertake limb re-attachments, and provided medical treatments to thousands injured during the Second World War.

After the War, the hospital continued as a centre of medical excellence and incorporated maternity services. Many baby boomers were born there, including me. Since 1971 it has been incorporated into Singapore medical services and university. Its lush gardens are treasured, especially the serene remembrance garden with its commemorative plaque.

References

1. **Bloch S, Green S,** and **Holmes J** (2014). *Psychiatry: Past, Present, and Prospect.* Oxford: Oxford University Press.

2. **Murphy E** (2015). Book Review. *British Journal of Psychiatry Bulletin* April, **39** (2) 104; DOI: 10.1192/pb.bp.114.048413.

3. <http://www.rcpsych.ac.uk/healthadvice/moreinformation/aboutourleaflets.aspx>.

Acknowledgements

This book exists thanks to its contributors, their writing, ideas, suggestions, edits, enthusiasm, and encouragement. Baroness Elaine Murphy discussed her book review (mentioned earlier) and my thoughts about the underrepresentation of women colleagues in psychiatry publications. She gave good advice: first, find a publisher.

Along the way I have sought advice from many people; I am grateful to Colin Gale, archivist of Bethlem Museum of the Mind for ideas, introductions, and access to that archive. To Alice White, Wikimedian in Residence, Wellcome Library, for guidance on finding images, locating Wellcome treasures, and warnings of 'weasel words' and 'peacock terms'. To Frances Maunze, Archivist and Librarian of the Royal College of Psychiatrists (RCPsych), for support and access to that archive, and to Vanessa Cameron, past Chief Executive of the RCPsych, for encouragement with the writing of this book.

A special thanks to Emily Wills for permission to use her poems; as a poet and general practitioner, she has a medical woman's observations and a poet's skill for using words that create mind-loops, imagery, and essence of emotions. Thanks also to Belinda Rathbone for tips and for drawing my attention to the allegory of truth and time as described in her book, *The Boston Raphael* (Boston, MA: Godine, 2014). Dr Miles Allison generously contributed text from his father, Anthony C Allison, in Profile on Helen Green Allison. I am indebted to Dr Koravangattu Valsraj, Consultant Psychiatrist and Associate Clinical Director, for his enthusiasm about this project and for giving generously of his time and knowledge on Chapter 8.

Helpful comments and corrections have been made to several of these chapters, thanks to Rose Rands, Annabel Rands, Jane Mellanby, Joanna Collicutt, Simon Adelman, Amy Enfield-Bance, Elinor Hynes, Emma Johnson-Gilbert, and Emily Wills.

My effusive gratitude also must be extended to Oxford University Press editors, Peter Stevenson and Lauren Tiley, who have been skilled midwives to this creation.

Gianetta Rands
2017

Contents

Abbreviations *xvii*

Contributors *xxi*

> **Poem**: Domestic Confessional *2*

1 Career Reflections of a 1970s Feminist *3*
Gianetta Rands

2 A History of Women in British Medicine *25*
Abi Rimmer

3 The Entry of Women into Psychiatry *39*
Fiona Subotsky

> **Profile**: The Life of Dr Helen Boyle (1869–1957) *50*
> *Fiona Subotsky*

> **Profile**: Dame Fiona Caldicott: An Inspirational Woman with
> an Astonishingly Impressive Career *52*
> *Katherine Kennet and Fiona Caldicott*

> **Poem**: My Small but Significant Body of Work *56*

4 History of the Royal College of Psychiatrists' Women's Mental
Health Special Interest Group *57*
Jane Mounty, Anne Cremona, and Rosalind Ramsay

5 Psychiatry and Patienthood *73*
Rosemary Lethem

6 Perinatal Psychiatry: Motherhood in Mental Health Services *91*
Jacqueline Humphreys

> **Profile**: Dora Black *104*
> *Rashmi Verma*

7 The Role of Women in Intellectual Disabilities: Clinicians,
Scientists, Parents *109*
Rupal Dave and Angela Hassiotis

> **Profile**: Helen Green Allison (1923–2011): A Story of Hope,
> Faith, and Charity *122*
> *Jane Mounty*

8 Are Women's Mental Health Units Needed? *125*
Aoife Rajyaluxmi Singh

9 Jail Birds: Challenges for Prisoners and Professionals *135*
Annie Bartlett

> **Poem**: Considering the Predictive Value of the Risk Assessment Score *148*

10 The Maternal Lap and the Mental Health Trust *149*
Jo O'Reilly

11 Historical Child Sexual Abuse *161*
Joanne Stubley, Victoria Barker and Maria Eyres

12 Old Age, Women, and Dynamic Psychotherapy *177*
Sandra Evans and Jane Garner

13 A Woman who Made a Difference: An Interview with Nori Graham *189*
Amanda Thompsell

> **Profile**: Eluned Woodford-Williams: 12 September 1913 to 25 November 1984 *202*
> *Itunuayo V. Ayeni*

14 A Woman the Government Feared: Barbara Robb (1912–76) *205*
Claire Hilton

15 Change and Continuity in Psychiatry: One Woman's Reflections *219*
Claire Murdoch

> **Poem**: The Disappeared *229*

> **Profile**: Lisbeth Hockey and Annie Altschul *230*
> *Nikita Hyare*

16 Reducing the Risk of Dementia *233*
Joanne Rodda

17 Whose Life is it Anyway? Life and Death in the Court of Protection *245*
Clementine Maddock

18 Women in Psychiatric Training *253*
Georgina Fozard and Philippa Greenfield

> **Poem**: The Art of Listening *264*

19 Women as Trainers in Psychiatry *265*
Hannah Fosker and Ann Boyle

20 How to Succeed in Psychiatry Without Really Trying: One
Woman's Accidental Pathway to the Top of Her Profession *277*
Wendy Burn

21 The Road Less Travelled *289*
Sue Bailey

    Poem: The Other Women in the Wardrobe *298*

    Index *299*

Abbreviations

ADHD	Attention Deficit Hyperactivity Disorder		CPN	Community Psychiatric Nurse
AEGIS	Aid for the Elderly in Government Institutions		CQC	Care Quality Commission
			CSIP	Care Services Improvement Partnership
AGENDA	Alliance for Women and Girls at Risk		DBT	Dialectical Behaviour Therapy
ALA	Alpha linoleic acid		DC-LD	Diagnostic Criteria for Learning Disabilities, RCPsych 2001
ASPD	Antisocial Personality Disorder			
BBC	British Broadcasting Corporation		DGH	District General Hospital
			DHA	Docosahexanoic acid
BDNF	Brain-derived neurotropic factor		DHSS	Department of Health and Social Security
BMA	British Medical Association		DLB	Dementia with Lewy bodies
BME	black and minority ethnic		DNAR	do not attempt resuscitation
BMI	Body mass index		DoH	Department of Health
BMJ	British Medical Journal		DOLS	Deprivation of Liberty Safeguards, under the Mental Capacity Act (2005); Schedule A1
BPD	Borderline Personality Disorder			
CAIDE	Cardiovascular risk factors, Aging and Dementia			
			DRCOG	Diploma of the Royal College of Obstetricians and Gynaecologists
CAMHS	Child and Adolescent Mental Health Services			
CASC	Clinical Assessment of Skills and Competencies		DSM	Diagnostic and Statistical Manual
CBT	Cognitive Behavioural Therapy		ECT	Electroconvulsive Therapy
CCT	Certificate of Completed Training		EFCAP	European Association for Forensic Child and Adolescent Psychiatry Psychology
CEMD	Confidential Enquiries into Maternal Deaths			
			EMDR	Eye Movement Desensitization and Reprocessing
CIA	Central Intelligence Agency			
CHAT	Comprehensive Health Assessment Tool		EPA	Eicosapentanoic acid
			EPDS	Edinburgh Postnatal Depression Scale
CMHT	Community Mental Health Team			
CoP	Court of Protection		ESMI	Effectiveness of Services for Mothers with Mental Illness
CPA	Care Programme Approach			
CPD	Continuing Professional Development		Exec	SIG Executive Committee

FCAMHS	Forensic Child and Adolescent Mental Health Services	MBRRACE	Mothers and Babies: Reducing Risk through Audits and Confidential Enquiries
FMFS	False Memory Syndrome Foundation	MBU	Mother and Baby Unit
FRCPsych	Fellow, Royal College of Psychiatry	MCA	Mental Capacity Act
		MCI	Mild cognitive impairment
FTD	Frontotemporal dementia	MDT	Multidisciplinary team
GABA	gamma amino-butyric acid	MH	Mental health
GDP	gross domestic product	MHA	Mental Health Act
GMC	General Medical Council	MHLT	Mental Health Liaison Team
GP	General Practitioner		
HC	House of Commons	MHT	Mental Health Trust
HCSA	Historical Child Sexual Abuse	MMC	Modernising Medial Careers
HL	House of Lords	MMHA	Maternal Mental Health Alliance
HMP	Her Majesty's Prison		
HO	House Officer	MoH	Ministry of Health
IAPT	Improving access to psychological therapies	MP	Member of Parliament
		MPS	Medical Protection Society
ICD	International Classification of Diseases	MRCGP	Member of the Royal College of GPs
ID	Intellectual Disability	MRCPsych	Membership of the Royal College of Psychiatrists
IMHA	Independent Mental Health Advocates		
		MTAS	Medical Training Application Service
IoPPN	Institute of Psychiatry, Psychology, and Neuroscience	MWF	Medical Women's Federation
IPT	Interpersonal Therapy	NAMH	National Association for Mental Health (later, Mind)
IQ	Intelligence Quotient		
IWL	Improving Working Lives initiative	NAS	National Autistic Society
		NaSSA	Noradrenergic and Specific Serotonergic Antidepressant
KQCPI	King's and Queen's College of Physicians of Ireland		
LEA	Local Education Authority	NET	Narrative Exposure Therapy
LMA	London Metropolitan Archives	NHS	National Health Service
		NHSE	National Health Service England
LMH	Lady Margaret Hall		
LSA	Licentiate of the Society of Apothecaries	NICE	National Institute for Health and Care Excellence
LSD	Lysergic acid diethylamide	NIMHE	National Institute for Mental Health in England
LTFT	Less than full-time (Training)		
		NTN	National Training Number
MAOI	Monoamine Oxidase Inhibitor	NWMRHB	North West Metropolitan Regional Hospital Board

OCD	Obsessive Compulsive Disorder		Section 12	Of the Mental Health Act (2007), conferring authority to instigate compulsory treatment
OOPE	Out-of-Programme Experience			
OSS	Overseas Special Service		SHO	Senior House Officer
OT	Occupational Therapist		SIG	Special Interest Group
PALS	Patient Advice and Liaison Services		SIG Exec	Special Interest Group Executive Committee
PAR	Population attributable risk		SNRI	Serotonin and Noradrenaline Reuptake Inhibitor
PEG	Percutaneous endoscopic gastrostomy			
PFI	Private Finance Initiative		SPL	Shared Parental Leave
PICU	Psychiatric Intensive Care Unit		SRN	State Registered Nurse
			SSRI	Selective Serotonin Reuptake Inhibitor
PIE	Paedophile Information Exchange		ST	sanitary towel
PHP	Practitioner Health Programme		STD	sexually transmitted disease
			SWH	Scottish Women's Hospitals Committee
PMP	Patient Management Problem			
PPP	Philosophy, Physiology, and Psychology		TCA	Tricyclic Antidepressant
			tf-CBT	Trauma Focused Cognitive Behavioural Therapy
PSS	Psychiatrists' Support Service		TNA	The National Archives
PTSD	Post-Traumatic Stress Disorder		TPD	Training Programme Director
RAE	Research Assessment Exercise		UCL	University College London
			UCLMS	University College London Medical School
RAMC	Royal Army Medical Corps		UK	United Kingdom
RCPsych	Royal College of Psychiatrists		USA	United States of America
			UWMRC	University of Warwick Modern Records Collection
RCT	Randomized controlled trial			
RFH	Royal Free Hospital		VAD	Voluntary aid detachment
RFHSM	Royal Free Hospital School of Medicine		WAAC	Women's Army Auxiliary Corps
RHB	Regional Hospital Board		WHC	Women's Hospital Corps
RIMA	Reversible Inhibition of Monoamine Oxidase Type A		WHO	World Health Organization
			WIPSIG	Women in Psychiatry Special Interest Group
RITA	Record of In-Training Assessment		WMHSIG	Women's Mental Health Special Interest Group
RMN	Registered Mental Nurse		WIST	Women in Surgical Training
RUI	Royal University of Ireland			
SAC	Society for Autistic Children		YOI	Young Offenders' Institute
SAIS	School for Advanced International Studies			

Contributors

Itunuayo V. **Ayeni** graduated from Kings College London and has an intercalated BSc in psychology. She is a Specialist Registrar in Old Age and General Adult Psychiatry in London, with a particular interest in the interface between mental and physical health.

Sue Bailey is a Child and Adolescent Forensic Psychiatrist, Past President of the Royal College of Psychiatrists, currently Chair of the Academy of Medical Royal Colleges, and Chair of the Children and Young People's Mental Health Coalition Research. Her clinical work has centred on delivering, as part of multi-agency teams, values evidence-based care and interventions for young people living at the margins of society, working in partnership with them and their families. She is helping policy-makers to make choices that will narrow the inequality gap for mental health.

Victoria Barker studied physiology at the University of St Andrews before going on to complete a PhD in Neuroscience at the University of Edinburgh. She qualified in medicine at the University of Manchester in 2006 and returned to Edinburgh to train in general adult psychiatry where she held a post as Clinical Lecturer in the Department of Psychiatry at the University of Edinburgh. Her research interests include early life programming and how developmental stressors perturb the development of the brain and contribute to the development of psychiatric illness, and the potential for reversal of these through psychotherapeutic treatment. She has a particular interest in childhood maltreatment and the impact of this on the development of psychotic symptoms and was awarded the British Medical Association's Margaret Temple grant in 2014 to investigate epigenetic changes in genes involved the stress response pathway in those with schizophrenia and schizoaffective disorder associated with childhood maltreatment. In 2015 she began a psychiatric training in psychodynamic psychotherapy at the Tavistock Centre in London.

Annie Bartlett is Professor of Offender Health Care at St George's, University of London, and an Honorary Consultant in Forensic Psychiatry. She is Deputy Head of the Graduate School at St George's, University of London and Clinical Director for the Health in Justice Clinical Network NHS England. She has published extensively on social exclusion and mental health (with particular reference to women and sexual orientation) and the culture of secure institutions.

Ann Boyle is a Consultant Old Age Psychiatrist in Leicestershire Partnership Trust. She is also a Specialist Advisor for the Foundation Programmes for the Royal College of Psychiatrists and Associate Postgraduate Dean at Health Education England.

Wendy Burn became a Consultant Old Age Psychiatrist in Leeds in 1990. She currently works in a community post. Her main clinical interest is dementia. She has held roles in the organization and delivery of postgraduate training since she started as a consultant. She set up the Yorkshire School of Psychiatry and was the first Head of

School. She was Dean of the Royal College of Psychiatrists from 2011 to 2016. In 2017 she was elected as President of the College and took office in June.

Fiona Caldicott is the Chair of the Oxford University Hospital NHS Foundation Trust. In 2014 Dame Fiona was appointed National Data Guardian of Health and Social Care by the Secretary of State for Health. As President of the Royal College of Psychiatrists (1993–96) she was also Chair of the Academy of Medical Royal Colleges (1995–96). From 1996–97 she chaired the Caldicott Committee on patient-identifiable data for the NHS, leading to the creation and appointment of 'Caldicott Guardians' in all providers of healthcare in the NHS. Since then she has led two further national reviews on the security and sharing of health and care data.

Anne Cremona was previously a Consultant Psychiatrist at the South London and Maudsley NHS Foundation Trust based at St Thomas's Hospital, and now works in the private sector, based at Nightingale Hospital and in the City of London. She was the founding Chairman of the Women in Psychiatry Special Interest Group at the Royal College of Psychiatrists. She has a long-standing interest in the equality of career opportunities for female psychiatrists and for all women doctors.

Rupal Dave is a Specialist Registrar in the Psychiatry of Intellectual Disability; she is currently a Clinician in the Westminster Learning Disability Service. Rupal has an interest in medical education and particularly enjoys teaching and mentoring medical students and junior trainees in London.

Sandra Evans is a Consultant in General and Old Age Psychiatry and has also trained as a group analyst. Her interest in psychological therapies has informed her work with older people in the City of London and Hackney, and in younger people in her role in student health and pastoral care at Bart's and the London Medical School, where she is a senior academic.

Maria Eyres qualified in medicine in 1991 and started working as a psychiatrist and psychotherapist in 1997, becoming a member of Royal College of Psychiatrists in 2002. She trained in medical psychotherapy and psychoanalytic psychotherapy at the Tavistock Centre in London between 2002 and 2008 where she was a member of the Trauma Unit. She joined East London Foundation Trust in 2002 where she continues to work with patients presenting with complex trauma. She received training in the number of therapeutic approaches to trauma, including tf-CBT (trauma focused Cognitive Behaviour Therapy), Narrative Exposure Therapy (NET), and DBT (Dialectical Behaviour Therapy), although she practises mainly using psychodynamic and psychoanalytic psychotherapy. Together with Dr Joanne Stubley she is a founding member and co-chair of the Historical Childhood Sexual Abuse task group at the Faculty of Medical Psychotherapy at the Royal College of Psychiatrists.

Hannah Fosker is a fourth-year Specialist Registrar in General Psychiatry with Leicestershire Partnership Trust. She has been committed to a career in Psychiatry since during her undergraduate training, and recently passed her RCPsych membership examinations.

Georgina Fozard studied preclinical medicine at the University of Cambridge, where she took her Part II examinations in philosophy, before going on to complete clinical school at King's College London School of Medicine. She completed her core training in psychiatry in North Thames Deanery where she became particularly interested in psychotherapy, personality disorders, and child and adolescent psychiatry. During the junior doctors contract dispute, she wrote on the subject for the *Independent* newspaper and *Grazia* magazine. She is currently a Specialist Registrar in Child and Adolescent Psychiatry on the Tavistock training scheme.

Jane Garner was a Consultant in Old Age Psychiatry in a team in North London for many years and then worked with students at University College London. She held honorary positions at the Royal College of Psychiatrists and is a founder member of the Older Adults Section of the Association for Psychoanalytic Psychotherapy in the NHS. Her academic and clinical interests include psychotherapy with older adults, institutional abuse, continuing care in dementia, and use of psychodynamic practice. She is currently retired from clinical work.

Philippa Greenfield is a Consultant Psychiatrist working in a psychosis service in inner London. She studied medicine at Queen Mary's University London (Barts and the Royal London) before undertaking her psychiatry training in North London. Her clinical interests are in first-onset psychosis and she has published work in this field. She also has interests in patient and carer engagement.

Angela Hassiotis is Professor of Psychiatry of Intellectual Disability at the University College London Division of Psychiatry and also has a clinical role as Consultant Psychiatrist in the Camden Intellectual Disability Service. Angela is committed to improving the lives of people with intellectual disabilities through evidence-based clinical practice and research, especially into clinical and cost-effectiveness of interventions. She strives to increase awareness of intellectual disability and associated issues on health and stigma through education and national and international appointments.

Claire Hilton was a consultant Old Age Psychiatrist in the National Health Service in north-west London from 1998 to 2017. She is also passionate about history. In 2014 she was awarded her PhD for her thesis: 'The development of psychogeriatric services in England, *c.* 1940–1989'. The chapter she has contributed to this book was written while on a Wellcome Trust-funded humanities sabbatical.

Jacqueline Humphreys is a Consultant Perinatal Psychiatrist working in Newham in east London. She graduated from Leicester Medical School in 2008 and completed her foundation medical years in the West Midlands. She moved to north London in 2010 to train as a psychiatrist, and decided to specialize in perinatal psychiatry in order to improve the health and well-being of women and their families.

Nikita Hyare is currently entering her final year of medical school at St George's University of London, and has always had a deep interest in mental illnesses and their wider impact on patients' quality of life. She has undertaken many special interest projects related to mental health, particularly its history and its relationship with the media and the lay public. Most recently, after undertaking an intercalated BSc in global health, she has become fascinated by the global distribution of mental illness, and how resources can reach the most deprived areas. Nikita hopes to pursue a career in psychiatry in the future.

Katherine Kennet is a core trainee in psychiatry based in north London. She sits on the Royal College of Psychiatry Sustainability Committee and is co-editor of *The Greening of Health; Healthcare, Health Systems and Wellbeing* (The Green Economics Institute, 2013. <http://www.greeneconomicsinstitute.com/>). She studied global health with history of medicine as an intercalated BSc and her professional interests include history of medicine and psychiatry, philosophy of psychiatry, and global health psychiatry.

Rosemary Lethem is a General Adult Psychiatrist who has suffered from bipolar 2 disorder for most of her life. In 2008, she retired early on grounds of ill health from her consultant post in Sheffield and since then has pursued a portfolio of activities in and out of medicine.

Clementine Maddock has trained in medicine and law. She completed psychiatric training at the Maudsley Hospital in London and was awarded the Laughlin Prize for the Highest Marks in the Royal College of Psychiatrists' membership exam. Dr Maddock became interested in law while conducting research into the incidence and predictors of mental capacity to make treatment decisions amongst psychiatric inpatients. Dr Maddock completed the Graduate Diploma in Law (GDL) at Swansea University in 2012 and was awarded a Prince of Wales Scholarship by Gray's Inn to study the Bar Professional Training Course at Cardiff University in 2013. Dr Maddock was called to the Bar of Gray's Inn in November 2014. She has a special interest in deprivation of liberty and was awarded the best GDL entry in the Bar Council Law Reform Essay Competition in 2012 for her essay entitled 'Are Deprivation of Liberty Safeguards Protecting Vulnerable Adults? The Case for Reform'. Dr Maddock currently works as a Consultant Psychiatrist at Abertawe Bro Morgannwg University Health Board and is an Honorary Senior Lecturer at Swansea University. She is a member of the Royal College of Psychiatrists Committee on Professional Practice and Ethics and their Specialist Advisor on Mental Health and Mental Capacity Law.

Jane Mounty is a Consultant Psychiatrist and Fellow of the Royal College of Psychiatrists, and she currently volunteers with the College and with Medical Justice. She worked at Greenwich District Hospital, was Clinical Tutor at South Buckinghamshire NHS Trust, and in 1997 was appointed Senior Lecturer in Rehabilitation Psychiatry at Lewisham Hospital, a borough of Lewisham within the South London and Maudsley NHS Trust. She became Lead Clinician and Champion for Carers in Low Secure Rehabilitation in the Avon and Wiltshire NHS Trust in 2006. She has always sought to promote the rights of minority groups.

Claire Murdoch is currently the National Mental Health Director at NHS England and the Chief Executive of the Central and North West London NHS Foundation Trust. Having trained as a Registered Mental Health Nurse in 1983, she has subsequently held a number of positions in the NHS in mental health and community services and has been active on various boards (currently Chair of the Cavendish Square Group), and is associated with raising the standard of mental health services and awareness of their vital contribution to twenty-first-century healthcare.

Jo O'Reilly is a consultant psychiatrist and a psychoanalyst. She completed medical and psychiatric training in London and undertook further training both at the Tavistock Clinic and the British Psychoanalytic Society in London. She works in the NHS in an inner city Mental Health Trust and has a keen interest in the application of psychoanalytic ideas to psychosis and severe psychiatric disorders.

Rosalind Ramsay is a Consultant Psychiatrist and Deputy Medical Director at the South London and Maudsley NHS Foundation Trust. She was a founder member of the Women in Psychiatry Special Interest Group at the Royal College of Psychiatrists, and previous Executive member with roles as secretary, newsletter editor, and from 2004 to 2007 she was the SIG Chair. She has worked to support the needs of women with mental illness and to develop the careers of women psychiatrists.

Gianetta Rands trained in Oxford and London and worked for 34 years in the NHS. She was Consultant in the Camden and Islington Mental Health Trust, Honorary Senior Lecturer at UCL, and Honorary Consultant at the Whittington and the Royal Free Hospitals. She now works with Recognition Health as a Consultant Psychiatrist with special interests in dementias and mental capacity. She has had many roles with the Royal College of Psychiatrists including College Tutor, Examiner, CPD Representative, Recruitment Committee Member, and Mental Capacity Adviser.

Abi Rimmer is the Deputy Editor of BMJ Careers. She has worked in medical journalism for a number of years, after completing a degree in Classical Literature and Civilization and Italian.

Joanne Rodda is a Consultant in Old Age Psychiatry in the North East London Mental Health Trust in north-east London and works primarily within the memory clinic. Her research interests include the identification of early symptoms of dementia, health, and lifestyle interventions for dementia, and initiatives to improve opportunities for people to be involved in dementia research. She is a keen triathlete and endurance runner.

Aoife Rajyaluxmi Singh trained at University of Leicester Medical School and is currently a Specialist Trainee in General Adult Psychiatry at the South London and Maudsley NHS Foundation Trust.

Joanne Stubley is a Consultant Psychiatrist in Psychotherapy at the Tavistock Clinic. She leads the Tavistock Trauma Service, and has considerable experience of working with individuals, groups, and organizations who have experienced trauma. She is actively involved in teaching and training in this field, with a particular interest in complex trauma. Dr Stubley is a member of the British Psychoanalytic Society, and is trained in Trauma Focused Cognitive Behavioural Therapy (tf-CBT) and Eye Movement Desensitization and Reprocessing (EMDR).

Fiona Subotsky was brought up on Denmark Hill in south London, near the Maudsley Hospital, where she later trained as a psychiatrist and subsequently became Medical Director. She has a long-standing commitment to promoting the interests of women as patients and as doctors, and was president of the Medical Women's Federation from

1999 to 2000. In retirement she pursues interests in medical history and literature, especially involving psychiatry.

Amanda Thompsell is the Chair of the Royal College of Psychiatry's Faculty of Old Age Psychiatry. She trained and worked as a general practitioner and then in old age medicine before meeting Nori Graham, who inspired her to retrain in old age psychiatry. As a consultant she now provides clinical leadership to a specialist care ward. She has a particular interest in care homes and for seven years was the clinical lead for a team working with care homes with nursing. Her other interests include, end-of-life care, the use of technology to support people who have dementia, and mental health tribunals.

Rashmi Verma is a Consultant Child and Adolescent Psychiatrist who graduated from The University of Sheffield Medical School in 2004. She completed her higher training in Child and Adolescent Psychiatry at The Tavistock Centre, London, achieving her MRCPsych and Diploma in Infant Mental Health. She works at The Tavistock Centre and, as a mother of three young children, she was particularly interested in learning about Dora Black's reflections on the work-life balance.

Emily Wills has two collections, *Diverting the Sea* (2000) and *Developing the Negative* (2008), and a pamphlet, *Unmapped* (2014), all published by The Rialto. She has won the Frogmore poetry competition three times and has been shortlisted for the Manchester prize. She works as a GP in Gloucestershire. www.emilywills.co.uk.

Domestic Confessional

I am trying to write a manly poem.

You would think, in this twenty-first century
postmodern have-it-all, this would be easy. You might say
that the programming of multiple white goods

has rendered obsolete words like *fairy* and *marigold* –
you might observe that we all have to eat –
but such concerns do not belong in the manly poem.

The manly poem may sit at a desk of managed forest
Or cheap laminate, brew unsourced coffee, stare out perceptively
At a pedestrian crossing, a rank of bins, a potted plant;

the manly poem has – presumably – a navel, with its fascinator
of blue fluff, but on these things both muse and man
must be silent. For the manly poem

is a crystal of pure thought, with no bodily needs,
apart from sex, of course – the consequences of which
may occasionally be permitted to enter

provided they wash their hands. Alas, there is no soap
or running water in the manly poem
and the children are hungry or sulky or tired.

For the manly poem, despite its umbilical scar, arrived
fully formed, punctuated with profound utterances,
a tendency to syllable count

and complex forms; also politics, apocalypses,
great themes. The manly poem
has a purpose, the manly poem must Lead The Way –

but with such rules, taboos, and no breakfast, the Inner Critic
– vestigial, but still lurking – convulses and dies,
not literally, you understand, with a lingering quotation,

but in the usual mess of grief and bodily fluids
which have to be dealt with, of course,
in another kind of poem.

Emily Wills
(Reproduced from *Unmapped,* published by The Rialto, 2014)

Chapter 1

Career Reflections of a 1970s Feminist

Gianetta Rands

In 1975, just over 40 years ago, I applied to medical school. That year Harold Wilson was the Prime Minister and Margaret Thatcher was elected Leader of the Conservative Party. In a televised interview, she said 'I doubt if we will see a female Prime Minister in my life time'.[1] The coal miners accepted a 35 per cent pay increase, 67 per cent of UK referendum voters chose to stay in the European Economic Community, there were Irish Republican Army bombings, Cod Wars, and football hooliganism. Newly released films included *Monty Python and the Holy Grail, One Flew Over the Cuckoo's Nest*, and *The Stepford Wives. Chicago: The Musical* opened on Broadway.

Our generation had adjusted to and enjoyed miniskirts and tights so the 1975 trend for maxi skirts and platform shoes was just another stage of fashion fun. We all had at least one item of clothing from Laura Ashley. The sports bra was invented in 1975 as 'the free-swing tennis bra'; in 1977 the 'jockbra' was created from two jockstraps sewn together. Examples are now in the Smithsonian Museum and the New York Metropolitan Museum of Art. The contraceptive pill was the big event of the 1970s and there were three choices—Microgynon, Eugynon 50, or Eugynon 30. It was prescribed for everything—moodiness, spots, heavy or irregular periods, pre-exam nerves, and as contraception. The only tampons available were Tampax which, we were told, should not be used until after a full-term pregnancy. This dogma lacked evidence so as the other option was sanitary towels (STs), which were attached to an ST-belt with loops and hence more restrictive than modern stick on pads, many young women of the 1970s chose tampons.

The National Health Service (NHS) was based on primary care services provided by general practitioners (GPs) and district general hospitals (DGHs); it was early days for specialist clinics such as family planning and sexually transmitted diseases (STD) clinics. On 29 December 1975 the Sex Discrimination Act 1975 and Equal Pay Act 1970 came into force aiming to end unequal pay and conditions for men and women.[2]

In this chapter, I describe some of my experiences as a doctor over the past 40 years. All events occurred but names, locations, and case stories may have been altered to protect identities. I have selected events that are relevant to trainee doctors, particularly women, and to the evolution of feminism. Some events are examples of the ways in which awareness, knowledge, and research develop.

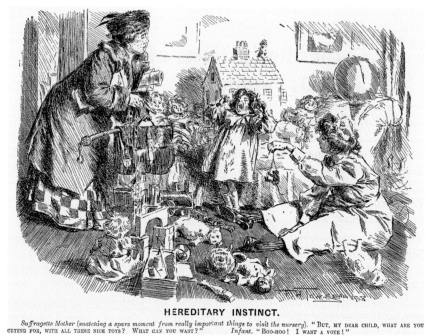

HEREDITARY INSTINCT.

Suffragette Mother (snatching a spare moment from really important things to visit the nursery). "BUT, MY DEAR CHILD, WHAT ARE YOU CRYING FOR, WITH ALL THESE NICE TOYS? WHAT CAN YOU WANT?" *Infant.* "BOO-HOO! I WANT A VOTE!"

Figure 1.1 *Punch* suffragette cartoon, 1909
© Punch Limited

This 1909 cartoon from *Punch* (Figure 1.1) shows a suffragette mother visiting her daughter's nursery to find that all her toys provide no comfort and what she wants is the same as her mother: the vote. Trainee doctors these days still want many of the things we strived for—equal opportunities, equal pay and conditions, the right to practice without harassment, and fair attribution.

1975: Undergraduate Studies

In 1975 I started my final year at Lady Margaret Hall, Oxford, where I was studying experimental psychology. I had matriculated in 1973 in PPP (Philosophy, Physiology, and Psychology) and swapped to experimental psychology which was a new and exciting science. In 1973, women undergraduates at Oxford could only go to women's colleges, of which there were five. There were about 35 colleges for men so the ratio of men to women undergraduates was about 10:1. In 1974, five men's colleges experimented with co-education ('co-ed') so women and men had a choice of single-sex or co-ed colleges. Nowadays all undergraduate colleges at Oxford are non-gendered.

My tutorial group at Lady Margaret Hall consisted of Joanna Collicutt, Jonquil Drinkwater, Georgina Ferry, and Gianetta Rands. We had tutorials in twos so the four of us could be combined in six different pairs. This caused confusion to many of our tutors who gave us each other's marked essays and end-of-term reports, which we still find hilarious. We were selected by physiology tutor, Professor Alison Brading

(1939–2011). As a student she contracted polio and her place at medical school was withheld. After being saved by an iron lung, she studied physiology. Her research into the functioning of smooth muscle, particularly bladder, made her a world-wide authority in this field. We have often wondered how she chose us: we had unusual backgrounds and disrupted educations; her selection changed our lives.

In our final year, we each completed a research dissertation. Dr Jane Mellanby supervised mine: 'An investigation of the effect of temporarily blocking inhibitory synapses in the hippocampus of rats by the injection of tetanus toxin.' Even then it was known that the hippocampus was important in memory storage and retrieval mechanisms. Tetanus toxin binds to presynaptic GABA (gamma amino-butyric acid) neurons blocking GABA release. GABA is the most ubiquitous inhibitory neurotransmitter in the human nervous system and modulates nerve and muscle activity. Whilst GABA was inhibited rats developed a syndrome with memory retrieval deficits, learning deficits, seizures, and behaviour changes. These all reversed after 8 to 12 weeks. Our electron microscopy slides showed neurons resprouting but other mechanisms such as toxin degradation were also probable. Our key finding was that a memory learned pre-intervention could not be retrieved whilst hippocampal GABA neurons were inhibited but could be retrieved after recovery. A second finding was that inhibiting GABA neurons in the CA3 area of the hippocampus caused a reversible impairment in the ability to learn a new task. It seemed that GABA was important for both retrieval and formation of memories.[3,4]

Forty years later, GABA is beginning to get attention as a possible treatment for some dementia symptoms,[5] and the hippocampi are routinely analysed in brain scans of people being investigated for memory and cognitive problems.[6] Dr Jane Mellanby now researches why women undergraduates underperform in university exams, despite their academic abilities, and has shown that one reason is lowered academic self-concept; that is, the belief in their own ability to achieve academically.[7]

The Royal Free Hospital School of Medicine (RFHSM)

I went to my interview at RFHSM by Tube to Russell Square. It was lunchtime and my carriage was not full. Most passengers were men in suits in various shades of grey, not the global collection of Londoners and tourists who use London Transport these days. They slowly migrated to the other end of the carriage when they noticed that the man opposite me was masturbating. He was in a trance, fingers fumbling his floppiness; he didn't pose a risk to me. I got out at Russell Square and went for my interview with a panel of men—in shades-of-grey suits—including Dennis Thatcher as the lay member.

In 1975 this sort of occurrence was not unusual. Many men leered at young women, fondled them if they could, flashed, frotteurized, whistled, and shouted at them. We all witnessed this sort of behaviour; it was one of the spurs to feminism. Most unfair, though, was that it was nearly always our fault—for wearing a shirt or skirt that was too short or tight or revealing or tantalizing; for wearing too much or the wrong kind of make-up; for looking too available; behaving provocatively. Our fault for being young women. These days, the term 'victim blaming' is helpful to describe these situations.

In 2016, this sort of occurrence was still not unusual; a YouGov survey of women found that nearly two-thirds had experienced some form of sexual harassment whilst in a public place, and that 35 per cent reported unwanted sexual touching. More than a quarter of these women were under 16 years old when the offence happened, and 75 per cent were under 21 years.[8]

As well as evidence, time unveils truth. In the news, we regularly hear about sexual behaviour towards non-consenting individuals, be they men, women, or children. We hear, retrospectively, about serial sex predators such as Jimmy Saville, Gary Glitter, and Frank Beck. In the last 40 years, attitudes towards non-consenting sexual behaviours have changed in most cultures. The extent of this problem may still be under-estimated and its devastating impact still under-researched (see Chapter 11).

The literary form of allegory has been used since Plato, and this artistic version of the allegory of truth and time from 1733 (Figure 1.2) is not only a beautiful painting

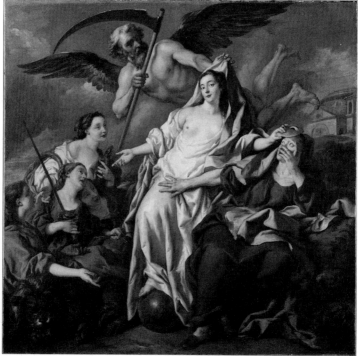

Figure 1.2 *Time unveiling Truth* (1733) by Jean-Francois Detroy
Time, the winged old man, flies. In so doing he unveils Truth, a beautiful woman, as she unmasks Deceit. Her companions, the Cardinal Virtues, are:
Fortitude, who rests by a lion, indicating her courage
Justice, who carries a sword and scales, symbolizing her power and impartiality
Temperance, with a pitcher of water, signifying abstinence
Prudence, who carries a snake, an allusion to her wisdom.
The Allegory of Truth and Time is that Time unveils Truth.
© The National Gallery, London

but also an optimistic one. It invokes the possibility that with the help of fortitude, justice, temperance, and prudence the truth, and deceit, will be revealed.

In 1875 the Royal Free Hospital (RFH) was the first hospital in London to admit women for medical training. In 1976, about a third of medical students were women; now the proportion is just over half. In the 1970s, the RFHMS was special because it led the way with mature student, or non-school leaver, entry to medical schools; my cohort was approximately 15 per cent mature students, including graduates.

In 1976, there were no student loans to fund degrees. Local Education Authority (LEA) grants were available and means tested according to parental income. Like other graduates not eligible for a second LEA grant, I had to fund myself with a collection of menial jobs until I successfully applied for a discretionary grant for clinical studies. It was a tough few years of flexible work, learning to do just enough to pass all those exams, very little socializing, and discovering just how many meals could be eked out of a bag of chickpeas and a cabbage. We didn't have loans or credit cards so money had to be earned up front.

Teaching was didactic, which required some adjustments after the Oxford tutorial system. A surgeon once said 'do not ask another question until you have looked it up in every book in the library and not found the answer'. Our cohort was the first to use problem-based medical records, a way of recording patient symptoms, medical history and physical signs, and analysing them in a problem list, each problem with its management plan outlined. The once-novel yellow student notepaper we used was still in use when I retired in 2015. The big student protest of our time was 'No Flowers for the Free' in which we successfully postponed a merger with University College London Medical School (UCLMS) until 1998.

1981: Junior Doctor

My first House Office (HO) job was at the RFH with the Renal and Diabetic teams. I was contracted to work 104 hours per week. That was 40 hours (office hours) plus 64 hours nights and weekends, which left 64 hours for the week's sleep ration and everything else. Even though our nights and weekend rate was about £1.92 per hour before tax, our hours were so long that funds soon built up. We had benefits, such as hospital accommodation, a doctors' mess, teamwork, control of our rotas, and the belief that we worked in a world-class system of social health care; most of these are not enjoyed by today's young doctors.

On my first morning at work in August 1981, a colleague put his hand up my skirt and pinched my bottom, an annoying memory of my first few hours as a doctor. I had to be defensive from the very start. In 2015, the Twitter storm '#DistractinglySexy' was a refreshing and humorous approach in response to this sort of attitude.[9] Over 50 per cent of all women still experience sexual harassment at work,[10,11] a sad reflection of its intransigence over the past 40 years. There is clearly a need to research the attitudes and behaviours, both individual and systemic, which perpetuate this problem.

We were told at medical school that 20 per cent of what we learned would be redundant or wrong a year after qualifying, and this would continue for each following year, exponentially. Medics are always aware that much of what we learn is provisional and changes with new evidence. We take our continuing professional development very seriously. It is after all, what we are interested in and how we make our living so it is no surprise that we enjoy keeping up to date.

Here are three lessons that have lasted from my GP training:

1. Pendleton's rules:[12] these define a process for giving and receiving feedback and are used for peer, trainee, and student clinical teaching. Other systems for giving feedback have subsequently been developed[13] but these have stood the test of time. The sequence is:

    1. Check that the learner wants and is ready for feedback.

    2. The learner presents material/case for discussion.

    3. The learner states what was done well.

    4. The observer(s) give their opinion on what was done well.

    5. The learner states what could be improved.

    6. The observer(s) give their opinion on what could be improved.

    7. An action plan for improvement is made.

2. Balint groups; these were devised by Michael and Enid Balint. Michael was a Hungarian psychoanalyst working at the Tavistock Clinic in north London. His third wife Enid was a social worker and psychoanalyst who had completed her training analysis with Donald Winnicott. In these groups, GPs discussed their feelings about patients and these were interpreted using psychoanalytic principles. Although the groups are usually attributed to Michael it is likely that Enid Balint (1903–94) had introduced him to a casework technique she already used to train social workers and that this was the basis of Balint groups.[14] She ran training courses for GPs at the Tavistock and continued to teach Balint techniques long after Michael died in 1976.

I remember attending a Balint weekend at Pembroke College, Oxford, in 1984 and witnessing Enid facilitate a group of about 100 GPs. These days Balint groups, sometimes called work support groups, are standard components of psychiatry and GP training and are included in most medical foundation programmes. Maybe it is time for fair attribution, which would be to acknowledge Enid.

3. Don't believe drug reps: in the 1980s 'drug reps', salespeople from pharmaceutical companies, had free access to doctors and GP practice staff. They provided food and drink for educational meetings and sometimes just wined and dined clinical and support staff. Free gifts included pens, tourniquets, sphygmomanometers, notepads, stickies, etc. An empty-handed young rep apologetically gave me his last remaining gift—a little screwdriver with four attachments, 'for the man in your life'. I still use it. These days this gift would be unacceptable as it displays the name of a specific drug. Most Royal Colleges[15] and NHS Trusts have guidance for clinicians about ethical interactions with pharmaceutical companies and most doctors choose to rely on their own analyses of available data.[16]

And so to Psychiatry

Around 1985 the first mobile phones became available, the first episode of 'EastEnders' was broadcast, the first heart–lung transplant was carried out at Harefield and Middlesex Hospitals, and the House of Lords ruled on Gillick competence,[17] namely that a person under the age of 16 may be competent to consent to contraception or other medical treatment without parental permission or knowledge. Comic Relief was launched, Lily Allen and Keira Knightley were born, and Philip Larkin and Laura Ashley died.

My psychiatry training started with the Royal Free Psychiatry Senior House Officer (SHO) training scheme. By then I had been a doctor for four and a half years and had achieved some post-graduate qualifications: MRCGP (Member of the Royal College of GPs), DRCOG (Diploma of the Royal College of Obstetricians and Gynaecologists), and a certificate in family planning. I was a savvy young doctor, competent and efficient, but politically idealistic and naïve; I believed the equality myth.

Around 1987/88 at Friern Hospital, a large asylum in North London, a young Muslim woman, admitted for assessment of first episode psychosis, complained she had been raped in the lift (see also Chapters 14 and 15). This was dismissed by colleagues (all men) as female fantasy, a sexual delusion. Didn't I know that mentally ill women had lots of sex fantasies? What the women reported couldn't possibly have happened as patients were 'supervised at all times'.

This was not satisfactory. Although this patient had some psychotic symptoms—delusions and auditory hallucinations—her report of rape was qualitatively different and did not seem delusional. I interviewed twelve other women patients and five had been sexually molested when acutely unwell; all were non-consenting, traumatized, did not tell, or had not been believed. I asked one of the more settled patients to show me the lift where the rape allegedly took place. It was the size of a small telephone cubicle with a sliding grill inner door which, if opened slightly, caused the lift stop. Thus, suspended between floors, this intimate cubicle became a private chamber ideal as a space in which abuse could occur; most patients knew about this and many preferred to use the stairs.

These patients also knew about the men, some ex-patients, some seeming very smart and professional, who cruised the hospital grounds picking up acutely unwell women, taking them off hospital grounds, to sexually assault them. This was clearly non-consenting and abusive behaviour. There was consensual sex amongst patients as well as 'fag shags' in which patients could trade sex for cigarettes. This was often easier than crossing the busy road to buy cigarettes, even when funds were available.

I discussed these findings with my two supervising consultants, both men, according to whom these were clearly female fantasies and delusions. I was naïve, they said, and they would train me to be a 'proper' psychiatrist.

What to do? First, patient care: I referred several women to the local sexually transmitted diseases (STD) clinic. As in-patients of an asylum many did not have home addresses and so could not independently access primary healthcare services including GPs and specialist clinics.

Second, secure the lift. I made a fuss and escorted several management staff to demonstrate the lift anomaly. Its mechanism was duly altered so it could only be used with a passkey held by staff. It was impossible to be certain how long the passkeys remained only with staff, but at least now this risk was known to exist.

Third, inform others about these findings. On good advice, I wrote an anonymous letter to the *British Medical Journal* (BMJ) in August 1988. It was printed and that same week quoted by the *Independent*[18] on their front page and page 4. Oliver Gillie, the medical editor of the paper, wrote: 'the doctor … He says … and He interviewed'. He assumed that the doctor was a man. My anonymity was guaranteed, but the content of my letter gained good publicity.

Finally, I encouraged one of the long-term patients to apply to the local council for a pedestrian crossing to be sited outside the hospital. It was, and I've always called it Kay's crossing. Patients had the option of going safely to local shops for cigarettes and no longer had to rely on their 'fag shag' system.

It was important to me that I did what I could to reduce risks for current patient victims, but also that the issue of non-consensual sex with people who were mentally unwell was not ignored or excused. However, this episode was useless in terms of my career progression. I spent time and effort investigating something that I could not put my name to, until now, and that therefore could not go on my CV. Also, I made a fuss and that was, and remains, largely unwelcome in organizations.

My anonymous letter to the BMJ marked the beginnings of a flurry of reports about sexual and violent crimes on psychiatry wards and about inappropriate behaviour of professionals. The Kerr–Haslam Inquiry (2005)[19] investigated two psychiatrists, William Kerr and Michael Haslam, working in York in the 1970s and 1980s, both of whom had been found guilty of indecent assaults against women psychiatric patients. The investigation found that numerous complaints had not been taken seriously, that professionals raising concerns (whistle-blowing) were not heard, and that raising concerns was detrimental to their careers. They found a culture of loyalty to colleagues and tolerance of sexualized behaviours in a predominantly male hierarchy of doctors and a predominantly female nursing cohort, which reinforced gender power relations.

Several good recommendations were made about education, promoting obligations to speak out, and protection of whistle-blowers. Information leaflets should be available to patients, so they knew what to expect when they saw their doctor, and complaints procedures in all Mental Health (MH) Trusts needed to be made clear to all who worked and were cared for there. They recommended Independent Mental Health Advocates (IMHAs) and Patient Advice and Liaison Services (PALS) which are now provided by MH Trusts. Their recommendations about policies for protecting vulnerable adults were incorporated into the Safeguarding Vulnerable Groups Act 2006.[20] All health and social services staff now have regular training about their responsibilities for safeguarding vulnerable people and local authorities take the lead in coordinating safeguarding procedures in their local organization partnerships.

This area has been getting more research attention. For instance, part of a national crime survey found that women with serious mental illness had a fourfold increase in odds of experiencing domestic violence, a tenfold increase in odds of experiencing community violence, and a fourfold increase in the odds of experiencing sexual violence.[21]

Psychiatry Trainees in the 1980s

Our main tasks as trainee psychiatrists were to learn psychiatry, pass our Membership exams, and provide around-the-clock medical care in our mental health services.

Personal safety was a big issue. The Royal College of Psychiatrists (RCPsych) had not yet published their book or DVD about violence awareness,[22,23] but we did receive some training in the management of violence. The most important message was that if you felt under threat then you should leave the room. Most of us experienced some form of personal attack during our duties and it was not unusual to be told that we must have been doing something to provoke this; violence towards staff was often denied or minimized.

On-call duties were still in addition to our office hours work and as the only doctor covering a psychiatry unit there were often medical emergencies such as heart attacks, septicaemia, accidents, self-harm attempts, burns, and haemorrhages, to name a few regulars. The on-call rota was crucial to our quality of life. Gaps in the rota tended to be filled by conscientious women trainees. We were super-efficient, very bright, mostly passing our exams first time, and over-conscientious about the quality of care we provided. It wasn't until after our Membership exams that it became evident that academic and prestigious jobs were not equally accessible to men and women doctors. The Medical Schools Council (2012) reports the gender balance in academic medicine as improving since 2004 but in 2011 only 42 per cent of lecturers, 30 per cent of senior lecturers, and 15 per cent of professors were women.[24]

The Equality Challenge Unit's Athena Swan charter was established in 2005 to recognize science departments that demonstrate gender equality policies.[25] The Sheffield Women in Medicine group are researching barriers to women's career progression in medicine.[26] Current experiences of women psychiatry trainees and trainers are described in Chapters 18 and 19.

More About Psychiatry Training

Later, as a new consultant, I was appointed College Tutor by the RCPsych and soon became an examiner for Membership exams, clinical and written papers, and a Training Programme Director (TPD). During my tenure as TPD (1999–2009) I witnessed many changes to the curriculum and exam structure. Like many colleagues I missed the 'long case' part of our exam, which was discontinued in 2008.[27] It assessed the very essence of our skills as psychiatrists—listening carefully, analysing thoroughly, and reporting accurately the history and mental state of a patient, then creating a personalized treatment plan using a bio-psycho-social framework.

Before MTAS (Medical Training Application Service, was introduced in 2007[28] we advertised for recruits to our training scheme twice each year, sometimes receiving over 500 applications. We valued diversity, welcoming those who changed specialty such as GPs, general physicians, or surgeons, as well as refugee doctors, part-time and job-sharing trainees, and an occasional trainee with special needs such as General Medical Council (GMC) rehabilitation. Of the 92 trainees in our programme over half were women and about a third were from ethnic minorities.

When I started as TPD there were two training posts to which our tutor committee chose not to allocate women trainees because of known risks of sexual harassment. Matching trainers and trainees was a skill and our aim was for both parties to have a good educational experience. Training needs were most important but personalities mattered too. Bullying within every medical specialty is now well recognized and women and ethnic minority trainees are especially vulnerable to it.[29,30] Even where policies about bullying existed, it was less clear how to manage some situations without becoming the shot messenger; having support from an employing establishment was not guaranteed.

Soon after the two-year foundation programme was introduced in 2005 an audit found that only 20 per cent of foundation doctors had any psychiatry training.[31] This evidence influenced the Collins Report (2010)[32] recommendations for greater emphasis on total patient care, long-term conditions, community care, and multi-professional teamwork, all of which could be provided in psychiatry placements. By 2015 about 51 per cent of foundation doctors had at least four-months training in psychiatry. This is very important for the quality of patient care and for reducing stigmatizing attitudes towards mental illness.

In 2015 the Royal College of Psychiatrists had 4,640 women and 6,015 men Members and Fellows, a ratio of 43.5 per cent to 56.5 per cent. Members and Fellows are doctors who have at least five-years post-qualification experience and have passed the RCPsych membership exams. Specialists registered with the GMC have completed higher training, usually another three to four years, in that medical specialty; in 2009 GMC data showed that one in seven non-GP specialists were psychiatrists.[31]

Throughout my career I have had several roles with the RCPsych, starting in 1989 with the inaugural chair of the senior trainees group of the Faculty of Old Age Psychiatry. This gave me a place on the Faculty Executive Committee and the opportunity to respond to one of the early Law Committee papers about mental capacity.[33] College committee work has been a good way to keep up to date, learn by osmosis, discover what goes on in services across the United Kingdom, and develop special interests such as recruitment, training, and mental capacity law.

In 1991 the purchaser/provider split was introduced by Margaret Thatcher's government and NHS expenditure rocketed. In 1988, it was 4.28 per cent of GDP (gross domestic product); in 2009 it was 8.8 per cent. An ethicist's view is that capitalist markets exist for humans to exploit each other; how could that benefit a publicly funded health service like the NHS? How many billions of pounds of taxpayers' money would be diverted to non-clinical administration, Private Finance Initiatives (PFIs), and private health companies? Pollock, and Davis and Tallis describe many deceptions in NHS reforms over the past twenty-five years.[34,35] Since devolution of UK governments, health expenditure has flat-lined at about £120 billion, the GDP percentage has fallen to one of the lowest in the European Union, and the amount spent on private providers has increased from 4.4 per cent in 2009 to 7.6 per cent in 2015.[36,37,38]

In the same year the Channel Tunnel was under construction and Freddie Mercury died from AIDS.

Unequal Pay

Salaries for men and women doctors are not equal. In 2004, in the United Kingdom, male doctors earned 21 per cent more than female doctors, and by 2013 this had increased to 40 per cent, with gender pay gap being less for trainees than for consultants.[39] The new contract for trainee doctors imposed in Autumn 2016 is likely to discriminate further against women.[40] For consultants there are discretionary incremental pay scales and clinical excellence awards, 85 per cent of which go to men.[41,42] Doctors in academic posts, disproportionately more men, retire later than those in clinical posts and more of them have higher clinical excellence awards, resulting in higher pay and hence higher pensions.[24] This is not a UK-specific finding; recent evidence shows that women doctors in the United States are paid an average of $20,000 per year less than their men colleagues.[43]

The Equal Pay Act 1970, implemented in 1975 and incorporated into the Equality Act 2010, stated the very simple concept that pay and work conditions should be equal for men and women.[44] Forty years later, a gender pay gap remains and in some cases, as in the case of NHS doctors, it has increased. If men and women in the United Kingdom had been paid equally in 2016 women would have worked unpaid every day after 10 November, Equal Pay Day.[45] In France Equal Pay Day in 2016 was 7 November. In Europe, only Germany, the Czech Republic, and Estonia have greater gender pay gaps than the United Kingdom and France.

Challenging Unequal Pay

Until recently the gender pay gap has been attributed to women's behaviour in the workplace—they are not confident, don't negotiate pay, don't apply for prestigious jobs, are too busy doing clinical work, work part-time, are distracted by non-work commitments, and so forth. It is beginning to be recognized that there are also powerful systemic forces in society and workplaces that resist changes to the status quo. Many women doctors have experienced this, including myself (see also Chapter 4).

In 2003 the new NHS consultant contract was implemented. My proposed contract was not equal to those offered to men colleagues doing similar jobs locally or nationally. Challenging this involved a series of negotiations, formal contract appeal, bullying from senior members of the Trust Board, an unsubstantiated fraud investigation, threats of a disciplinary investigation, and intimidation with a report that read like a tabloid newspaper article—a few half-truths slung together with derogatory innuendos. In the end, women managers resolved this with a second appeal, the outcome of which was almost identical to the first appeal, but now acceptable to the Trust Board. This process took five years by which time a large amount of back-pay had accrued.

Throughout these negotiations, I experienced a degree of revelry and sadism from some colleagues, offensive texts supposedly sent by mistake, a willingness by some colleagues to believe gossip, an apparent endorsement to be unhelpful, and an obvious lack of respect for confidentiality. To me, it seemed the person being 'attacked' was not me but a replica, an effigy, a straw (wo)man called Dr Rands that took on an identity distinct from my persona.

Feminist interpretations of witch trials[46] argue that women healers and midwives were a threat to men doctors and hence they were tried as witches, or scolds. If they drowned on the ducking stool they were innocent and if they survived they were guilty and burnt to death.[47] Either way, they died. Many women doctors seem to have been on the metaphorical ducking stool and had our careers damaged as a result (see Figure 1.3).

The concept of yin and yang, from ancient Chinese philosophy, is that opposite forces such as male and female are equal, need to be in balance and in perpetual motion to maintain a stable and harmonious unit. In 1982, Carol Gilligan wrote about masculine and feminine moral voices which were qualitatively different but both important in modern workplaces. Whilst some women authors, such as Sheryl Sandberg , have suggested ways that women can survive in a male dominated workplace by adopting male type strategies, others such as Anne-Marie Slaughter return to the complex issue of equal value for stereotypical male and female roles in modern society. Our organizations appear to have inertia that has resisted implementing

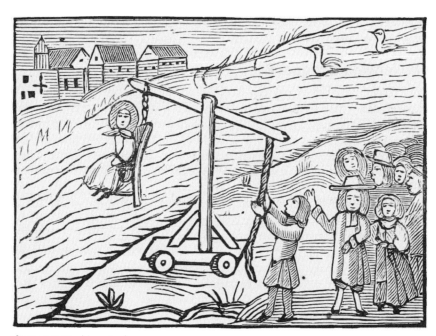

Figure 1.3 Ducking stool

the Equality Act 2010 and its predecessors for over 40 years. Research is needed to identify systemic, socio-political, and behavioural factors that perpetuate gender inequality.

Duties of a Doctor

In 1993, with great rejoicing, our local asylum closed. The last wards to close contained the asylum dregs; patients who had been there for decades, were complicated cases, often without families or friends, and who had not been selected for any of the new community and nursing homes. The patients who transferred to my wards needed full assessment, review of diagnoses, and new treatment plans. Our target was to assess one case per week, in addition to routine clinical work. Gradually we found the right place for each person and made good discharge plans.

On another site, patient transfers had been made without arrangements for their medical care. A colleague had been saying for months that these patients would need doctors; it may be unbelievable but there was no provision for doctors to treat these patients. There was no nominal consultant cover and no ward doctors. Patients discharged to community facilities would have access to GPs; patients transferred to hospital facilities needed access to doctors too. All credit to her; she repeated this almost daily until the transfers happened, yet still no doctors were employed to look after these patients. A non-psychiatry colleague complained 'your patients are filling the mortuary'. They weren't our patients but they were people transferred from the asylum.

We conducted an urgent audit of deaths amongst transferred patients and found that there had been too many. Our results caused fury. A second opinion was sought from a professor of medicine at University College London. He agreed with our findings. This was not what the establishment wanted to hear. His report was destroyed and I was sternly spoken to about my role in instigating this audit.

Changes did happen, however. There was an urgent review of medical staffing for these wards and consultant, junior doctors, and out-of-hours cover were all arranged. Soon, an incident precipitated a formal inquiry in 1999.[48] Lessons learnt were shared, which was useful because asylums were closing all over the country. I still suspect that this inquiry was a decoy and know that some nursing colleagues suffered terribly during its process, which often seems to be the effect of bad planning for service changes.

The GMC Duties of a Doctor[49] (see Box 1.1) had not yet been published but I was certain that if patient care—the services we provided for vulnerable ill people—was not good enough then one needed to make a fuss. This audit proved to be a small fuss using a professionally endorsed process which had a huge impact and a good outcome overall because patient care improved.

Around the same time in the early 1990s, it was considered reasonable to employ as a colleague a convicted paedophile who had been investigated four times by the GMC, not struck off but told to work only with older people. He would be fine for our services, wouldn't he? We didn't think so. We needed colleagues to provide safe services and not expose any patients, carers, or their families to unnecessary risk.

Box 1.1 GMC Duties of a Doctor

Patients must be able to trust doctors with their lives and health.

To justify that trust you must show respect for human life and you must:

♦ Make the care of your patient your first concern

♦ Protect and promote the health of patients and the public

♦ Provide a good standard of practice and care

♦ Treat patients as individuals and respect their dignity

♦ Work in partnership with patients

♦ Be honest and open and act with integrity

You are personally accountable for your professional practice and must always be prepared to justify your decisions and actions.

© General Medical Council

It seems extraordinary that this sort of attitude towards the employment of doctors could have existed so recently.

Later in my consultant career, I had the misfortune to have contact with PIE (Paedophile Information Exchange)[50] members again. By this time systems for protecting vulnerable adults and policies for sharing information with other agencies were established. The Safeguarding Vulnerable Groups Act (2006) was being effectively implemented. However, the issue of hospital patients consenting to see visitors is sometimes not taken seriously. It may be assumed that all in-patients want visitors but some visitors may not be welcome. As in so many situations, the only valid consent is positive affirmation and this should be routinely sought from patients with regard to their hospital visitors.

Feminist Themes

Several feminist themes are repeated in patients' histories. Most notable have been abuse, consent, and pathologizing normal functions. Taking the last group first, a memorable 90-year-old woman reported giving birth to at least two babies per day. They were different ethnicities and none were given names. It seemed that any abdominal discomfort she experienced heralded another baby. She was permanently post-partum and exhausted. This was a psychotic interpretation of normal somatic experiences—probably wind—and responded well to antipsychotics. When she stopped having babies she went home where she was followed up by a community psychiatric nurse (CPN) and any talk of having babies was taken as a sign that her medication and compliance with taking it needed reviewing.

Some women with dementia were comforted by caring for 'babies'. A cushion or a doll may be fed, nursed, and cradled, and carried around in a shopping-bag bassinet. This behaviour could last for months, sometimes occurred in women who had not been mothers (as far as we knew), and sometimes resulted in very smelly cushions and dolls needing sensitive management, such as surreptitious washing or substitution.

At times, it seemed that over half my in-patients had experienced abuse in their childhoods. It is possible that this predisposed them to not coping well with adjustments needed as they aged and entered a second phase of dependency. It was not unusual for patients, mostly women, when they became demented to recall incidents of childhood sex abuse which they had not disclosed to their families. As staff we needed to respect their choice to keep secrets and find ways to manage their distress confidentially. A patient in her 90s, very demented and unable to tell us her history, wailed every evening, causing distress to all around her by the sadness of her keening. We discovered that her mother had died when she was about ten years old and she had had to look after six or seven younger siblings, several of whom died. Her father was an alcoholic. We could only speculate about the abuses she might have experienced in childhood and how they might be replaying in her final days. All we could do was make sure female nurses cared for her, keep a dim light on overnight, talk quietly and reassuringly to her, and give her night sedation so she could get some respite in the form of sleep. This approach could be used in care homes and general hospitals. I remember a renal unit successfully looking after one of their elderly dialysis patients who had been abused in a children's home; she became distressed in the evenings by intrusive memories. Rather than use sedation someone sat with her for a few hours reading stories, listening to the radio, or colouring in pictures until she was sleepy and her demons had receded.

As a doctor, one witnesses both the best and worst of humanity. The cases I dreaded most were women who had been brought up in Irish orphanages. I had to brace myself for the saddest stories of torture, abuse, loss, neglect, sadism, and inhumanity. I would rationalize to myself that I only had to listen; they had had to live these experiences, and relive them as memories resurfaced in later life. What could we offer 70 years later except understanding and care?

Experiences of domestic violence were not unusual. Most old-age psychiatrists have had several patients with 'dementia pugilistica' as part of their caseloads: cognitive impairment due to repeated brain injury, also called 'boxer's brain', but in these cases due to domestic violence. Sometimes safeguarding policies resulted in separations and taking vulnerable adults into care. Sometimes a perpetrator developed dementia and the victim-spouse then felt it was payback time, as they were now the individuals who could wield power. Again, intervention might be needed. Sometimes ways were found to care for both parties that respected their choice to stay together.

In the early years of my time as a consultant it was not unusual to receive referrals from the general hospital along the following lines: 80-year-old woman complains of vaginal bleeding; Professor Jay, gynaecologist, recommends hysterectomy; patient refuses—refer to psychiatrist!

So the psychiatrist (in this case, myself) visited patient and found a friendly alert woman who talked clearly about her life, her illnesses, and her views about treatments. The patient knew the possible diagnoses and her options for assessment and management. She had no mental illness or cognitive impairment and would only consent to an ultrasound scan of her pelvis to investigate the cause of her bleeding. She did not want a general anaesthetic or major surgery but would accept medical management and pain relief if those were needed. I reassured the referrer that this patient was not mad and that her informed decision should be accepted.

These days we all benefit from the GMC guidance about consent: Doctors and Patients making decisions together[51] and the Mental Capacity Act (2005),[53] which clearly set out processes for decision-making, especially for people who do not have the mental capacity to make their own decisions. The increase in Mental Health Liaison Teams in general hospitals has helped teamwork and care of patients who are incapacitous or have fluctuating mental capacity due to mental or physical illnesses (see Chapter 17).

Decisions about resuscitation of patients often make headline news, especially if they seem to have been made carelessly. Early in my consultant days we were required to complete DNAR (do not attempt resuscitation) forms within 24 hours of every patient admission. This would be monitored with other routine activity data. In my professional judgement, this was unethical. How could I discuss resuscitation with someone who had just cut their throat or taken an overdose? They were suicidal; of course they didn't want resuscitating. Nor could these discussions be had with the many people admitted when confused, disorientated, delirious, or psychotic. All my patients were to be resuscitated (apologies to data collecting managers) until we had had the relevant discussion with them.

If someone had dementia and was not going to regain mental capacity their views were discussed with family or legally appointed advocates. Occasionally, the response was 'we're not quite ready to make this decision, can we think about it?' Two weeks later the decision might be to take medical advice and choose DNAR, which we advised if, for medical reasons, resuscitation was unlikely to be successful.

Community Work

As I worked mainly with older people living in one London borough I gradually learned its twentieth-century social history. I learnt about the wallpaper printing factory, the flour mill, the workshops for milliners, tambour-beaders, and cigar-rollers, and where the wooden crosses for Second World War graves had been made. I understood that many people lived in the same street, and sometimes the same house, in which they had been born, and where young women could go 'for help' if they 'got in the family way'; some of my patients had personal stories about their abortion skills, usually with some gruesome highlights. At least five of my patients had been brought up as their mother's sibling. In their youth, this was not an uncommon solution to the shame of illegitimacy. Another accepted action was to give excess children to Barnardo's charity where, it was believed, they would get a better childhood than in a poor family. Both situations had lifelong consequences in terms of personal identity, happiness, and resilience to mental illnesses; but this was a biased sample.

As a community psychiatrist my local knowledge was specific. I knew which bus stop had been selected by a Russian princess for her monthly rendezvous with one of our CPNs. She had developed late onset psychosis and was kept well for years by depot antipsychotic injections administered as she pinged down her elasticated waistband to expose the upper outer quadrant of chosen buttock, for safe injection. This was her choice and no other venue, or treatment, was acceptable to her. I knew which corner shop had our team phone number and whose staff called us if one of our patients had not been seen for a few days or had seemed distressed. I remembered the park bench where I'd sectioned a patient and which cafes were good for patient reviews and writing up notes. One particularly family-orientated 'greasy-spoon' café did wonders helping us treat and rehabilitate a grieving, depressed, and self-harming elderly man. They remained his source of community care long after we had discharged him.

Never Give Up; There is Always Something Else That Might Help

It sometimes seemed that my most important role as a consultant was never to run out of ideas for options that might help improve a patient's mental state or reduce their distress. Sometimes I resorted to the adage that time will heal; we just had to keep that patient safe until they were ready to heal or settle themselves.

In 1999, the National Institute for Clinical Excellence (NICE) was set up with the aim of standardizing quality of care and treatments provided by the NHS. It is now the National Institute for Health and Care Excellence (still NICE) and includes guidance about social care. Guidelines are important and have been used well in commissioning services, but they are only guidelines and based on appraisal of current best evidence, which is sometimes very poor. In psychiatry, our diagnostic categories are provisional, based on symptom clusters and rational, though rarely evidence-based, classification systems, and drug trials are often poorly designed, biased, and exclude complex cases and older patients. Doctors specializing in dementias quickly learned to diagnose all dementias as Alzheimer's so they complied with guidelines for prescribing dementia drugs that sometimes benefitted some of our patients.

If guidelines worked our wards would be empty and that would be a wonderful success. When patients have complex illnesses and following guidelines has not worked we then research other options. When a middle-aged woman, Elle, who had been an in-patient for six years, was moved to my ward 'for bed management reasons', our skills were tested. We reviewed her diagnoses and researched medications that had not been tried. She was fully informed about her options and had mental capacity to share in decision-making. We introduced memantine, a dementia drug, but theoretically of benefit to people with unstable psychotic or affective symptoms.[53,54] She stabilized sufficiently to be discharged and that year sent a Christmas card saying 'this is to thank you very much for trying me on memantine! It certainly does seem to be the thing to help me.' The fact that this intervention changed this patient's life, with no additional side effects, was sufficient justification to try it, despite us having to undergo an investigation for prescribing outside guidelines (see Figure 1.4).

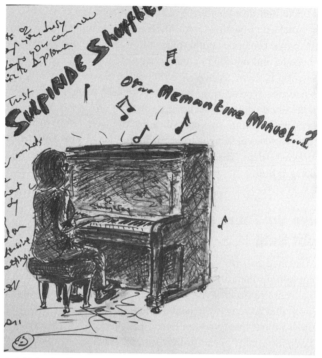

Figure 1.4 Sulpiride Shuffle, Memantine Minuet—a colleague's view of my prescribing habits.

Time to Retire from the NHS

In 2012 mental health services were restructured. Many experienced, non-medical mental health professionals were made redundant and bed numbers were slashed. In-patient and community teams were stripped down to minimum staffing levels and roles for unqualified staff were expanded. On a weekly basis there were near misses. Unqualified or junior staff were doing their best to assess and treat but were missing serious mental illnesses such as psychosis, suicidal intentions, cognitive impairment, and delirium. Training needs were excessive, with eight or more students and trainees attending ward reviews which were meant for seeing patients and their relatives, and deciding care plans. We all know that best healthcare is provided when there are enough trained and experienced professional staff working in small multi-professional teams. It takes years to build these teams[55] and they can be destroyed by decisions made in minutes.

There came a point when, for me, the quality of care that we could provide in my areas of work was no longer good enough. Although there are many explanations for the 21 per cent rise in deaths of patients in mental health services recorded between 2012 and 2015,[56] it was, sadly, unsurprising.

At this stage of my career, I spoke out about anything that was unfair, discriminatory, unsafe, or otherwise ethically and morally unacceptable such as inadequate staffing levels, poor clinical assessments, deficits in our clinical database, bed management decisions that disrupted patient care, cold wards, cold water on the wards, editing medical letters, prescribing restrictions, uncritical acceptance of guidelines and their ubiquitous implementation, no staff canteen or onsite refreshments, and so on. When things go wrong and there is a public inquiry—for example the Francis Inquiry—there is always the question: 'what were the consultants doing about this?'[57] I would ask myself, what if I did nothing? Are vulnerable people at risk? Are there other ways to solve this problem? What are my duties as a doctor? Sometimes the only option was to make a fuss. Women professionals seem more likely to do this than men and at some personal cost despite the Whistle-blowers charter.[58] One of the Francis Inquiry recommendations was to appoint a national guardian of the NHS, to ensure the right of NHS staff to speak up without fear of reprisal; the first appointments were made in 2016.[59] As the allegory foretells, time will reveal the true effectiveness of this provision.

In this chapter, I have selected examples from 40 years as a medical student and doctor working in the NHS. The focus has been on women's experiences as professionals and patients. Over those years many things have changed in terms of technology, illnesses, treatments, laws, fashion, workplaces, policies, and procedures. But many women scientists still rely on hidden learning (Figure 1.5) and networks

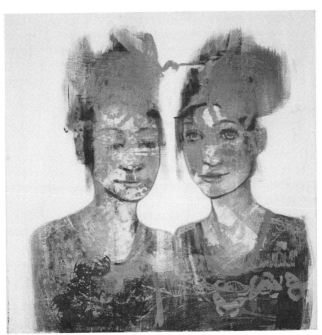

Figure 1.5 *Hidden Learning* by Sophie McKay Knight (2016); created as part of 'Chrysalis', an initiative designed to bring together women at all stages of their careers in science research to talk about issues and to seek advice and inspiration.

to survive in their workplaces. Equality and equal opportunities seem resistant to change. Women these days still want what we wanted—gender equality, the right to live and work without harassment, fair attribution, and equal pay. My cohort of 1970s feminists consolidated some advances made by the first and second wave pioneers but feminist mantras continue to be needed until equality and human rights legislation is effective.

References

1. **Singleton V** (1973). Interview with Margaret Thatcher on BBC1 'Val meets the VIPs'; 5 March. <http://www.margaretthatcher.org/document/101992>.
2. **The Equality Act** 2010 (incorporates Equal Pay Act 1970). <http://www.legislation.gov.uk/ukpga/2010/15/pdfs/ukpga_20100015_en.pdf>.
3. **Mellanby J, Renshaw M, Cracknell H, Rands G**, and **Thompson P** (1982). Longterm impairment of learning ability in rats after an experimental epileptiform syndrome. *Experimental Neurology* **5**, 690–9.
4. **Mellanby J, Strawbridge P, Collingridge GI, George G, Rands G, Stroud C,** and **Thompson P** (1982). Behavioural correlates of an experimental hippocampal syndrome in rats. *Journal of Neurology, Neurosurgery, and Psychiatry* **44**, 1083–92.
5. **Yanfang L, Hao S, Zhicai C, Huaxi X, Guojun B,** and **Hui Z** (2016). Implications of GABAergic neurotransmission in Alzheimer's disease. *Frontiers in Aging Neuroscience* **8**, 31. <https://www.ncbi.nlm.nih.gov/pmc/articles/PMC4763334/>.
6. **Barkhof F, Hazewinkel M, Binnewijzend M,** and **Smithuis R** (2012). *Dementia: Role of MRI Radiology Assistant.* <http://www.radiologyassistant.nl/en/p43dbf6d16f98d/dementia-role-of-mri.html>.
7. **Mellanby J, Zimdars A,** and **Cortina-Borja M** (2013). Sex differences in degree performance at the University of Oxford. *Learning and Individual Differences* **26**:103–11.
8. **Dahlgreen W** (2016). Over a third of British women have received unwanted, sexual physical contact in public—and most take precautionary measures to stay safe at night. <https://yougov.co.uk/news/2016/03/08/third-women-groped-public/>.
9. **Richards V** (2016). #DistractinglySexy: Female scientists take to Twitter to mock Sir Tim Hunt's sexist remarks. 9 November, *The Independent.* <http://www.independent.co.uk/news/uk/home-news/distractinglysexy-female-scientists-mock-sir-tim-hunts-sexist-remarks-on-twitter-10313435>.
10. **Trades Union Congress, in association with Everyday Sexism Project** (2016). Still just a bit of banter–sexual harassment in the workplace in 2016. London: Trades Union Congress.
11. **O'Grady F** and **Bates L** (2016). Sexual Harassment at work is getting worse. We need to stamp it out. 11 August, *Guardian.* <https://www.theguardian.com/commentisfree/2016/aug/10/sexual-harassment-at-work-getting-worse?>.
12. **Schofield T** (1984). In Pendleton D and Hasler J (eds). *Doctor–Patient Communication.* London: Academic Press.
13. **Choudray RR** and **Kalu G** (2004). Learning to give feedback in medical education. *The Obstetrician and Gynaecologist* **6**:243–47.
14. <https://en.wikipedia.org/wiki/Enid_Balint>.

15. **Royal College of Psychiatrists** (2008). *Good Psychiatric Practice, Relationships with Pharmaceutical and Other Commercial Organisations*. London: Royal College of Psychiatrists, College Report CR148.

16. **Goldacre B** (2008). *Bad Science*. London: Fourth Estate.

17. <https://en.wikipedia.org/wiki/Gillick_competence>.

18. **Gillie, O** (1988). Doctor highlights sexual harassment in mental hospitals. *The Independent*, 20 August.

19. **The Kerr/Haslam Inquiry Report** (2005). <https://www.gov.uk/government/publications/the-kerrhaslam-inquiry-report>.

20. **Safeguarding Vulnerable Groups Act** 2006. <https://www.legislation.gov.uk/ukpga/2006/47/pdfs/ukpga_20060047_en.pdf>.

21. **Khalifeh H, Johnson S, Howard LM, Borschmann R, Osborn D, Dean K, Hart C, Hogg J,** and **Moran P** (2015). Violent and non-violent crimes against adults with mental illness. *British Journal of Psychiatry* **206**:275–82.

22. **Safety in Psychiatry—The Mind's Eye (DVD Training Pack)** (2008). London: Royal College of Psychiatrists, September.

23. **Kidd B** and **Stark C** (1991). *Management of Violence and Aggression in Health Care*. London: Royal College of Psychiatrists.

24. **Fitzpatrick S** (2012). A Survey of Staffing Levels of Medical Clinical Academics in UK Medical Schools as at 31 July 2011. A report by the Medical Schools Council, London. London: Medical Schools Council.

25. <http://www.ecu.ac.uk/equality-charters/athena-swan>.

26. Sheffield Women in Medicine personal contact Stephanie Moore, medical student; lecture to Medical Women's Federation conference, 2016 'Barriers to female career progression in medicine'.

27. **Benning T** and **Broadhurst M** (2007). The long case is dead—long live the long case; Loss of the MRCPsych long case and holism in psychiatry. *Psychiatric Bulletin* December:441–2. DOI:10.1192/pb.bp.107.014951.

28. **Medical and Dental Recruitment and Selection in the United Kingdom**. <https://specialtytraining.hee.nhs.uk>.

29. <https://en.m.wikipedia.org/wiki/Bullying_in_medicine>.

30. **Quine L** (2002). Workplace bullying in junior doctors: questionnaire survey. *British Medical Journal* **324**:878.

31. **Lowe J** and **Rands G** (2012). The current position of psychiatry in the UK foundation schools. *The Psychiatrist* February (36):65–8. DOI:10.1192/pb.bp.109.026419.

32. **Collins J** (2010). Medical Education England Foundation for Excellence; an evaluation of the foundation programme, October 2010. London: National Health Service.

33. **Benow SM, Jones R, Rands G,** and **Wattis J** (1992). Mentally incapacitated adults and decision making: Implications of the Law Commission consultation paper for old age psychiatrists. *Psychiatric Bulletin* **16**:740–2.

34. **Pollock A** (2005). *NHS PLC: The Privatisation of Our Health Care*. London: Verso.

35. **Davis J** and **Tallis R** (2013). *NHS: SOS How the NHS was Betrayed—And How We Can Save It*. London: Oneworld Publications.

36. <https://www.kingsfund.org.uk/projects/nhs-in-a-nutshell/nhs-budget>.

37. <https://www.kingsfund.org.uk/blog/2016/01/ how-does-nhs-spending-compare-health-spending-internationally>.

38. **Iacobucci G** (2017). The long arm of government. *British Medical Journal* **356**:j41. DOI:10.1136/bmj.j41.

39. **Rimmer, A** (2014). Why do female doctors earn less money for doing the same job? *BMJ Careers* 15 September.

40. **Rimmer, A** (2016). Doctors slam junior contract for discrimination against women. *BMJ Careers* 4 April.

41. **Rimmer A** (2015). Under a fifth of CEA applicants in 2013 and 2014 were women. *BMJ Careers* 25 June.

42. Advisory Committee on Clinical Excellence Awards, Department of Health. <https://www. gov.uk/government/organisations/advisory-committee-on-clinical-excellence-awards>.

43. **Jena AB, Olenski AR**, and **Blumenthal DM** (2016). Sex differences in physician salary in US public medical schools. *JAMA Internal Medicine* **176**(9), 1294–304. DOI:10.1001/ jamainternmed.2016.3284.

44. **Devlin K** (2015). Battle of the sexes: 'Radical' laws reach 40th birthday. BBC News, 29 December. <http://www.bbc.co.uk/news/uk-england-35174688>.

45. <http://www.fawcettsociety.org.uk Equal Pay Day>.

46. <https://en.m.wikipedia.org/wiki/Feminist_interpretations_of_the_Early_Modern_witch_ trials>.

47. <https://en.m.wikipedia.org/wiki/Cucking_stool>.

48. **Andrews S** (1996). Beech House Inquiry: Report of the Internal Inquiry Relating to the Mistreatment of Patients Residing at Beech House, St Pancras Hospital, During the Period March 1993 April 1996. London: Camden and Islington.

49. **GMC** (2013). Good medical practice. <http://www.gmc.org.uk/guidance/good_medical_ practice.asp>.

50. <https://en.m.wikipedia.org/wiki/Paedophile_Information_Exchange>.

51. **GMC** (2008). Consent: Patients and doctors making decisions together. London: General Medical Council.

52. **Mental Capacity Act** (2005). <http://www.legislation.gov.uk/id/ukpga/2005/9>.

53. **Rands G** (2005). Memantine as a neuroprotective treatment in schizophrenia: Correspondence. *British Journal of Psychiatry* **186**:77.

54. **Taylor D, Paton C**, and **Kapur S** (2012). *The Maudsley Prescribing Guidelines in Psychiatry*, 11th edn. Oxford: Wiley-Blackwell.

55. **Rands G, Ford M, Okeowo A, Matthew-Bernard C, Kapfumvuti J**, and **Skinner A** (2009). How Consultation Liaison Meetings improved staff knowledge, communication and care. *Nursing Times* 27 October, **105**(42):18–20.

56. **Iacobucci G** (2016). Rise in deaths of mental health patients needs investigating, says MP. *British Medical Journal* **352**:518.

57. **Francis R** (2013). The Mid Staffordshire NHS Foundation Trust Public Inquiry. London: The Stationery Office.

58. <https://www.gov.uk/whistleblowing/who-to-tell-what-to-expect>.

59. **Hughes H** (2016). Enabling staff to speak out. *British Medical Journal* 355. <https://doi.org/ 10.1136/bmj.i5943>.

Chapter 2

A History of Women in British Medicine

Abi Rimmer

This chapter will explore the history of women in medicine, and more specifically women doctors, from the first registration to present day. It will explore women's changing role within medicine, as well as the foundation and work of the Medical Women's Federation.

Gaining Qualification

The General Medical Council (GMC), the body responsible for regulating doctors in the United Kingdom, was established in 1858. That same year, Parliament passed a statute requiring every legally qualified medical practitioner to be recorded in a register held by the GMC. At the time, women were not accepted as students in UK medical schools and although women practiced midwifery this was not deemed to fall into the category of medicine.[1]

The GMC register began the following year and it was stipulated that any doctor with a degree in medicine from a British university and any doctor with a foreign medical degree who was practising in England in 1858 was allowed to be entered onto it.

In 1858 Elizabeth Blackwell (1821–1910) became the first woman to receive a medical degree in the United States.[2] The following year Blackwell came to England to lecture on 'medicine as a profession for ladies' and an application was made on her behalf to be included on the GMC register.

After serious deliberation, the GMC conceded that Blackwell could be registered, even though she was not actually practising in England at the time, making her the first woman to appear on the medical register.[3] Prior to this achievement, however, one British woman had already succeeded in practising as a doctor, by disguising herself as a man. Margaret Ann Buckley (1795–1865), otherwise known as James Barry, was a British Army surgeon whose secret was only discovered after she died.[4]

It was Blackwell's successful entry onto the register that would truly mark the beginning of the fight by British women to practise as doctors. While travelling in America in 1861, Sophia Jex-Blake (1840–1912), a young English woman from Sussex, met Dr Lucy Sewall, a disciple of Blackwell. This meeting convinced Jex-Blake that she too could become a doctor (Figure 2.1).[5] In 1869, Jex-Blake sought the right to attend classes at the University of Edinburgh and although she received little support from

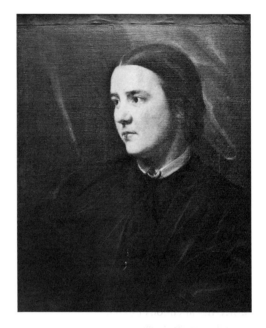

Figure 2.1 Sophia Jex-Blake
(1840–1912) founded the first
medical school for women in 1874.
© Wellcome Library, London.
Reproduced under the Creative
Commons Attribution Licence
CC BY 4.0

her male peers she was eventually allowed to attend medical classes under certain conditions.[6] Jex-Blake was later followed by four other women into that medical school.

Despite this success, Jex-Blake and the other female students went on to meet with great opposition and they failed to gain the right to qualify.[7] However, they raised the profile of their cause and gained many supporters.

In 1878 the Medical Act was redefined by Parliament to confirm that women were eligible to attend medical education, allowing Jex-Blake and her fellow Edinburgh trainees to enter prescribed examinations and become registered doctors.

It was Elizabeth Garrett (1836–1917), later Garrett Anderson, who would become the first British woman to be registered with the GMC (Figure 2.2). At the age of 23, Garrett Anderson had heard Blackwell speaking and, like Jex-Blake, became determined to become a doctor.[8]

Unable to gain a medical degree at a UK university, Garrett Anderson achieved the Licentiate of the Society of Apothecaries (LSA) in 1865. This enabled her to be entered on to the GMC register, a major step forward for British women in medicine. Following her success, the Society of Apothecaries passed a resolution that candidates for their diploma must have worked in a recognized medical school, effectively baring other women from attaining the LSA.

Despite her GMC registration Garrett Anderson still wanted to gain a medical degree, something she achieved in Paris in 1870 after Paris University opened its medical course to women.[9] Garrett Anderson went on to become the first female member of the British Medical Association (BMA), which had been founded in 1832, when she joined in 1873.[10] Following her membership, the association voted against the admission of further women.[11]

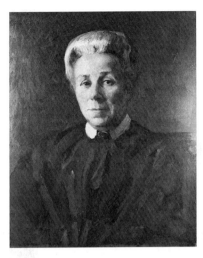

Figure 2.2 Elizabeth Garrett Anderson (1836–1917) was the first woman to achieve the Licentiate of the Society of Apothecaries (LSA) and was the first female member of the British Medical Association.
© Wellcome Library, London. Reproduced under the Creative Commons Attribution Licence CC BY 4.0

Meanwhile, following her failure to gain a medical degree in Edinburgh, Jex-Blake turned her attentions to opening a medical school for women in London. Although Garrett Anderson was not wholly supportive of the idea, on 22 August 1874 she attended the provisional committee of Jex-Blake's planned new school.[12]

In its first year, 1875–76, 23 students enrolled at the London School of Medicine for Women (it became the Royal Free Hospital School of Medicine).[13] The period of study covered three years and the curriculum included four subjects, more than those required by most medical examining boards at the time.[14]

Although students of the school were initially refused examination by the 19 London Examining Bodies, in 1876 the Irish College of Physicians and Queen's University of Ireland agreed to admit students to their examinations and diplomas.[15] In 1878 Jex-Blake, along with a fellow student Edith Pechey (1845–1908), sat examinations in Dublin and passed.

By 1887, the London School of Medicine for Women had 77 students, in 1889 enrolment was 91, and 3 years later it was 133. In 1896, an unprecedented entry of 50 new students brought the total enrolment to 159, by 1903 there were 318 students, and in 1917 the number had grown to 441.[16]

In May 1876, Russell Gurney (1804–78), the Recorder of London, proposed the Medical Act (Qualifications) Bill 'to remove restrictions on granting of qualifications under the Medical Act on the grounds of sex and extend the power to grant qualification to all bodies under the Medical Act'.

The first women to benefit from Russell Gurney's Enabling Act were Pechey and Edith Shove (1848–1929) when they applied for admission to the Irish College of Physicians and were accepted in September 1876.[17]

In 1888 Jex-Blake complied and published, through the National Association for Promoting the Medical Education of Women, a pamphlet entitled 'Medical education of Women; a comprehensive summary of present facilities for education, examination and registration'. It listed the 60 women who, between 1859 and 1888, had taken medical diplomas which entitled them to enter their names on to the GMC register.[18]

Over the next few years, women continued to make progress in medicine and by 1916 it was apparent that women doctors needed a body to speak on their behalf and represent their interests. The Medical Women's Federation (MWF) was founded in 1917. One immediate stimulus for its creation was the government's attitude towards women doctors who wished to offer their professional skills to the war effort.[19]

Women in the First World War

In 1907 Mabel St Clair Stobart (1862–1954) formed the Women's Sick and Wounded Convoy Corps (Figure 2.3). In 1912, during the first Balkan War, Stobart and a unit of 16 women including 3 doctors were asked to set up a hospital at the headquarters of the Bulgarian army.[20]

On 4 August 1914, the day that Britain declared war on Germany, Stobart spoke at a peace meeting in London. The following day, she founded the Women's National Service League.[21] Although Stobart's offers of help were rebuffed by Sir Frederick Treves (1853–1923), chairman of the British Red Cross, the League was asked by the

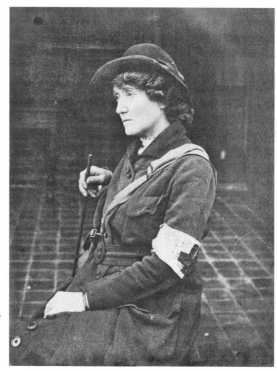

Figure 2.3 Mable St Clair Stobart formed the Women's Sick and Wounded Convoy Corps in 1907 and helped care for soldiers throughout the First World War.
© IWM

Belgian Red Cross to establish a hospital for French and Belgian soldiers in Brussels. Subsequently, Stobart served on the Balkan Front where she commanded the Serbian Relief Fund's Front Line Field Hospital. In 1915 she and her medical staff accompanied the Serbian Army's retreat through the Albanian mountains.[22]

Many women doctors wanted to play their part in the war effort but the War Office refused to accept that women doctors could serve with the armed forces abroad and they were not accepted into the Royal Army Medical Corps (RAMC).[23] Instead, like Stobart, several women doctors set up their own voluntary organizations.

In August 1914, Louisa Garrett Anderson (1873–1943), daughter of Elizabeth, and fellow doctor Flora Murray (1869–1923) founded the Women's Hospital Corps (WHC). The women's initial efforts were also rebuffed by the War Office and the British Red Cross so they went to Paris at the request of the French Red Cross.[24]

In September 1914, the WHC established a hospital in Hotel Claridge in Paris which was eventually so successful that the RAMC came to regard it as a British Auxiliary hospital. The War Office also eventually invited the WHC to establish a hospital in Wimereux in France.[25]

Also in September 1914, Elsie Inglis (1864–1917), who had previously trained the Sixth Edinburgh voluntary aid detachment (VAD), went to London to offer the services of herself and fellow women doctors to the War Office (Figure 2.4). She was told by the departmental chief whom she approached, 'My good woman, go home and sit still!'[26]

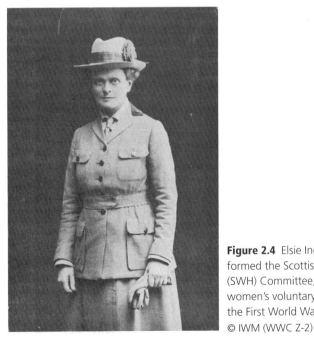

Figure 2.4 Elsie Inglis (1864–1917) formed the Scottish Women's Hospitals (SWH) Committee, the largest of all the women's voluntary organizations during the First World War.
© IWM (WWC Z-2)

Determined to do quite the opposite, in October 1914 Inglis formed the Scottish Women's Hospitals (SWH) Committee, the largest of all the women's voluntary organizations during the First World War.

In December 1914 an SWH unit established a hospital in Calais to nurse French soldiers with typhoid. In the same month two further units were dispatched to Serbia. The SWH went on to set up the Royaumont military hospital in France which did not close until 1919. They also established hospitals in Serbia, Salonika, Corsica, Russia, and Romania.

Despite the achievements of women's voluntary units abroad, the War Office maintained that the front was not a place for women doctors. However, the success of the WHC hospital in Wimereux prompted Sir Alfred Keogh (1857–1936), Director General of the Army Medical Services, to offer the women a large military hospital in Endell Street in London. The WHC accepted the offer and took control of the hospital on 22 March 1915.[27]

Progress at Home During the First World War

While many women were serving overseas during the War, others were making progress at home. An acute shortage of male doctors in civilian hospitals meant that women were recruited in their place. They were also needed in military hospitals and were known as Civil Medical Practitioners, but they were not granted a rank or a uniform and were paid less than their male counterparts, which caused some resentment.[28,29]

In 1916 the War Office sent volunteer women doctors to serve with the RAMC in Salonika, Egypt, India, and Malta but they were refused commissions and had to travel third class while all army nurses and VADs in uniform travelled first class.[30]

Fighting for Parity

In 1917 the Medical Women's Federation signed its articles of association and was incorporated as a limited company with an office in London (Box 2.1).[31] In the same year, Alexandra Chalmers Watson (1872–1936), chief controller of the Women's Army Auxiliary Corps (WAAC), wrote to the MWF to ask for help in recruiting women doctors to carry out medical examinations of women entering the WAAC.[32,33]

Box 2.1 The Medical Women's Federation

Founded in 1917, the Medical Women's Federation has been working for the advancement of women doctors for 100 years

By 1925 membership had passed the 1000 mark.

In 1970, the MWF was designated as eligible for charitable status.

Today the MWF has around 1500 members.

Initially, women doctors employed in connection with the WAAC medical boards did not receive the same pay as their male colleagues. However, in 1917 the War Office ruled that the women should be 'paid for each day worked at the local rates obtained for men doctors similarly employed'.[34]

In 1918, the SWH saw it finest hour. With the Germans advancing on Aisne in France, the SWH unit in Villers Cotterets provided relief for the wounded. During the period of fighting, between 31 May and 13 July, the hospital was one of the only facilities working and its three operating theatres ran day and night.[35]

When the war broke out, male medical students close to qualification were urged not to enlist into the forces due to fears of a shortage of doctors.[36] By 1915, there were 1000 fewer medical students than at the same time the previous year and by the autumn of 1917 there was growing concern about the depletion of student numbers.[37] If the war had continued until 1919 and beyond, historians have suggested that opportunities for women doctors would have increased due to an undersupply of male doctors.[38]

Post-War Attitudes

Despite their notable contribution to the war effort, women doctors had still not gained equality. In the 1920s, a number of medical schools which had opened their doors to women during the First World War closed them again, and the principle of medical co-education came under serious threat.

Women over the age of 30 gained the right to vote in 1918 (the age limit was lowered to 21 in 1928), and in response various legislative enactments had thrown professions open to women. However, marriage continued to act as a bar to women wishing to enter professions.[39]

During this time the MWF began to place less emphasis on the professional struggles faced by its members but women doctors were by no means having an easy time. In January 1923 a letter was submitted to the *British Medical Journal* (*BMJ*) by a doctor who identified himself as 'Grammatista' argued forcibly against the use of the expressions 'women doctors' and 'Lady Doctor'. Instead, the writer called for a feminine form of 'doctor' to be used—'doctress'—so that women doctors could be distinguished from their male colleagues.

Two years later, in January 1925, WM Robinson wrote to the *BMJ* to warn of a 'glut' of women doctors.[40] In response to Robinson's letter, Mabel Ramsey, a surgeon of obstetrics and gynaecology, said that women accounted for one in every five newly qualified doctors. She said that the total number of registered medical women in 1925 was around 2000 while the number of men was around 25,000, and she called for selection committees to treat women more fairly.[41]

Despite this perceived glut of women doctors, or perhaps because of it, in 1930 women broke through a number of barriers: the first women Commissioner was appointed to the Board of Control, and the first female Chief Medical Officer of a London Borough and the first female Regional Medical Officer took up their posts. Three years later, following a long campaign, Christine Murrell (1874–1933) became the first woman doctor to be elected to the council of the GMC, but she died before she could take her place. As well as being the president of the Medical Women's Federation between 1926 and 1928, Burrell was also the first woman to be appointed to the central council of the British Medical Association (BMA) in 1924.

Women in the Second World War

In 1937 the MWF wrote to the War Office to request that women doctors were allowed to serve in the Army in the event of war breaking out. At the time, the Director General of Army Medical Services, Sir Alexander Hood (1888–1980), thought that any employment of women doctors within the army should be strictly limited. Twelve months later, the BMA raised the issue again. This time Hood conceded that women doctors could be employed in the Axillary Territorial Service with the pay and rank of lieutenant, or as replacements for RAMC officers in the blood transfusion services. However, it was the Army Council's policy that there should be only one female Corps with the Axillary Territorial Service and women doctors were excluded from the RAMC for the duration of the War.[42]

In 1940 the BMA published a notice entitled Medical Women in the Forces.[43] It stated that the General War Committee had 'authorised a scheme for the employment of women practitioners with the armed medical services in time of war. They are now eligible for employment either as civilian medical practitioners or medical officers attached to the RAMC with a military status.'

In 1947 a committee was launched to look at equal pay for equal work for men and women under the new National Health Service (NHS). With the inception of the NHS in 1948 all medical schools were finally opened to women, although for several decades a quota system of around 20 per cent was applied by most of them.[44]

Medicine and Women in the 1950s and Beyond

In 1943 Jane Scott Calder, who identified herself as a doctor, wrote to the *BMJ* about post-war planning for medical education and the future of women in the medical profession. She warned that women were losing their dignity by becoming doctors.[45] She also called for women to be allowed to treat only women and children patients, and for there to be no birth control clinics in hospitals. 'Medicine is not for any and every woman; it is for the inspired, the gifted, the special few', Scott Calder wrote.[46]

It is perhaps unsurprising that Scott Calder's letter prompted a number of strong reactions. Catherine Swanston, a senior medical officer at the Royal Ordnance Factory, wrote in reply in the *BMJ* 'Dr Calder wishes ... to undo all the good work put in by her predecessors who fought for and eventually obtained a measure of equality, and to put back the clock at least 100 years.'[47] Joan Walker wrote, 'I trust no-one will ever seriously consider suggestions that medical women revert to such a narrow-minded medieval status as that mapped out by Dr Scott Calder.'[48]

Although much headway was made by women doctors by the late 1950s, questions continued to be raised about their dedication to medicine after marriage. In 1958, a joint working party on medical staffing structures said it expected '1,730 medical students to qualify in 1964, 1,330 of these being men and 40 women. Allowing for two-thirds wastage of women due to marriage, this will leave us about 1464 working doctors.'[49]

In 1962 an Advisory Service was established to deal with the problems of married women seeking part-time work or returning to practise after a break. Particular attention was devoted to the questions of postgraduate education and higher qualifications.[50] In 1966, Kenneth Robinson, the Minister of Health, said that arrangements were being made to help medical women to return to work.[51] A scheme for the re-employment of married women was eventually set up in 1969.[52]

In 1966 Jean Lawrie, Muriel Newhouse, and Patricia Elliot wrote an article in the *BMJ* which highlighted that marriage and having children was still perceived as a barrier to women working in medicine.[53] At that time 25 per cent of medical students were women. Looking at two surveys of qualified female doctors, carried out by the Medical Practitioners Union and the MWF, the authors found that 80 per cent of respondents actively worked as doctors and nearly 50 per cent of them were in full-time work. The researchers concluded that 'the overall wastage of women doctors is not as alarming as is suggested'.

In 1972 a retainer scheme was launched for doctors who were unable to work more than two sessions, enabling them to remain professionally active by subsidising their subscriptions to the GMC and the Medical Protection Society.[54]

Two years later, in 1974, the then health secretary Barbara Castle (1910–2002) expressed her intention to improve opportunities for women working part-time in the NHS.[55] In July of that year a special conference was held specifically to address problems faced by women doctors.

In 1976, Rita Henryk-Gutt and Rosalie Silverston wrote an article that appeared in the *BMJ* about career problems faced by women doctors.[56] There were around 19,000 women doctors in Great Britain, accounting for 22 per cent of the workforce. Women accounted for 35 per cent of medical students who started training in 1975. Through a survey of 61 women doctors, the authors found that women faced two main problems during their careers. 'Firstly, it was difficult to obtain a part-time post in training grades, despite official provision of supernumerary posts for this purpose,' the authors said. 'Secondly, when training was complete, and if the doctor was still unable to undertake full-time work, she was likely to find that there were virtually no permanent part-time posts available in the hospital specialties or above the basic grade in the community health service.'

In 1978 the Medical Act, which consolidated the Medical Acts 1956–1978, stipulated that majority of GMC Council members should be elected. This led to five women being elected to council. In the previous 30 years there had been a maximum of three women on the Council at any one time.[57]

Two years later, in 1980, Swerdlow, McNeilly, and Rue wrote to the *BMJ* about the problems faced by women entering medical training.[58] Perhaps surprisingly, whether a women doctor was married or not was still of interest. They wrote: 'In 1978 nearly 38% of medical school entrants were women and by 1985 this could rise to 50%.' They added: 'The increasing proportion adds uncertainty to current attempts to plan medical manpower because little is known about which specialties women doctors now in training will enter as career posts and how many sessions they will work.'

The authors carried out a survey of 231 women doctors and they found that women still had problems with conflicting loyalties—between work and children—and with reactions from senior doctors.

The authors concluded that more needed to be done to encourage women doctors into specialties which had high levels of out-of-hours and night work. They suggested that one incentive could be financial. 'The size of the medical manpower pool could probably be increased rapidly, were this desired, by greater financial incentives to work (either direct or via tax relief) for women doctors.'

During the 1980s the BMA established an advisory service for women to look at part-time working, the retainer scheme, maternity benefits, and superannuation, as well as women's careers.[59] The BMA Under Secretary for membership and recruitment, Dr Ian McKim Thompson, said: 'This is the first time that a determined effort has been made to coordinate advisory services to doctors at a regional level. With the number of women entrants to medical schools reaching nearly 50% there will obviously be a demand for a special service within the next five years and we intend to be geared up for it.'

In 1997 a survey of 1000 GPs and consultants found that women doctors believed that medicine was still a male-dominated profession in which they had to work harder than men to compete successfully and they had less status than them.[60] The research also found that women doctors felt that they got passed over for promotion and they found it more difficult to get a GP partnership.

Women doctors continued to face difficulties into the 2000s, including accusations that medicine had become 'feminized'. In 2004, the then President of the Royal College of Physicians in London, Carol Black, was quoted as saying, 'We are feminizing medicine. It has been a profession dominated by white males. What are we going to do to ensure [the profession] retains its influence?'[61]

In 2009 the Chief Medical Officer published a report called 'Women Doctors: Making a Difference', which highlighted obstacles that prevented women doctors' career progression.[62] Recommendations included improving access to child care, part-time working, and flexible training.

Despite the obstacles, women continued to make progress. In 2005, the *BMJ* appointed Fiona Godlee as its first woman editor since the journal was founded in 1840. In 2011, Sally Davies became the first female Chief Medical Officer for England. In 2016, a record number of women were presidents of Royal Medical Colleges, with women holding these positions in the Faculty of Intensive Care Medicine, the Royal College of General Practitioners, the Royal College of Surgeons, the Royal College of Obstetrics and Gynaecology, the Royal College of Paediatrics and Child Health, the Royal College of Physicians, the Royal College of Pathologists, the Royal College of Ophthalmologists, and the Royal College of Radiology. Dame Sue Bailey, recent past President of the Royal College of Psychiatrists, became chair of the Academy of Royal Colleges.

Despite the achievements of women in medicine over the last 150 years, there is still progress to be made. Women doctors still do not receive the same pay as their male colleagues—in 2004 male doctors earned 21 per cent more than their female colleagues, but by 2013 they earned 40 per cent more—and recent changes to doctors contracts threaten their ability to work part time.[63,64] The Medical Women's Federation still actively promotes issues affecting women in healthcare and has a membership of around 1500. There are currently 127,498 women on the GMC register, accounting for 45 per cent of the total.

References

1. **Lutzker E** (1959). *Medical Education for Women in Great Britain*. Master's thesis. New York: Columbia University, p. 5.

2. **Moberly Bell E** (1952). *Storming the Citadel*. London: Constable.

3. **Moberly Bell E** (1953). *Storming the Citadel*. London: Constable, pp. 44–5.

4. <http://www.sciencemuseum.org.uk/broughttolife/people/jamesbarry>.

5. **Moberly Bell E** (1953). *Storming the Citadel*. London: Constable, pp. 65–6.

6. **Lutzker E** (1959). *Medical Education for Women in Great Britain*. Master's thesis. New York: Columbia University, p. 6.

7. **Moberly Bell E** (1953). *Storming the Citadel*. London: Constable, pp. 62–83.

8. **Moberly Bell E** (1953). *Storming the Citadel*. London: Constable, pp. 46–54.

9. **Moberly Bell E** (1953). *Storming the Citadel*. London: Constable, pp. 62–83.

10. **British Medical Association** (1881). The British Medical Association. A brief account of its origin, objects, and progress. *British Medical Journal* (2):1. <https://www.jstor.org/stable/25258437?seq=1#page_scan_tab_contents>.

11. **Manton, J** (1965). *Elizabeth Garrett Anderson*. London: Methuen, p. 258-60.

12. **Moberly Bell E** (1953). *Storming the Citadel*. London: Constable, pp. 92–3.

13. **Moberly Bell E** (1953). *Storming the Citadel*. London: Constable, p. 94.

14. **Lutzker E** (1959). Medical Education for Women in Great Britain. Master's thesis. New York: Columbia University, p. 50

15. **Moberly Bell E** (1953). *Storming the Citadel*. London: Constable, p. 97.

16. **Lutzker E** (1959). Medical Education for Women in Great Britain. Master's thesis. New York: Columbia University, p. 50.

17. **Moberly Bell E** (1953). *Storming the Citadel*. London: Constable, p. 99.

18. **Jex-Blake S** (1888). Medical Education of Women: a comprehensive study of present facilities for education, examination and registration. Edinburgh: National Association for Promoting the Medical Education of Women.

19. <http://www.medicalwomensfederation.org.uk/about-us/our-history>.

20. **Powell A** (2009). *Women in the War Zone*. Stroud: Sutton, pp. 18–19.

21. **Powell A** (2009). *Women in the War Zone*. Stroud: Sutton, p. 19.

22. <http://www.iwm.org.uk/collections/item/object/205022514>.

23. **Whitehead I** (1999). *Doctors in the Great War*. London: Leo Cooper, p. 107.

24. **Powell A** (2009). *Women in the War One*. Stroud: Sutton, p. 14.

25. **Whitehead I** (1999). *Doctors in the Great War*. London: Leo Cooper, p. 107.

26. Wellcome Library. SAMWF/C/1/3. Pioneers: Campbell, Julia Cock, MB Douie, D Hare, F Hoggan (nee Morgan), E Inglis, S Jex-Blake.

27. **Whitehead I** (1999). *Doctors in the Great War*. London: Leo Cooper, p. 111.

28. **Powell A** (2009). *Women in the War Zone*. Stroud: Sutton, p. 15.

29. **Whitehead I** (1999). *Doctors in the Great War*. London: Leo Cooper, p. 110.

30. **Powell A** (2009). *Women in the War Zone*. Stroud: Sutton, p. 16.
31. <http://www.medicalwomensfederation.org.uk/about-us/our-history>.
32. **NATS 1/822**. Woman medical practitioners: employment of women to leave men free for active service. The National Archives (TNA), Kew.
33. NATS 1/822. TNA.
34. WO 162/35. Payment of women doctors: Minutes and correspondence. TNA.
35. **Whitehead I** (1999). *Doctors in the Great War*. London: Leo Cooper, p. 109.
36. **Whitehead I** (1999). *Doctors in the Great War*. London: Leo Cooper, p. 91.
37. **Whitehead I** (1999). *Doctors in the Great War*. London: Leo Cooper, p. 92.
38. **Whitehead I** (1999). *Doctors in the Great War*. London: Leo Cooper, p. 97.
39. <http://www.medicalwomensfederation.org.uk/about-us/our-history>.
40. **Robinson M** (1925). Women doctors. *British Medical Journal*, 17 January, pp. 140–1. <https://doi.org/10.1136/bmj.1.3342.140-b>.
41. **Ramsay ML** (1925). Women doctors. *British Medical Journal*, 24 January, p. 192. <https://doi.org/10.1136/bmj.1.3343.192-a>.
42. **Harrison M** (2004). *Medicine and Victory: British Medicine in the Second World War*. Oxford: Oxford University Press, p. 34.
43. **Souttar HS** (1940). BMA Notices. *British Medical Journal* 1(4137):51–64. <http://www.jstor.org/stable/20316244>.
44. **Laurie JE, Newhouse ML**, and **Elliot PM** (1966). Working capacity of women doctors. *British Medical Journal* 1:409. <https://doi.org/10.1136/bmj.1.5484.409>.
45. **Calder JS** (1943). Future of women in medicine. *British Medical Journal* 1(4288):329–30. <http://www.jstor.org/stable/20325614>.
46. **Calder JS** (1943). Future of women in medicine. *British Medical Journal* 1(4288):329–30. <http://www.jstor.org/stable/20325614>.
47. **Swanston S** (1943). Future of women in medicine. *British Medical Journal* 1(4292):461. <http://www.jstor.org/stable/20325872>.
48. **Walker J** (1943). Future of women in medicine. *British Medical Journal* 1(4291):429. <http://www.jstor.org/stable/20325813>.
49. **Morgan JAU** (1962). Women doctors. *British Medical Journal* 1(5279):714. <http://www.jstor.org/stable/20357021>.
50. <http://www.medicalwomensfederation.org.uk/about-us/our-history>.
51. <http://hansard.millbanksystems.com/written_answers/1966/jan/26/married-women-doctors-part-time-work#S5CV0723P0_19660126_CWA_98>.
52. **Arie T** (1975). Married women doctor as part-time trainees. *British Medical Journal* 3(5984):641–3. <http://www.jstor.org/stable/20406796>.
53. **Laurie JE, Newhouse ML**, and **Elliot PM** (1966). Working capacity of women doctors. *British Medical Journal* 1(5484):409–12. <http://www.jstor.org/stable/25406694>.
54. <http://www.medicalwomensfederation.org.uk/about-us/our-history>.
55. MH 149/1647. Promotion of employment of married women doctors. 1974–75. (TNA).
56. **Henryk-Gutt R** and **Silverstone R** (1976). Career problems of women doctors. *British Medical Journal* 2(6035):574–7. <http://www.jstor.org/stable/20411271>.
57. **Scott JM** (1984). Women and the GMC. *British Medical Journal* **289**:1764–6.

58. **Swerdlow AJ** et al (1980). Women doctors in training: problems and progress supplement. *British Medical Journal* **281**(6242):754–8. <https://www.jstor.org/stable/25441369?seq=1#page_scan_tab_contents>.

59. BMA Advisory Service for Women Doctors. *British Medical Journal* **19** February 1983, **286**:661. <https://doi.org/10.1136/bmj.286.6365.661>.

60. **Dobson R** (1997). Women doctors believe medicine is male dominated. *British Medical Journal* **315**:75. <http://www.bmj.com/content/315/7100/75.12>.

61. **Khan M** (2012). BMJ Careers. Medicine—a woman's world? <http://careers.bmj.com/careers/advice/view-article.html?id=20006082>.

62. **Oxtoby K** (2009). BMJ Careers. Women in medicine. <http://careers.bmj.com/careers/advice/Women_in_medicine>.

63. **Rimmer A** (2014). BMJ Careers. Why do female doctors earn less money for doing the same job? <http://careers.bmj.com/careers/advice/Why_do_female_doctors_earn_less_money_for_doing_the_same_job%3F>.

64. **Rimmer A** (2016). BMJ Careers. Doctors slam junior contract for discrimination against women. <http://careers.bmj.com/careers/advice/Doctors_slam_junior_contract_for_discrimination_against_women>.

Chapter 3

The Entry of Women into Psychiatry

Fiona Subotsky

Introduction

While Henry Maudsley is principally remembered by his professional successors for the hospital he founded, his hostile remarks on the higher education of women in 1874 are also well-known.[1] These were responded to robustly by Elizabeth Garrett Anderson, Britain's major pioneer in the medical education of women.[2] This chapter examines how the debate and its participants may have affected the admission of women into the profession of psychiatry, at that time largely reflected by participation in the Medico-Psychological Association (MPA), founded in 1841 as the Association of Medical Superintendents of Lunatic Asylums, and later becoming the Royal Medico-Psychological Association and then the Royal College of Psychiatrists.

The Participants: Henry Maudsley (1835–1918)

Born in 1834, Maudsley (Figure 3.1) qualified as a doctor at University College London. He became involved in psychiatry by chance when he sought mental hospital experience as required by the East India Company medical service. However, after a brief spell at the Essex County Asylum, he became a successful medical superintendent at Manchester Royal Lunatic Asylum, Cheadle, at the age of 24. After three years he became restless and moved to London.[3] He was elected to the MPA in 1858,[4] where he doubtless distinguished himself by his assertiveness and intellectual cogency, impressing John Conolly, a foremost psychiatrist of his day, who was known for his 'non-restraint' policies. Soon Maudsley was engaged to one of his daughters. Conolly did not live long after the wedding and Maudsley seems to have been the successful son-in-law, inheriting both the small private asylum Lawn House, Hanwell, and private visiting positions.[5] An obliquely negative obituary article on his late father-in-law included a comment germane to his views of women:

> His mind seemed to be of the feminine type, capable of momentary lively sympathy, which might even express itself in tears ... and prone to shrink from the disagreeable occasions of life.[6]

Maudsley became joint editor of the *Journal of Mental Science* (JMS) of the MPA in 1863, contributing many articles and reviews over the ensuing years, and he became president of the association in 1871.

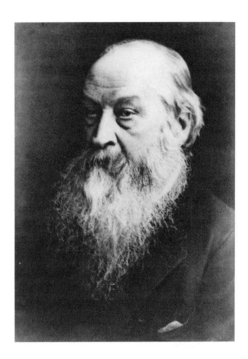

Figure 3.1 Henry
Maudsley (1835–1918)
© Royal College of
Psychiatrists

The Participants: Elizabeth Garrett Anderson (1836–1917)

Elizabeth Garrett Anderson (see Chapter 2, Figure 2.2) was also a well-established figure in her field by the time of the debate. She had started medical studies in 1860 at the Middlesex Hospital, technically as a nursing student, until in 1861, the medical students presented a petition against her and she had to withdraw. Although it was possible to gain qualifications abroad, Garrett did her utmost to gain admission to courses in Britain, but was refused. Eventually she found that the rules of the Society of Apothecaries did not prevent a woman from being granted their qualification and found people to teach her the required courses privately. She achieved the Licentiate of the Society of Apothecaries in 1865 and as a result was allowed on to the Medical Register in 1866 and was admitted as a member to the British Medical Association in 1874. However, all three organizations subsequently amended their regulations to prevent women being admitted. In 1870, Elizabeth Garrett became the first woman to gain MD from Paris: her dissertation was on migraine.[7]

The Debate: Maudsley

Maudsley's article 'Sex in Mind and Education' was published in a lay rather than professional magazine, and was surprisingly direct in its discussion of the physiology of women, particularly menstruation, although this word is not used.[1] His motives are not obvious, although he may have been keen to prevent the admission of women into his own hospital, St Mary's, and also the University of London.[8] Maudsley's key points against the higher education of women were: that the education of women would be detrimental to their health; that women, having 'periodic functions', were incapacitated for a quarter of the time; that education would particularly impair their reproductive function; and that this would show (and in the United States) in loss of menstruation, infertility, underdeveloped breasts, and inability to breastfeed. Women would try too hard (being conscientious) and impair their health through excessive study; adolescent girls were particularly at risk; men would not stand for it; no women had asked for it before, and those pressing for this were not representative; women should be educated only for their roles as mother and man's helpmeet.

Maudsley's style is often evangelistic in the sense of somehow threatening hellfire— in this case a risk to the nation:

> It would be an ill thing, if it should so happen, that we got the advantages of a quantity of female intellectual work at the price of a puny, enfeebled and sickly race.[1]

For effect, rather than consistency, he allows that 'without doubt there are women who ... will ... distinguish themselves' and that women should be allowed to try, although they would certainly fail. High-blown phrases are also often used—'it will not be possible to transform a woman into a man'; 'there is sex in mind as distinctly as there is in body'; 'you may hide nature but you cannot extinguish it ... the result may be a monstrosity'—statements which are difficult to disagree with because of inherent vagueness and yet which forcefully imply that the higher education of women is a waste of time.

Maudsley's approach here is not peculiarly misogynistic but rather typical of generally accepted ideas of the time and his own very biological approach. His view was that girls should not be educated either by the same methods or for the same ends as boys because their biological makeup and biological purposes were different. Maudsley's arguments are to a large extent a priori, but he also draws from American physicians who had observed the co-education available in the United States and who had drawn negative conclusions. The preoccupation of contemporary scientists with measurement and ranked categories appears to have made them more hostile to women's progress, more so even than other members of the educated classes.

The Debate: Elizabeth Garrett Anderson

Elizabeth Garrett Anderson replied to medical arguments with medical reasoning.[2] She noted that Maudsley's article was a reproduction of a lecture by Dr Clarke adapted with additions for an English audience. As it was originally given to an audience of women, perhaps a great degree of frankness was forgivable even if the argument was not accepted; however, as Maudsley had gone so far she herself had to 'use plain language':

> Dr Maudsley's paper consists mainly of a protest against the assimilation of the higher education of men and women, and against the admission of women to new careers; and this protest is founded upon the physiological peculiarities of women.[1]

Her argument is that there had been no aim to 'assimilate the female to the male mind' as 'women cannot choose but to be women'. She argues that Maudsley's use of American evidence is misleading as what is being advocated in England is different. For instance, higher education started later in Britain. However, if a course of education is excellent (like beef and bread) why should it not be good for both boys and girls irrespective of differences? Such a matter could be put to the test, not just assumed to be correct. There was, anyway, no reason why the final examination should not be the same. Meanwhile women, far from going through the same courses equally, had faced much opposition and difficulty.

The arguments that periodic functions always interfere with work was disproved by domestic servants, who were expected to carry on as usual. It was also illogical to argue that a function could be 'a cause of weakness when present and also when absent'. She argued that for women in good health and well nourished there was normally no loss of strength. Nevertheless, in early womanhood, there could more often be a temporary sense of weakness and teachers had to allow for this. However, this could be arranged as well in schools as in homes; physical education was no longer neglected as gymnastics and games had been introduced. Garrett Anderson pointed out that boys were also affected by pubertal changes and were liable to taxing their strength in different ways, for instance 'by drinking, smoking, unduly severe physical exercise, and frequently by late hours and dissipation generally'. A more real danger than study to young women in her view was the lack of worthwhile occupation, on the one hand leading to vanity and frivolity such as theatre-going and novel-reading, and on the other hand depressing dullness, which could lead to hysteria. She also thought that discouraging early marriage was likely to promote health. Other sources of harm were heavy skirts and over-heated rooms (i.e. a lack of fresh air and exercise). Overall, in Maudsley's argument the 'projectiles … are miscellaneous and obsolete'. She concludes that '[w]e may be guided by the general principles of equity and common sense, while waiting for the light of a larger experience'.

Garrett Anderson's reply is thus an effective one, appealing to justice, finding inconsistencies, putting forward alternative explanations and remedies for educated women's alleged ill health, and only having a little side-swipe about the energy dissipated by boys.

Maudsley, Women, and the Medico-Psychological Association

An anonymously written article in the *JMS* in 1866 entitled 'Sisters In Asylums' criticizes asylum attendants as, in the main, 'coarse, harsh, passionate, untrustworthy, intemperate', wanting in 'self-control, common-sense and co-operation', and praises the services of the sisterhood of a Rome asylum.[9] The author remarks: '[t]here is a cry for women's emancipation and her rights. Here is offered her hereditary right—to care for the wounded, the stricken, the fallen', and recommends asylum work as an opportunity for a life of 'cares and anxieties, duties and rewards'.[9] As Maudsley was editor of the *JMS* he either wrote or approved this. Maudsley thus envisaged 'caring' roles for women, but subordinate ones.

In 1871, after Maudsley's presidential address to the Medico-Psychological Association, there was a debate whether to enlarge the membership by admitting 'non-medical men'. Dr Batty Tuke inquired if the proposal was meant to include ladies, as it used the word 'person' at one point, and it was quickly agreed to substitute the word 'gentlemen'. Maudsley dominated the issue by concluding that 'persons who … have peculiar views—Swedenborgians and Spiritualists' would attempt entry and must be kept out, so the proposal was rejected.[10] For the next few years Maudsley continued to edit the journal and contribute to it. However, by 1877 there was a move (apparently led by his brother-in-law Harrington Tuke) to remove him from the editorship for not having the interests of the Association in mind. He resigned the following year. After 1881 Maudsley rarely attended MPA meetings, and by 1890 seems to have left the organization.[11] However, in terms of reputation outside the MPA, Maudsley's was still at its height. He continued to write books and did extremely well at his private practice; he was able to move to Mayfair, buy a mansion in Bushey Heath, and leave a substantial estate on his death.

Women Training as Doctors in the 1870s and 1880s

What had happened to women aspirants in the interim? For several years Sophia Jex-Blake (Figure 2.1) and other women had attempted to be allowed to enter, study, and graduate in medicine at Edinburgh, but had failed.[12] Jex-Blake reported that she received a letter from Thomas Laycock, an Edinburgh professor and a former president of the MPA, that 'he could not imagine any decent woman wanting to study medicine—as for any lady, that was out of the question'.[13] Eventually several of these women achieved graduation overseas (which at this point did not allow access to the British Medical Register, but did not necessarily preclude practice). However, following Gurney's Enabling Act of 1876, the General Medical Council (GMC) conceded that this meant that women could potentially graduate in the United Kingdom and Ireland and have their qualifications recognized for the Medical Register. The Irish institutions were the first to allow this and Edith Pechey and Sophia Jex-Blake obtained licentiateships there in 1877, thus gaining access to the Medical Register. By 1886, out of 50 women on the GMC register, 44 had entered it as licentiates of the King's and Queen's College of Physicians of Ireland (KQCPI).[14] The Royal Free Hospital in 1877 became the first London hospital to offer facilities for clinical instruction to female medical students and began its close association with the London School of Medicine for Women. At the University of London in 1877 the Senate proposed the admission of women to medical degrees, but the Convocation, with many vocal doctors, opposed this unless all degrees were considered, which was achieved the following year.[14]

The MPA Thinks Again

In 1879, there was a discussion of new rules at the annual general meeting of the MPA. Dr Stewart suggested that the wording about membership eligibility should be altered from 'qualified medical practitioner' to 'medical men'. Dr Orange suggested that this decision could be made at election but he was overruled, and the original amendment was agreed.[15]

Thomas S Clouston of Edinburgh, Maudsley's proposer for presidential office and for several years his co-editor, also gave public lectures on female education in 1882.[16] He is duller but more explicit than Maudsley, claiming that excessive education of adolescent girls led to anaemia, growth impairment, scrawniness, nervous over-sensitivity, head-aches, a tendency to take alcohol or drugs, and the impairment of fertility. Clouston appears however to have changed his mind to some degree later as when President himself in 1888, he announced to the MPA annual meeting that 'they had granted the certificate to forty-five gentlemen and one lady, all of whom had passed most satisfactory examinations'.[17] He also later supported the admission of ladies to membership.[18]

A Qualification in Lunacy (MPC)

The 'Certificate in Psychological Medicine of the Medico-Psychological Association of Great Britain' (MPC), was established by the MPA in 1885 as a qualification in lunacy. There were no stipulations about gender, as the word 'candidate' is used, but it is clear from the discussions that only men were being considered and indeed on the application and certificate forms the name to be filled in appears next to 'Mr'.[19]

Nevertheless, a woman—Jane Waterston (1843–1932) (Figure 3.2)—acquired the MPC in 1888; she was also the second woman to be elected a member of the MPA, in 1895. Waterston was a Scottish missionary based in South Africa who had returned to Britain seeking medical qualifications in 1874, and was in the first cohort of 14 women at the London School of Medicine for Women. She gained further clinical experience at Elizabeth Garrett Anderson's New Hospital for Women, at the Rotunda Lying-In Hospital, and at the Royal Free Hospital. She also took the Irish route, and was allowed registration when she passed the licentiate examination of the KQCPI in 1879. She returned to Africa, joining a mission for a while and later in 1883 establishing a private

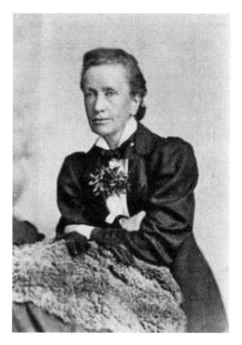

Figure 3.2 Jane Waterston (1843–1932)

practice in Cape Town. She did not take up exclusive psychiatric practice; indeed at the time, it was usual in South Africa for such problems to be dealt with by generalists. She was well-known for her philanthropic activities and was highly regarded both by patients and by the establishment, medical and non-medical.[20]

In the United States

There had been women doctors in asylums for some time in the United States, as the MPA was aware. In 1888 reporting on a visit to America, Dr Yellowlees stated that he had gone through the whole of these asylums, but had not met a single lady medical officer, although he had been told that they were there. Dr Clark said that his impression was that they were not liked, but nevertheless they were still appointed. In 1890, Fletcher Beach, commenting on American journals noted that 'impartial testimony from hospital superintendents has proved that women who have held hospital positions have not been able to perform their duties as satisfactorily as men' and hoped himself that 'women physicians will not be appointed Assistant Medical Officers in English Asylums for many years to come'.[21] Elsewhere in the same journal a much more positive view is reported by an American, Dr Gerhard: as legislation had enabled the appointment of female physicians to be in charge of female inmates of asylums, his view was that this should be encouraged and the medical needs, especially gynaecological, of women should be in the hands of women.[22] Hirshbein gives an account of this process: appointments were made largely because of concerns about preserving the modesty of women patients, and coincided with theories that gynaecological problems were the cause of much insanity. About half of all asylums in the United States employed women physicians at the beginning of the twentieth century. However, women were not allowed to become asylum superintendents and were not admitted into the professional organization until well into the twentieth century.[23]

In 1886 Dr Withers Moore in his presidential address to the British Medical Association (BMA) repeated the usual arguments against the education of women with a moving flourish:

> Unsexed it might be wrong to call her, but she will be more or less sexless. And the human race will have lost those who should have been her sons. Bacon, for want of a mother, will not be born.[24]

At the British Medical Association

In 1892, the BMA agreed to re-admit women as members at a specially held meeting. A Dr Stuart remarked that 'throughout Ireland (women doctors) were respected and admired, and were regarded as most helpful in the profession'. Elizabeth Garrett Anderson was present and spoke to the cause, using the argument that as all were disciples of Darwin 'here before their eyes was the great evolution of women out of one stage into another'. There were now 140 women in the profession.[25] The tide seemed to have turned, despite Withers Moore being President of Council and chair of many important committees. Psychiatrists such as Clouston are also named as sitting on BMA committees and so were part of this process.[26]

A Woman Proposed for the MPA

The following year in 1893 the issue of female membership arose again at the MPA. A woman's name had been put forward, a situation described by the President, James Murray Lindsay, as 'an innovation, a revolution'. 'Hole-in-corner' methods were suspected. Conolly Norman, the Irish President-elect, admitted to being behind this move and argued that recent legislation had deemed that the words 'man' and 'men' when used in a general sense could be understood to include members of both sexes. He was in favour of admitting women to the Association 'the female graduates whom the speaker had met were decidedly superior to the average of male graduates', and there were already women medical officers in asylums, of whom the nominee was one: 'he could say from personal knowledge, that at the meetings of the various sections … of the Academy of Medicine in Ireland female graduates and students were constantly present, and no difficulty arose'.

The President was inclined to support this interpretation of the rules, but a motion was insisted upon. Dr Whitcombe pointed out that there was already a lady doctor holding the Certificate, and that women were being received into various medical associations. The eventual motion passed was that 'according to the rules of the Association women are not eligible'. This was declared to be 'a victory for good grammar'.[27] The Rules Committee considered the situation in January the following year, with opposing views: there still appeared to be some muddle over whether the terminology was 'men' which might include women, or 'practitioners', before which Mr Richards suggested the word 'male' should be put. Dr Yellowlees' firm opinion was that it was time for women to be admitted, as the BMA had done. Dr Ireland felt that there would be matters 'which it would be very disagreeable to have to discuss before women'. Drs Benham, Whitcombe, and Bonville Fox thought that the Annual Meeting resolution was not designed to keep out women, but was instead a question of procedure and grammar; they were now all in favour.

It was then agreed to alter the wording (for eligibility) to 'registered medical practitioner', which allowed for the admission of women.[28] Later in 1894 Conolly Norman was in the chair as President in his home town of Dublin and put forward a woman candidate, Eleonora Lilian Fleury (Figure 3.3). It was moved that the adoption of the

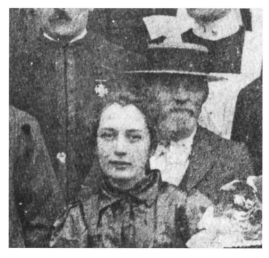

Figure 3.3 Eleonora Lilian Fleury
© St Brendan's Hospital

candidates should not be en masse, so individual votes were taken. As there were 23 votes for and 7 against, Conolly declared that constitutionally Fleury was elected.[29]

Eleonora Fleury was in a good position for this, apart from her gender. She was born in Dublin in 1860, daughter of Dr Charles Fleury. She was the first woman medical graduate of the Royal University of Ireland (RUI), coming first in order of merit with first-class honours and an exhibition. She had been a student at the Richmond Hospital in Dublin and the London School of Medicine for Women. She worked at the Homerton Fever Hospital in London for a year before returning to Ireland to work at the Richmond Asylum for 27 years. Although she became deputy medical director she was always passed over for male colleagues for the most senior post.[14]

Career Progress

Bearing in mind the extreme difficulties early women doctors had first in getting qualified and second in getting jobs, it is interesting to consider their possible pathways. Many would have known each other through attending the London School of Medicine for Women, gaining clinical experience at the New Hospital and studying for the Irish examinations. As a forum for mutual support the forerunner of the Medical Women's Federation—the Association of Registered Medical Women—was formed in London in 1879, supported by Elizabeth Garrett Anderson. Her brother-in-law, Henry Fawcett, as Postmaster General introduced equal pay for women doctors when appointing a female medical officer to the Post Office, a principle followed by the London County Council when appointing to their new asylums.[30] It is of interest that three of the later candidates were put forward from Claybury, presumably with the support of the superintendent, Sir Robert Armstrong-Jones. These were Emily Louisa Dove (1897), Margaret Orange (1898) possibly related to a previous president of the MPA, and Helen Boyle (1898) (Figure P1.1), who much later in 1939 became the first woman President of the Royal Medico-Psychological Association.[31] By 1899, in addition to these women, the following had been elected members: Elizabeth Jane Moffett (1895), Margaret Cochran Dewar (1896), Norah Kemp (1898), and Amelia Grogan (1899).[32] In the same year women listed as having obtained the MPC were: Jane B Henderson; Annie B Jagannadhan; Elizabeth J Moffett; Lucia Strangman, and Jane Elizabeth Waterston.[33]

While women psychiatrists had begun to emerge by the end of the nineteenth century, they remained in lower positions in the public hospitals, being placed in charge only of female wards; in private and voluntary hospitals, especially if established by themselves, they had more autonomy.[34] Showalter's view is that as the twentieth century progressed, even though there were many more women psychiatrists in Britain 'they remained a powerless minority'.[35]

Conclusion

The Maudsley/Elizabeth Garrett Anderson debate on female education in 1874 occurred at a tipping point for the participants and the argument. Maudsley essentially became preoccupied elsewhere, but Garrett Anderson, now married and with a growing family, persisted in her missions to provide better care for women and children and to support women in entering the medical profession. This she did primarily in London with powerful political, social, and professional support and direct lobbying herself, such as by writing to *The Times*. She claimed to favour a gradual, quiet approach. The more militant but equally persistent group connected with Sophia Jex-Blake, failing initially in Scotland, achieved the opening up of the 'Irish route'. Being on the Medical Register, however, did not necessarily gain admittance to Societies and Colleges. Garrett Anderson's involvement in the 1892 BMA debate was successful in getting women re-admitted, a decision which clearly influenced the MPA.

Maudsley's personal style has been emphasized here because it may well have been counterproductive for his views. While he could be a powerful speaker and writer, he evidently had an increasingly negative effect on his colleagues. By 1896, in a review of the second edition of *The Pathology of Mind*, the author commented that 'Dr. Maudsley's philosophy is frequently unsound, his psychology prohibitive of truth, and his sociology repulsive and unsuited to average humanity'.[36] Thus, while his views against the education of women carried considerable weight in the 1870s, this was much less the case later when both public and professional opinion had begun to shift, and he himself was not attending many meetings of the MPA. One might have expected that none of the existing members would have shifted their views but that a younger generation would have different ideas. However, the well-minuted debates make it clear that several medico-psychologists including Clouston, Maudsley's co-editor, did indeed change their minds about the acceptability of women entering the profession, even though the method was somewhat circuitous, with political manoeuvring and distracting arguments about wording. It is interesting to speculate whether, in the later years, when Frederick Mott, the main activist behind the founding of the Maudsley Hospital, and keen to point out Maudsley's positive social qualities,[36] ever discussed with him the employment of women at Claybury Asylum where Helen Boyle collaborated with him on research.[37]

References

1. **Maudsley H** (1874). Sex in mind and education. *Fortnightly Review*, **15**, 467–83.
2. **Garrett Anderson E** (1874). Sex in mind and education: a reply. *Fortnightly Review*, **15**, 582–94.
3. **Maudsley H.** Autobiography (1988). *Journal of Mental Science*, **153**, 736–40.
4. Annual meeting of the Association: Election of new members (1858). *Journal of Mental Science*, **4**, 57.
5. **Scull A, Mackenzie C,** and **Hervey N** (1996). *Masters of Bedlam: The Transformation of the Mad-Doctoring Trade.* Princeton: Princeton University Press, p. 245.
6. **Maudsley H** (1866). Memoir of the late John Conolly, M.D. *Journal of Mental Science* **12**:151–74.
7. **Crawford E** (2002). *Enterprising Women: The Garretts and their Circle.* London: Francis Boutle.
8. **Collie M** (1988). *Henry Maudsley: Victorian Psychiatrist. A Bibliographical Study.* Winchester: St Paul's Bibliographies.
9. **Anon.** (1866). Sisterhoods in Asylums. *Journal of Mental Science*, **12**, 44–63.
10. (1871). Notes and News: Alteration of the Rules. *Journal of Mental Science* **17**:445–6.

11. **Turner T** (1988). Henry Maudsley: psychiatrist, philosopher, and entrepreneur. *Psychological Medicine* **18**:551–74.

12. **Blake C** (1990). *The Charge of the Parasols: Women's Entry to the Medical Profession.* London: Women's Press, pp. 91–155.

13. **Jex-Blake S** (1886). *Medical Women: A Thesis and a History.* Edinburgh: Oliphant, Anderson and Ferrier.

14. **Bewley B** (2005). 'On the Inside Sitting Alone': pioneer Irish women doctors. *History Ireland* **13**:33–6.

15. (1879). Notes and News: Report of the Thirty-Fourth Annual General Meeting of the Medico-Psychological Association. *Journal of Mental Science* **25**:431–42.

16. **Clouston TS** (1882). *Female Education from a Medical Point of View. Being Two Lectures Delivered at the Philosophical Institution.* Edinburgh: Macniven & Wallace.

17. (1888). Notes and News: The Admission of Lady Members to the Association. *Journal of Mental Science* **34**:452.

18. (1893). *Journal of Mental Science* **39**:600–1.

19. (1885). Notes and News: Report of Committee appointed by Council on Certificate in Psychological Medicine. *Journal of Mental Science*, **31**, 432–3.

20. **Van Heyningen E** (1996). Jane Elizabeth Waterston—Southern Africa's first woman doctor. *Journal of Medical Biography* **4**:208–13.

21. **Beach F** (1888). Psychological Retrospect. *Journal of Mental Science* **36**:100.

22. **Gerhard Dr** (1888). Female physicians and the state hospitals for the insane in the United States. *Journal of Mental Science* **36**:151–2.

23. **Hirshbein LD** (2004). History of women in psychiatry. *Academic Psychiatry* **28**:337–44.

24. **Withers Moore W** (1886). Presidential Address. *The Lancet* **II**:314–15.

25. (1892). Extraordinary General Meeting. *British Medical Journal* **II**:62–3.

26. (1892). Committee List. *British Medical Journal* **II**:ii.

27. (1893). *Journal of Mental Science* **39**:598–601.

28. (1894). *Journal of Mental Science* **40**:156–7.

29. (1894). *Journal of Mental Science* **40**:690–1.

30. **Moberley Bell E** (1953). *Storming the Citadel.* London: Constable, pp. 178–9.

31. (1957). Obituary, Helen Boyle M.D. *British Medical Journal* **II**:1310.

32. (1899). Membership list. *Journal of Mental Science* **45**:v–xxii.

33. (1899). Certificate list. *Journal of Mental Science* **45**:xxiii–xxv.

34. **Mackenzie C** (1983). Women and psychiatric professionalization, 1780–1914. In: **Feminist History Group** (ed.). *The Sexual Dynamics of History: Men's Power, Women's Resistance.* London: Pluto Press, pp. 107–19.

35. **Showalter E** (1985). *The Female Malady: Women, Madness and English Culture, 1830–1980.* London: Virago Press, p. 203.

36. (1918). Obituary of Henry Maudsley. *Journal of Mental Science* **64**:116–29.

37. **Boyle AH** (1899). A case of juvenile general paralysis. *Journal of Mental Science* **45**:99–104.

The Life of Dr Helen Boyle (1869–1957)

Fiona Subotsky

'No-one should join any profession without being determined to contribute something new, of value to that profession.'

Helen Boyle (Figure P1.1), was born in 1869 in Dublin, where she spent her first 13 years. She then lived on the Continent with her family and was educated in France and Germany. She trained at the London School of Medicine for Women from 1890, qualifying in 1893 with the Scottish triple qualification, becoming licentiate of the Royal College of Physicians of Edinburgh, the Royal College of Surgeons of Edinburgh, and the Royal Faculty of Physicians and Surgeons of Glasgow. In 1894 she achieved her MD in Brussels with distinction.

Her first post was as assistant medical officer at the London County Council Claybury Asylum where Sir Robert Armstrong Jones was the Medical Superintendent. While there, she collaborated with the pathologist Sir Frederick Mott. At that time, she was the first psychiatrist to identify bacillary dysentery among mental patients.

Later, while medical superintendent at Canning Town Mission Hospital in the east end of London, she observed that nervous and mental disorders in their early stages were scarcely recognized and impossible to treat until they became so severe that certification became necessary. It became her mission to improve this situation, and she visited various clinics abroad to see how other societies dealt with this.

In 1897 she set up in general practice in Hove in Sussex with her friend Dr Mabel Jones. They were the first women doctors in Hove, and their practice was at 3 Palmeira Terrace, 37 Church Road, mostly attended to by Mabel Jones. Helen Boyle started the Lewes Road Dispensary for Women and Children in Brighton which in 1905 became the Lady Chichester Hospital (Figure P1.2) for the Treatment of Early Mental Disorders, the first of its kind. This was a successful pioneering venture, with Helen Boyle its 'head and heart' for 50 years, seeing it through several moves and expansions. She continued to work there until the National Health Service took over in 1948.

In the First World War she served for five months in Serbia with the Royal Free Hospital Unit, and was decorated with the order of St Sava.

Helen Boyle was actively involved in the founding of several major societies:

- The Brighton Guardianship Society (1913), which aimed to keep 'mental defectives' within the Community.
- The Medical Women's Federation (1917)
- The International Medical Women's Federation (1922)
- The Child Guidance Council (Figure P1.3)
- The National Council for Mental Hygiene (later the National Association for Mental Health, now MIND) with Sir Maurice Craig, paying the rent of its office herself for the first three years

After becoming a member of the Medico–Psychological Society in 1898 Helen Boyle was always actively involved in its meetings and committees, and in 1939 became its first woman President. In 1955, the spring meeting of the Royal Medico–Psychological Association took place at Hove in her honour on the occasion of the Jubilee celebrations of the Lady Chichester Hospital.

Helen Boyle died one day after her 88th birthday, in 1957.

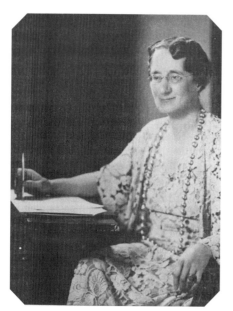

Figure P1.1 Dr Helen Boyle, President of the Medico-Psychological Society, 1939–40.
© Royal College of Psychiatrists

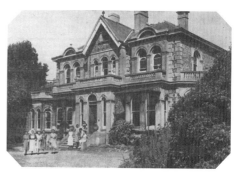

Figure P1.2 The Lady Chichester Hospital.
© Royal College of Psychiatrists

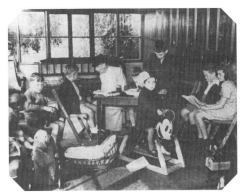

Figure P1.3 Child Guidance Clinic, The Lady Chichester Hospital.

© Royal College of Psychiatrists

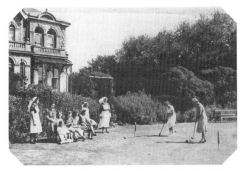

Figure P1.4 Staff and Patients in the Gardens, The Lady Chichester Hospital.

© Royal College of Psychiatrists

The Principles of the Lady Chichester Hospital

1. It is not reserved for nervous cases
2. The patients are not kept in bed unless needful (Figure P1.4)
3. The medical supervision is done by people who have had some experience of both insanity and neurology
4. Numerous patients should be treated together
5. There should never be too many patients for the medical staff to know them thoroughly personally
6. There should be provision for the treatment of women by women
7. There should be an entire absence of red tape

Quotations

'Insanity begins before a person is insane, and it is then that recognition and skilled treatment are most valuable.'

'I saw mental patients ... neglected and maltreated until after days, months or years ... they were turned into the finished product—lunatics—and were certified.'

'I saw the impecunious and harassed mother of five ... with a nervous breakdown after influenza ... apply for treatment, wait many weary hours, and get a bottle and the advice not to worry ... No hospital would take her because she had no organic disease; no asylum because she was not certified.'

'If anyone needs entire change of life and surroundings in order to get better surely it is the poor.'

'I have seen differences of opinion and treatment far wider and more radical than is apparent in other diseases, and the management of such cases undertaken by all and sundry.'

'If all neurologists were alienists too, and all alienists were also neurologists, in fact, neuro-alienists, we should begin to get a healthier and more intelligent public opinion on these vital matters.'

'Never will these early nervous and mental cases be efficiently understood until there are wards in the general teaching hospitals for them.'

Major Papers

- A Case of Juvenile General Paralysis. *Journal of Mental Science* 1899;45:99–105.
- Some points in the early treatment of mental and nervous cases (with special reference to the poor). *Journal of Mental Science* 1905; 51:676–81.
- Account of an attempt at the early treatment of mental and nervous cases (with special reference to the poor). *Journal of Mental Science* 1909;55:683–92.
- Some observations on early nervous and mental cases, with suggestions as to possible Improvement in our methods of dealing with them. *Journal of Mental Science* 1914;60:381–98.
- The ideal clinic for the treatment of nervous and borderline cases. *Proceedings of the Royal Society of Medicine* 1922; 15:39–48.
- 'Watchman, what of the night?' Presidential address delivered at the ninety-eighth annual meeting of the Royal Medico-Psychological Association held at Brighton, July 12, 1939. *Journal of Mental Science* 1939;85: 0–870.

Other Sources

Dr Helen Boyle, 1869–1957. <http://womenofbrighton.co.uk/helenboyle.htm>.

East Sussex Record Office

Hingston CL (1955). The Jubilee of the Lady Chichester Hospital, Hove, Sussex. *Journal of the Medical Women's Federation* 80–4.

Hingston CL and Vince C (1958). Death of a pioneer: Helen Boyle. *Journal of the Medical Women's Federation* 72–5.

Milliken E (2004). Helen Boyle (1869–1957), physician and specialist in the treatment of mental illness. *Oxford Dictionary of National Biography*. Oxford: Oxford University Press p. 11.

(1957) Obituary: Helen Boyle, MD. *British Medical Journal* **2**:1310.

Dame Fiona Caldicott

An Inspirational Woman with an Astonishingly Impressive Career

Katherine Kennet and Fiona Caldicott

Dame Fiona is the first woman to be President of the Royal College of Psychiatrists, has been Principal of Somerville College, the University of Oxford, and is the pioneer behind the Caldicott Principles. These principles are used throughout the National Health Service (NHS) to guide confidentiality in the age of newly computerized data. These are just three of her numerous notable achievements. Dame Fiona's continuing career spans so many successes that her accomplishments are dazzling. Her work on confidentiality enhances the daily practice of all clinicians and patients in the NHS. On meeting her in preparation for this profile, I found her inspirational in person, humble, and above all a deeply family orientated woman.

Key list of achievements and roles[2]

- Represented St Hilda's College, University of Oxford, in the 2016 Christmas University Challenge as part of an all-female team which won the competition (see Figure P2.2).

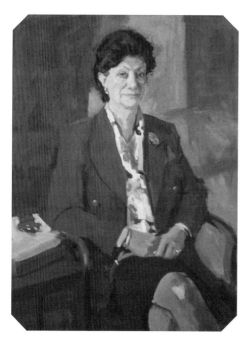

Figure P2.1 Portrait of Dame Fiona by Susannah Fiennes on permanent display at the Royal College of Psychiatrists, London.

© Susannah Fiennes

- Led Review of Data Security and Consent / Opt-Out, 2015–16
- National Data Guardian, 2014–present.
- Led an independent review of information governance, 2012–13
- Chaired the National Information Governance Board, 2011–13
- Chair, Oxford University Hospitals NHS Foundation Trust, 2009–present
- Elected Member General Medical Council, 1997–2001
- Chaired the Caldicott Committee on patient-identifiable data in the NHS, leading to the creation of 'Caldicott Guardians' in all NHS Trusts, 1996–97
- Principal of Somerville College in the University of Oxford, 1996–2010
- Chair of the Academy of Medical Royal Colleges, 1995–96
- President of the Royal College of Psychiatrists, 1993–96, the first woman to hold this position
- Dean of the Royal College of Psychiatrists 1990–93, the first woman to hold this position
- Consultant and Senior Clinical Lecturer in Psychotherapy for the South Birmingham Mental Health NHS Trust, 1977–96

Life

Fiona Caldicott was born in Troon in 1941 to a civil servant mother and barrister father. Her paternal grandparents were greengrocers and 'didn't believe in education'. As a result, her father was encouraged to leave school in his mid-teens. He later returned to

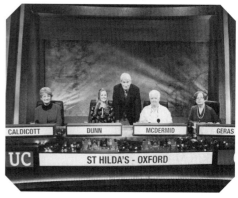

Figure P2.2 Dame Fiona representing St Hilda's College, Oxford on Christmas University Challenge, 2016.

education to complete a chemistry degree at night school, and subsequently completed a law degree via correspondence. Her father passed this work ethic, and his ethos of education being an utmost priority in life, on to his daughter. Her mother, a civil servant, gave up her professional life once married, as was required at the time. Fiona was awarded a local authority scholarship to attend the City of London School for Girls, where the philosophy was one of achieving potential through dedication and hard work. She became head girl and went on to St Hilda's College, Oxford University, where she read medicine. During her medical studies (see Figure P2.3) she married her husband, who ran a family wine merchant company, and moved to the Midlands. She completed her clinical training and worked as a doctor in the area, and in subsequent years had two children. She describes her personal and family life as the foundations for her career and reported that she couldn't have achieved these accomplishments without the support of her husband.

In 1990 tragedy struck Dame Fiona's family. The younger of her children, her son Richard, was involved in a car crash which resulted in his early and unexpected death aged just 19. Six weeks after this devastating event Dame Fiona was elected the Dean of the Royal College of Psychiatrists. Dame Fiona described this moment as a turning point in her life; clearly both these events were profoundly significant.

Dame Fiona currently lives in Warwickshire with her husband Robert.

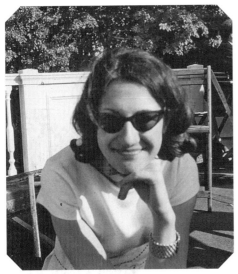

Figure P2.3 Dame Fiona as an undergraduate in 1963.

Career

After her 'house jobs' in Coventry, including working in Accident and Emergency while heavily pregnant with her first child Lucy, she briefly considered a career in hospital medicine but instead opted for a period at home with her new baby. After three months she began work as a part-time general practitioner (GP) and she maintains that 'every doctor should do some work as a GP'. After her second child, Richard, was born she decided to train as a psychiatrist, drawn to the specialty by a fascination since her undergraduate days in neuroscience and the workings of the brain, but deeply attracted to the medicine of the whole person. Psychiatry, with its ability to not just acknowledge but embrace these sometimes conflicting aspects of medical science, was therefore a natural choice for her.

At the time of her specialization, psychiatry was a male-dominated profession, and she was one of only three female part-time trainees in the Midlands. Part-time working in medicine and the Royal College of Psychiatrists (RCPsych) membership had both been only recently introduced, and it was unclear if full membership of the RCPsych would even be possible for a less than full-time psychiatrist.

In 1976 Dame Fiona was offered and accepted a position on the Department of Health and the British Medical Association's (BMA) Central Manpower Committee. In this role she succeeded in shedding light on the need for the provision of far more psychiatrists not only as junior doctors but also at consultant level. This was a defining moment in the work of the Royal College of Psychiatrists and a triumph for Dame Fiona.

In 1990, working as a consultant psychiatrist in Birmingham, she was elected to the prestigious position of Dean of the RCPsych. Coming at a time of personal tragedy, Dame Fiona had carefully considered the impact that standing for this prominent position could have on her career, and the different path it would lead her to follow. After three years she stood for the Presidency of the Royal College. When elected to this position, she became the first woman president of the RCPsych (see Figure P2.1). This historic appointment stands as a clear testament to Dame Fiona's dedication to hard work, achievements thus far, and the skill of balancing both career and family responsibilities.

Dame Fiona's presidency involved work at a national and international level, and the question of what should follow professionally when her term was completed was answered by her appointment as Principal of Somerville College, Oxford University (see Figure P2.4).

Caldicott became a household name amongst doctors following the Caldicott Report, which resulted

Continued on next page

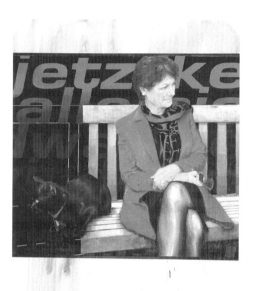

Figure P2.4 Portrait of Dame Fiona by Thomas Leveritt on display at Somerville College, Oxford.

© Tom Leveritt

from the committee she chaired investigating data confidentiality in the NHS. This came at a time when the use of information technology was expanding exponentially and its use in healthcare was becoming inevitable. This committee was appointed to explore the conflicting views of the BMA that all personal patient information should be encrypted to ensure privacy, and the Department of Health's view that the cost of this would mean that data collection and maintenance would be non-viable. The now famous 'Caldicott Principles' (see Box P2.1) guide all NHS employees on how to use patient data safely and confidentially. Initially there were six principles but the second Caldicott Report in 2013 introduced an additional one which highlighted the duty clinicians have to share clinically important information.

Dame Fiona reflected that although all doctors use these principles of confidentiality and consent in their work, it is psychiatrists who often deal with the most complex issues. Her earlier career experiences as a consultant psychiatrist and her RCPsych roles helped to inform her pioneering work in this area.

Since 2009 Dame Fiona has been Chair of the Oxford University Hospitals NHS Foundation Trust,

---

Box P2.1 *The Caldicott Principles for Information Governance when Handling Patient Information*[6]

1. Justify the purpose(s)

Every proposed use or transfer of personal confidential data within or from an organisation should be clearly defined, scrutinized and documented, with continuing uses regularly reviewed, by an appropriate guardian.

2. Don't use personal confidential data unless it is absolutely necessary

Personal confidential data items should not be included unless it is essential for the specified purpose(s) of that flow. The need for patients to be identified should be considered at each stage of satisfying the purpose(s).

3. Use the minimum necessary personal confidential data

Where use of personal confidential data is considered to be essential, the inclusion of each individual item of data should be considered and justified so that the minimum amount of personal confidential data is transferred or accessible as is necessary for a given function to be carried out.

4. Access to personal confidential data should be on a strict need-to-know basis

Only those individuals who need access to personal confidential data should have access to it, and they should only have access to the data items that they need to see. This may mean introducing access

controls or splitting data flows where one data flow is used for several purposes.

5. Everyone with access to personal confidential data should be aware of their responsibilities

Action should be taken to ensure that those handling personal confidential data—both clinical and non-clinical staff—are made fully aware of their responsibilities and obligations to respect patient confidentiality.

6. Comply with the law

Every use of personal confidential data must be lawful. Someone in each organisation handling personal confidential data should be responsible for ensuring that the organisation complies with legal requirements.

7. The duty to share information can be as important as the duty to protect patient confidentiality.

Health and social care professionals should have the confidence to share information in the best interests of their patients within the framework set out by these principles. They should be supported by the policies of their employers, regulators and professional bodies.

Reproduced from Williams Lea for the Department of Health, Information; to share or not to share, The Information Governance Review, pp. 20–21, Copyright (2013), Crown copyright

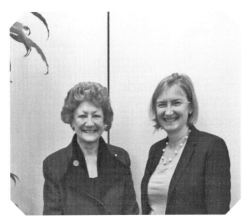

Figure P2.5 Dame Fiona meeting with Sarah Wollaston MP, Chair of the Health Select Committee to discuss data sharing in the NHS.

© Sarah Wollaston

the fourth largest NHS Trust in England. She continues her work on confidentiality and is currently on the National Information Board as the National Data Guardian (see Figure P2.5).[1]

Dame Fiona's evolving legacy is an epic one; every NHS Trust in the United Kingdom has a 'Caldicott Guardian', entrusted with ensuring patient confidentiality and the Caldicott Principles are upheld. This work has impacted on every patient in the country. Due to the ever-increasing importance of technology and the prominent role it plays in healthcare, 19 years after the publication of the first Caldicott Report, Dame Fiona's work remains as relevant as ever.

Favourite quotations

- 'No surprises', for people regarding the use of their data

Most notable works and major papers

- Report on the review of patient-identifiable information: 'The Caldicott Report', 1997
- Information; to share or not to share by the Information Governance Review: 'Caldicott 2', 2013

- Review of Data Security, Consent and Opt-Outs by the National Data Guardian for Health and Care, 2016

Sources and Bibliography

Dame Fiona Caldicott was interviewed by Dr Katherine Kennet at the Department of Health 19 September 2016.

1. Fiennes S (1997). *Dame Fiona Caldicott, DBE, President of the Royal College of Psychiatrists (1993–1996)*. [Oil on canvas] London: Royal College of Psychiatrists.
2. Biography of Dame Fiona Caldicott, National data Guardian. <https://www.gov.uk/government/people/fiona-caldicott>.
3. Tweet from Twitter account: <http://www.google.co.uk/url?url=http://topsy.one/hashtag.php%3Fq%3D%2523UniversityChallenge&rct=j&frm=1&q=&esrc=s&sa=U&ved=0ahUKEwiv5Naf-fPRAhVBRhQKHWTXC304PBDBbgggMAU&usg=AFQjCNE3ElpszXV7CO-O7EJj64ujjjGY6g>.
4. Unknown (unpublished). *Fiona Caldicott in 1963*. [photograph] Fiona Caldicott's personal collection.
5. Leveritt T (2002). *Dame Fiona Caldicott, Principal of Somerville College (1996–2010)*. [Oil on canvas] Oxford: Somerville College, University of Oxford.
6. Caldicott F (2013). The Information Governance Review, Department of Health. Information; to share or not to share. London: Department of Health, pp. 20–1. <https://www.gov.uk/government/uploads/system/uploads/attachment_data/file/192572/2900774_InfoGovernance_accv2.pdf>.
7. Wollaston S. <https://www.google.co.uk/url?sa=i&rct=j&q=&esrc=s&frm=1&source=images&cd=&cad=rja&uact=8&ved=0ahUKEwj287TCye3RAhWLtBoKHWt5AjwQjRwIBw&url=https%3A%2F%2Ftwitter.com%2Fsarahwollaston%2Fstatus%2F666761837862592512&psig=AFQjCNE7L11dK5M4q4xt0a3Niamv3kBZAw&ust=1485992962470214>.

My Small but Significant Body of Work

Eyes watering with formaldehyde, some would-be
Surgeon will swallow her nausea, green-cloth
my face to stop me watching, make her first cut
through my outdated covering. Once under the skin
she'll neatly slice through yellow adjectival fat,

already over-edited, pared down to twinge
of ligament and bone. I can't hide anything
from her: the tripe, the lack of guts, the bile
and vented spleen, my once inspiring
bags of wind, my silenced sounding box.

She'll learn by rote the vessels where my blood
ran hot, the grey roots threaded through
my chilling spine. Word-perfect, she'll recite
my intricate syllabic arteries, derivative veins,
the chain rhymed branching of my nerves.

She'll probe and scalpel my biography,
until it hangs together, lucid, fleshless, merely
a standard diagram in her classic text. And after that
she'll turn the page to my remaindered heart.

Emily Wills
(Reproduced from *Developing the Negative,* published by The
Rialto, 2008)

Chapter 4

History of the Royal College of Psychiatrists' Women's Mental Health Special Interest Group

Jane Mounty, Anne Cremona,
and Rosalind Ramsay

The Women's Mental Health Special Interest Group (WMHSIG) of the Royal College of Psychiatrists, re-established in 2015, has a number of aims and objectives relevant to both female psychiatrists and female patients. These include:

◆ to build on previous initiatives around women and mental health, whilst taking the Group in a more outwardly-facing direction;

◆ to provide a space for psychiatrists to learn from, and network with each other;

◆ to take a cross-disciplinary approach to women's mental health;

◆ to engage with women including healthcare professionals *outside* psychiatry, and the wider public—and in doing so showcase psychiatry by raising awareness of and interest in it, as a specialty and career;

◆ to forge cross-disciplinary links with fellow mental health workers within the Royal College of Nursing, the British Psychological Society, Alliance for Women and Girls at Risk (AGENDA), and other medical specialities;

◆ to counteract discrimination against women patients;

◆ to raise awareness of the effects of abuse: childhood sexual abuse, trauma, and domestic violence, on the development of mental illness in all patients, especially women.

WMHSIG developed from the Women in Psychiatry Special Interest Group (WIPSIG), set up in 1996 with the dual objectives of improving the working lives of women psychiatrists and improving the provision of care to women using mental health services.

In this chapter we describe the journey of WMHSIG (formerly WIPSIG) over the last 21 years. We look at the how the Group began, its early initiatives, the taking stock and alignment with College work around the time of its tenth anniversary, and the increasing focus on women patients. Radical changes for both women psychiatrists and women patients have taken place in this time. As authors of this chapter and members of WIPSIG, we participated in many of the changes. From 1997 to 2007

Jane Mounty served on the Executive in the various roles of Treasurer, Secretary, and Conference organizer, while Anne Cremona is the Founder and first Chair (1996–2002), and Rosalind Ramsay a former Chair of the Group (2004–07). We refer to the Group throughout this chapter as the SIG (Special Interest Group), until the time it became WMHSIG.

How the Group Began

After the birth of her fourth child in 1994, Dr Anne Cremona was refused permission to job-share the consultant post that she had previously carried out full-time for ten years, despite the intervention of the British Medical Aassociation (BMA) and her identifying a number of psychiatrists interested in job-sharing with her. The wisdom of the day was that no woman doctor could carry the responsibility of an adult psychiatry consultant post putting in the long hours required while also caring for a large family. Comments such as 'part-time work means part-time commitment' were frequently bandied about.

In the mid 1990s, flexible medical/psychiatric training was a new concept.[1] Little thought had been given to ways of working part-time. Although there were a few early examples of women psychiatrists job-sharing or working part-time, this was uncommon. Only a very small number of part-time consultant posts were available in specialties such as Child and Adolescent Mental Health (CAMHS). In General Adult psychiatry—where people were appointed to consultant posts at an older average age (35–40 years)—part-time consultant posts were rare. Was it assumed that women would have already passed their child-bearing days by the time they became consultants? Or, more likely, that little thought had been given to the needs of women consultants in their child-bearing years? Although it was theoretically possible to apply for a full-time consultant post on a part-time basis (as part-time consultant posts were almost never advertised), in practice suitable full-time applicants would always be given priority.

Ten years earlier, Dr Julie Hollyman had written to the then President of the Royal College of Psychiatrists, Dr Thomas Bewley, asking 'why should career breaks for family reasons have to jeopardise promotion?' She also recommended that women trainees be counselled about their careers from the start of training. Later, Dr Ann Gath, Registrar of the Royal College, had suggested a change to the career structures of all psychiatrists, men and women, citing growing evidence that *all* wanted a better work–life balance. She advised that few women ultimately drop out of medicine, despite the considerable practical difficulties when their children were young. Traditions were also beginning to change in other medical specialties with the creation of the first ever part-time surgical training posts.

In the 1990s, because of long working hours due to on-call requirements, the average number of hours worked per week in all medical specialities often exceeded 80. Thus, even in 'part-time' arrangements, doctors worked 40-plus hours per week. Trainees who applied through the National Approval Scheme PM79 (Part III)[2] for supernumerary posts encompassed a wide variety of people with a range of reasons for wanting to work only 40 hours per week; not only those with domestic and caring roles, but some with health issues, some with alternative aspirations, which required a substantial time commitment, such as would-be Olympians.

Clinical and medical directors and deans across the country wanted to assist but the lack of funding attached to the Scheme caused financial difficulty. Even after funding for a post was found from within a Trust, there were further problems when part-timers were added to on-call rotas because this sometimes reduced the level of remuneration for all by changing the banding allocated to a particular rota.

Interestingly, there was a considerable number of consultants who effectively worked part-time in the National Health Service (NHS) with 'maximum part-time' contracts, which allowed them to drop some of their NHS sessions. These were usually male consultants who combined a full-time NHS workload in reduced hours with their private practice. The maximum part-time contract was a concession dating back to the days of Aneurin Bevan, founder of the NHS, and the political necessity of winning doctors' agreement to work in the NHS without having to relinquish private practice.

Dr Cremona decided the only solution was to resign from her full-time post to retrain as a child psychiatrist because flexible training was better established within that field. This seemed to her to be the only way for her to resume working as a consultant—albeit in a new specialty, CAMHS. In the event, Dr Cremona managed to find a consultant post in General Adult psychiatry that she could job-share. This unusual application to retrain from an already established Consultant brought her to the attention of Professor Fiona Caldicott (first female President of the Royal College of Psychiatrists) and Dr Catherine Oppenheimer (who had a particular interest in equality of career opportunities for women psychiatrists). Instead of retraining, they encouraged her instead to continue in her chosen specialty and to help others by making a proposal to set up a special interest group within the College for women psychiatrists. This group would promote job-sharing and part-time working for all psychiatrists if needed, and to offer support if they were having difficulties in doing so. In 1994 Dr Cremona proposed the new Women In Psychiatry Special Interest Group (WIPSIG). It was approved in 1995 with over 100 College members, men and women, in support. The Executive Committee was elected and met for the first time in 1996.

Early Years: Focus on Part-Time Working

One of the first initiatives of the SIG was to set up a Job Share Register to facilitate flexible working. The Job Share Register was a popular concept with College Members, though in practice it was little used. However, it did promote a culture of women networking locally to see what sharing arrangements they might be able to make. The regular meetings of the SIG gave more support to women networking and keeping themselves informed of developments with their specialty and in the wider medical establishment that might affect their working lives.

In 2003, two founder members of the SIG, Alicia Etchegoyen and Jane Marshall, were appointed to the post of National Director of NHS Flexible Training as a job-share. Their appointment provided a direct link between the group and national initiatives on flexible training. In the same year Mr Eric Waters, a surgeon, was appointed to champion doctors in achieving a better work–life balance because of the lethargy of the medical establishment in adopting the goals of the Department of Health's (DoH) 'Improving Working Lives' initiative.[3]

Academic Development of Women Psychiatrists

Professor Mary Robertson, Emeritus Professor of Neuropsychiatry, succeeded Dr Cremona as the second SIG Chair. She established an annual essay prize for trainees on a topic related to women's health. She also set up the tradition of a regular spring and autumn conference for SIG members and others, and proposed a SIG lecture. The SIG Executive Committee (Exec) regularly submitted topics for academic sessions at the College Annual Meeting. At the 2002 Annual Meeting in Cardiff the SIG had proposed a debate on gender awareness, with the motion that 'single sex services (are) the way forward'. Contrary to the DoH's recommendation[3] to put in place single-sex in-patient mental health wards throughout the United Kingdom, the motion was defeated. It seems that audience members from specialties such as Old Age and Rehabilitation favoured balanced mixed sex environments, and they outnumbered members from acute general psychiatry and psychiatric intensive care units (PICUs) who argued the need for segregation was greater.

SIG Exec members produced teaching materials for the College CPD (Continuing Professional Development) online and further raised the profile of gender issues by providing gendered exam questions including PMPs (Patient Management Problems).

Professor Robertson also encouraged members of the SIG to publish. We can see the range of issues covered over the next ten years in Table 4.1. This time coincided with

Table 4.1 The Following Topics were Researched and Published by Members of the SIG Over an 11-year Period Between 2002 and 2013.[26,27,28,29,30,31,32,33]

Title	Year
The female psychiatrist: professional, personal, and social issues	2002
Women in academic psychiatry	2003
Making a difference. Invited commentary on effects of domestic violence and sexual abuse on mental health	2008
Developing a policy to deal with sexual assault on psychiatric in-patient wards	2009
Addressing the sexual and reproductive health needs of women who use mental health services	2010
Domestic violence: its relevance to psychiatry	2012
Teamwork: the art of being a leader and a team player	2013

the establishment of the first Chair of Women's Mental Health, when Dora Kohen, a founder member and first Secretary of the Exec, was appointed Professor at Lancashire Postgraduate School of Medicine and Health. The Athena Swan Charter (supporting women's academic development within medicine and other scientific specialities) was also established improving the prospects for equality of all women academics including psychiatrists.[4]

Data About Women in Psychiatry and WIPSIG

By November 2003, 47 per cent of core trainees, 53 per cent of higher trainees, 55 per cent of staff grade and associate specialists, and 36 per cent of consultants in psychiatry were women. Twenty-two per cent of College Fellows were women, and there were twenty-one women professors of psychiatry. One in five higher trainees was undergoing flexible training.

Tenth Anniversary Year and Beyond

This was a period of growth and development for the Group with increasing alignment with the College and further clarification of the objectives of the SIG.

Tenth Anniversary, July 2005

By 2005, SIG membership had increased to over 1,250, including 85 men. Sixty per cent of medical students in the United Kingdom were women. Women's performance in the College membership exams exceeded that of their male counterparts. The posts of President, Registrar, and Treasurer of the Royal College of Psychiatrists as well as Chief Executive were all held by women, an indication of the changes in career progression for women psychiatrists and women employees of the College. The SIG represented the interests of women psychiatrists within the College and beyond; this broad appeal supported the continuing growth of its membership.

The SIG marked its tenth anniversary with a celebratory meeting at 17 Belgrave Square (the Royal College premises), hosted by the College President, Dame Professor Sheila Hollins, and with a number of eminent women speakers including Professor Isobel Allen and Dr Geraldine Strathdee, MBE. Isobel Allen, Emeritus Professor of the Policy Studies Institute, demonstrated that women doctors with children tended to have an 'M'-shaped pattern of performance, with a second peak of achievement after their children reached 12 or so. Dr Strathdee recommended to all part-time trainees and consultants male and female that they have clear three-year goals, as she had done—with a 'portfolio' career covering five key areas: clinician, policy and regulation, research, training and teaching, and service and practice development. She also felt that full-time working for both men or women would be increasingly rare in the future.

Professor Robertson celebrated the anniversary with a poem (Box 4.1).[5]

Box 4.1 The Triumphal March of WIPSIG

The overture was played just ten years ago,
Now over a thousand members in full song.
The conductors' batons waving—rightly so –
Being Cremona, Ramsay and poet Robertson.
We have our first Professor of Women's Mental Health:
Dora Kohen's been one of us, since our opening tune.
The WIPSIG prize was then born, showing our great stealth
But a WIPSIG lecture, as well, would be a real boon.
We've published many papers, and written books too,
The Divas doing well for the dreaded RAE.
We have now got sessions at the AGM: that's new.
Just watch us in the future and you will see.
More of our amazing alto Triumvirate now in post:
Women President, Registrar and Treasurer too,
Perform at our November encore, of which we will boast.
So come join our WIPSIG chorus, singers me and you.

Poem by Mary Robertson
to celebrate the 10th Anniversary of the Group

© Mary May Robertson

Work on Gender Equality in the College

The SIG supported Dame Professor Sheila Hollins in a Presidential working group on gender equality throughout the College. The Statement from the working group, commented that the core attributes for good psychiatric practice included full sensitivity to gender, with a commitment to equality, anti-discriminatory practice, and working with diversity (RCPsych Gender Equality Statement of Intent, 2005).[6]

WIPSIG's Mission Statement

Following the tenth anniversary celebrations, the SIG issued a questionnaire to members lobbying them on priorities for the next ten years. The strategy meeting proposed and hosted by Dr Fiona Mason in Spring 2006 produced a mission statement and clarified the values of the Group (Box 4.2).

National Interest in Women Doctors and Their Careers

The SIG took guidance from the Department of Health ('Improving Working Lives'[3]), and the Medical Women's Federation on 'Making Part-time Work',[7] which aimed to overcome attitudinal barriers to part-time working and which supported the career development of part-time doctors. The SIG raised awareness among its membership

Box 4.2 Mission Statement and Values of the SIG, 2005

The Mission

- Promote mental health services for women, their families, and carers, and to enable women psychiatrists to achieve their potential across the NHS, academic institutions and the independent sector

- Support services that are holistic, comprehensive, equitable, responsive, empowering, and evidence-based

- Recognize the need for work life balance for psychiatrists and consider those working across all areas relating to women's mental health including clinical services, service development, management, teaching, and research

The Values

- Understand the complexity of women's lives

- Recognize the needs and experiences of women service users, their families, and carers

- Value the commitment of clinicians working with women

- Work with diversity and facilitate equality of opportunity

- Challenge stigma and discrimination

- Promote gender awareness

- Value choice

- Be open to change

that women doctors prefer specialties with more predictable hours and more patient contact.[8] Research published by Sir Liam Donaldson[9] revealed that later in their careers many women doctors had regrets about entering medicine because they had encountered barriers to career progression. SIG members, however, felt empowered to challenge situations which did not comply with guidance about discrimination from the Royal College.[10]

Professor Dame Carol Black, President of the Royal College of Medicine, in an interview with the *Independent* newspaper in August 2004, publicly questioned the glass ceiling for women doctors: why weren't women progressing into managerial, executive, and leadership roles within the medical profession? Was it because women lacked the commitment of their male colleagues in taking on additional roles? Were they opting out of serving on committees and refusing to take on the additional non-clinical commitments as their male colleagues undertook? The evidence was inconclusive. The proportion of women Fellows in the College was still relatively low, possibly reflecting the lower numbers entering psychiatry 15 years earlier. The number of women medical directors in mental health remained low. Fewer women consultants were awarded clinical excellence awards than their male colleagues. Even though women achieved more distinctions in medical school than men, later in their careers they failed to reach the same levels of achievement.[11]

The SIG networked informally with other women doctors' organisations, such as Women in Medicine (WIM), the Medical Women's Federation (MWF), and Women in Surgical Training (WIST). There were joint discussions with other relevant organisations, such as the Mental Health in Primary Care group of the Royal College of General Practitioners and the Royal College of Obstetricians and Gynaecologists.

National Changes to Training

The Modernising Medical Careers initiative[12] introduced run-through training, which meant that a trainee in psychiatry might spend the whole six years of specialty training in the same part of the country. Little thought had been given to the possibility of transfers between Deaneries if one half of a couple wished to relocate to live with, or near to, their partner. There was also an official shift from supernumerary flexible working towards a pattern of working called 'Less than Full-time Training' (LTFT). Funding was guaranteed for LTFT flexible training for the first time, because as well as job-sharing it allowed slot shares: two flexible trainees could share a full-time post working between six and eight sessions each, and Deaneries would top up the difference in terms of extra cost.[13] Working part-time within pre-existing funded full-time training posts was difficult to negotiate with some supervisors so it was still not ideal.

Discrimination in Practice for Trainees and Psychiatrists in Consultant Posts

For women psychiatrists there was a lack of role models and of career mentoring. A report from the BMA[14] pointed to a failure in the appointment of women to editorial boards or grant-giving panels. It commented that when flexible working was unavailable to women this significantly impeded career advancement. In a meeting for part-time trainees in 2007 Dr Jane Marshall quoted Dr Fiona Subotsky: 'Only when enough women hold leadership roles, will women in general be able to follow the careers they choose and in the manner that needs dictate they follow them.' Yet biases against women, particularly from surgical specialties, continue.

John Black, the President of the Royal College of Surgeons, suggested that women might lack the technical skills and flexibility necessary for a surgical career, saying: 'Managing surgical cases is both highly unpredictable and technical, which goes some way to explain why there are fewer women going into surgery'. The theme continues with a commentary in the *Mail Online*: 'Why having so many women doctors is hurting the NHS'.[15]

The SIG was not a union but it offered support to its members as well as members of the wider psychiatric community (Table 4.2).

Table 4.2 Examples of Those Who Received WIPSIG Support Because of Discrimination

Gender differences in pay	In a Trust where male consultant psychiatrists were paid 20 per cent more, the women consultants won a court case granting them equal pay but subsequent ill-will made it impossible for them to continue working in that Trust; in effect, constructive dismissal.
Loss of dedicated perinatal service	An academic consultant specializing in perinatal care was supported by the SIG for 12 years after her dedicated service was closed and she was transferred to a generic post. The perinatal service was reinstated as it had previously existed but she was by then very close to retirement.
Health problems	A male trainee with serious health problems suggests that the SIG's campaigning for flexible training was helpful in enabling him to work part-time as a Senior Registrar. Not having to step down from his chosen career was vital to his coping. With residual disabilities he continues to practise to this day as a part-time Consultant.
Sexual harassment, bullying, and defamation	For several years a mid-career Consultant psychiatrist, post-divorce and opposing cuts to her rehabilitation service, was supported by the SIG while subject to sexual harassment and defamation by her (female) lead clinician, and later when she left to take up another post.
Stigmatization of a forensic psychiatrist by the media	A female forensic Consultant psychiatrist was supported informally when she received hostile press following one of her patients having harmed a member of the public.
Constructive dismissal and ageism	A near end-of-career psychiatrist was supported by the SIG, the BMA, and her defence union when harassed for a year by a female nurse manager and male lead clinician with the aim of forcing her to retire early. She retired but suffered financial detriment. She received practical support from the SIG in finding work in retirement.

Support for Psychiatrists

There is evidence that the suicide rate for women doctors (especially anaesthetists and psychiatrists), although lower than that of male doctors, is overall double that of the female population. The SIG does not offer psychiatric/psychological help to sick doctors, but it is alert to those who are at risk of adverse practice, and directs them to appropriate sources of help.[16] The death of Dr Daksha Emson postnatally, referred to later in this chapter, directly led the Royal College to develop the Psychiatrists' Support Service (PSS)[17] and to the development of the Practitioner Health Programme (PHP) initially for London practitioners but now available in other cities in the United Kingdom.

The mental health of women service users, their families, and carers

Dora Kohen, Professor of Women's Mental Health at Lancashire Postgraduate School of Medicine and Health, had a real interest in improving services for women with psychiatric problems. With the backing of the SIG she flagged up the specific needs of female psychiatric patients within the Royal College of Psychiatrists.

Half of the patients in mental health services are women, although in Old Age services women outnumber men by 2:1. Anxiety, depression, and eating disorders are all more common in women. Socio-economic and psychological factors associated with poverty, unemployment, and social isolation play a considerable part in female mental illness. Other disorders such as puerperal psychosis, postnatal depression, and premenstrual dysphoric disorder are specific to women.

From its inception, the SIG focused on the specific physical and mental health needs of women relating to pregnancy, childbirth, and motherhood, eating disorders, and those suffering the consequences of violence, particularly sexual violence. Research demonstrated a strong link between mental ill health and earlier child sexual and domestic abuse (as we now know this is true for men too). Gender-sensitive facilities that would maintain family links began to be developed within services, such as family units on acute wards and more mother and baby units. *Women's Mental Health: Into the Mainstream* (2002)[18] remains the only guidance available to this day on the provision of comprehensive equitable mental health services for women. It provides an evidence base to inform the need for gender-sensitive and gender-specific services. The SIG also raised awareness of the biological differences in the side effects of drugs existing between men and women. In 2009 it co-hosted a conference with the Psychopharmacology Society, entitled 'Gender Differences in Prescribing'.

Following the tragic postnatal death of a trainee forensic psychiatrist and her baby in 2000 and subsequent deaths of other mothers with postnatal mental health problems, the findings of the UK Maternal Deaths Enquiry (North East London Strategic Health Authority, 2003)[19] led to the Postnatal Special Interest Group at the College becoming a full Faculty. The SIG continued to maintain close links with the Perinatal Faculty as it had with the Postnatal SIG, with continuing interest in perinatal mental health, reducing depression, and suicide risk postpartum, and connecting maternal health and mental health. The priorities of the SIG for women's mental health included women as parents, and as carers for other family members including their own parents.

The SIG Autumn conference in 2009 was concerned with women carers and the impact of caring on their mental health. The Department of Health (2005),[20] CSIP (Care Services Improvement Partnership)[21] and NIMHE (National Institute for Mental Health in England (2006)) recommended supporting families, tackling violence, and empowering women from black and minority ethnic communities. They also recommended that women who were victims of violence would be referred to as victims of 'domestic abuse', rather than 'domestic violence', as this included both physical and sexual abuse. Marginalized women have significant levels of distress, with women in poverty suffering the greatest levels of domestic abuse; 40 per cent of those in poverty who have been abused attempt suicide.

Women Patients in Forensic Services

Dr Fiona Mason's appointment to the SIG Chair in 2007 coincided with tremendous progress in the provision of women's forensic services. She brought extensive experience and skill in health service management, medical leadership, and representing the needs of women patients within secure services to the SIG. She widened its influence through her membership of many influential committees in the field of Forensic Psychiatry, including the National Programme Board for Gender Equality on Women's Mental Health, the Working Party of the Solicitor General on Rape Prosecution, and the Mental Health Expert Reference Group on Women in the Criminal Justice system. Her first SIG conference as Chair was 'Women in Contact with the Criminal Justice System', while the following year she arranged workshops by SIG members at the College Annual Meeting on Domestic Violence: 'Justice for Rape Victims' and the 'Mental Health of Refugees and Trafficked Women'. The United Kingdom had recently signed up to the Council of Europe Convention on Action against Trafficking in Human Beings[22] which meant that the SIG workshop could educate College members about trafficked women who, for the first time, would have rights to care, including therapy, protection, and greater access to asylum.

Changes in the SIG: A New Name

In 2014 the SIG Executive Committee endorsed the name WMHSIG, (Women's Mental Health Special Interest Group) to increase its emphasis on women patients. There followed a reduction in activity by the SIG with no Executive meetings for almost a year. The College cited poor financial viability and questioned the continuation of the SIG. There was a call for new nominations to positions on the Executive Committee.

WMHSIG: The Future

The appointment of Dr Nicola Byrne as the new Chair in 2015 heralded the re-emergence of the Group which by now had over 3000 members.

The relaunched WMHSIG has a commitment to organize 'Women in Mind' meetings two or three times a year: these are events in collaboration with the Institute of Psychiatry, Psychology, and Neuroscience (IoPPN) at King's College London which aim to engage health professionals and the public in discussion on challenges to women's mental health across the life cycle. The events centre around interviews with inspirational women about professional or personal experiences that have shaped their views on women's mental health both in terms of difficulties and resilience. The guest speakers from health, media, politics, and the arts will raise gender awareness and help inform and guide the direction of travel for WMHSIG.

There is a continuing commitment to communication and networking for members through the additional means of social media; WMHSIG will provide updates on research, service development, medical careers, and articles of interest from journals, newspapers, and magazines.

Current Issues for Women Psychiatrists' Careers

Doctor parents who are single, separated, or divorced in sole charge of children, or having other care demands or limitations on their stamina are now acknowledged, and have the right to request reduced hours, although this still inevitably leads to a slowing

Box 4.3 Why the Need for Part-Time Working is Reduced, Compared to 21 Years Ago

The Consultant Contract of 2003[34] allowed for specific planned activities to be delineated in each consultant's job plan so that there would be protected time for teaching, committee work and research work in every consultant contract.

- In 1998 the European Working Time Directive limited doctors' hours to 48 hours per week
- The switch to LTFT (Less Than Full-time) training posts in 2006
- Childcare more widely available—for longer and more flexible hours
- Financial pressures—meaning a pressing need for both partners to work longer hours
- Increasing involvement of partners in child and home care and society's acceptance of such
- Shared maternity and paternity leave
- A specified minimum amount of on-call to meet training requirements rather than continuing on-call commitments throughout training
- National Training Numbers for Trainees (NTN) meant that once on a specialist register pathway trainees were able to take career breaks
- There were also changes in working patterns with a move to shorter working weeks[35]

of career progression. In earlier years, our survival as part-time trainees and viability as future consultants was in jeopardy, but now with the Gender and Age Discrimination Acts firmly in place (2005 and 2010) part-time doctors are on a more secure footing. WMHSIG acknowledges that as the number of women doctors continues to rise, we need to make appropriate adjustments and take active measures to counteract the slowing of career progression due to the social pressures of the demanding and challenging years (Box 4.3).

At the first Women in Mind networking event in 2016, a talk by Dr Clare Gerada, former Chair of the Royal College of GPs, considered the current proposals for a seven-day working NHS week, and questioned whether the disadvantages for doctor caregivers within the new contract simply reflected a societal lack of awareness of the needs of those workers, rather than deficits specific to the NHS and DoH as institutions.

Work–life Balance for All

Within the medical profession, it is important for women and men to have a reasonable work–life balance. There are real questions about how best to support women and men in achieving their potential as doctors, researchers, and managers without undermining their other important roles as parents and carers. WMHSIG will continue to promote flexible working and role models with whom women particularly can identify at different stages of their careers, and who can offer mentoring and coaching. Campaign groups can take an organizational approach to bringing about the necessary changes in the profession. Many men aspire to work more flexibly. We look forward to the day when flexible working patterns are the norm for both men and women, allowing all doctors to achieve a healthy work–life balance.[23]

Current Issues for Women Patients

AGENDA: the alliance for women and girls is a cross-sector alliance of organizations and individuals who believe that current systems and services are failing to protect, and divert some women and girls from repeated experiences of inequality, violence, abuse, and trauma, and offer them adequate support, with the result that they can face lifelong, severe, and multiple disadvantage. AGENDA, one of several organizations with which our SIG is recently linked, launched a new campaign in 2016 to address the findings of a survey that only one in 35 Trusts in the United Kingdom has a specific women's mental health strategy, and in half of all Trusts there was no policy requiring practitioners to ask about any history of sexual or physical abuse.

WMHSIG acknowledges that wherever there is gender discrimination in mental health services, whether in acute or long-term services, patients get a raw deal. Within forensic psychiatry there is a tradition of providing services for men. Because the numbers of women are relatively small and presentation of women patients can be complex, services for them are often left for the independent sector to provide, which means that the NHS lacks expertise here. Women are similarly under-represented in clinical research trials; women and men are not biologically the same but published trials invariably concern male or mixed groups.[24]

Eighty per cent of people admitted to hospital with personality disorder are women. There may be gender biases in secondary services with Borderline Personality Disorder (BPD) diagnosed more in women and Antisocial Personality Disorder (ASPD) in men. Diagnoses are made on constellations of symptoms and may be defined by symptoms which are more characteristic of either gender. The diagnosis of BPD is unpopular with some women[25] who say they would prefer a diagnosis including the word trauma, thereby acknowledging it as a key factor contributing to their condition. Others are grateful for the diagnosis enabling them to access therapies—DBT and CBT (Dialectical Behaviour Therapy and Cognitive Behaviour Therapy)—recommended by the National Institute for Health and Care Excellence to address specific difficulties associated with the condition.

International View

WMHSIG supports the World Health Organization (WHO) which advocates gender equality in health and supports gender mainstreaming, stating that gender equality is not only a fundamental human right but a necessary foundation for a peaceful, prosperous, and sustainable world. Gender equality does not mean that women and men will become the same but that their rights, responsibilities, and opportunities will not depend on whether they are born male or female.

Acknowledgments

Dr Elaine Arnold, Dr Nicola Byrne, Dr Jane Marshall, and Dr Fiona Mason

References and Notes

1. **Royal College of Psychiatrists** (1995). Annual Census of Psychiatric Staffing: Occasional Paper 34. London: Royal College of Psychiatrists.

2. This scheme was initiated by the Department of Health and Social Security in 1979, offering guidance on opportunities for part-time training in the NHS for doctors and dentists with domestic commitments, disability, or ill-health. Personal Memorandum (PM(79)3). DHSS; 1979.

3. NHS Executive (2002). 'Safety, privacy and dignity in mental health units: guidance on mixed sex accommodation for mental health services'. London: Department of Health.

4. **Equality Challenge Unit** (2005). Athena Swan Charter. <http://www.ecu.ac.uk/equality-charters/athena-swan/>.

5. **Robertson, M** (2005). 'The Triumphal March of WIPSIG' (poem). Data supplement to Ramsay R. Women in psychiatry: Ten years of a special interest group. *Advances in Psychiatric Treatment* **11**(6):383–4.

6. **Professor Sheila Hollins, President of the Royal College of Psychiatrists from** 2005, issued a Gender Equality Statement of Intent. <http://www.rcpsych.ac.uk/policyandparliamentary/miscellaneouscollegepolicies/equalityanddiversity.aspx>.

7. **Medical Women's Federation** (2008). (Government Equalities Office). Summary Report: Making part-time work. Nottingham: Russell Press. <http://www.medicalwomensfederation.org.uk/images/Download_-_MWF_-_Making_Part_Time_Work.pdf>.

8. **Royal College of Physicians** (2009).Women and medicine: the future. Summary of findings from Royal College of Physicians Research. London: Royal College of Physicians. <https://www.rcr.ac.uk/sites/default/files/RCP_Women_%20in_%20Medicine_%20Report.pdf>.

9. **Donaldson, L** (2007). Chapter Two—On the State of Public Health: Annual Report of the Chief Medical Officer, 2006. <http://webarchive.nationalarchives.gov.uk/20130107105354/http:/www.dh.gov.uk/en/Publicationsandstatistics/Publications/AnnualReports/DH_076817>. See also neeed author and weblink for this one xxx (2007). Chapter Seven—Women in Medicine: Opportunity Blocks. London: DoH

10. **Royal College of Psychiatrists** (2009). Council Report. *CR154: Good Psychiatric Practice*, 3rd edn. London: Royal College of Psychiatrists.

11. **Deech R** (2009). 'The Deech Report. Women Doctors: Making a Difference. Report of the National Working Group on Women in Medicine Presented to Sir Liam Donaldson, Chief Medical Officer'. London: Department of Health.

12. **Tooke J** (2007). *Aspiring to Excellence: Findings and Recommendations of the Independent Inquiry into Modernising Medical Careers*. London: MMC Inquiry.

13. **Marshall J** (2008). Flexible training. In: Bhugra D and Howes O (eds). *Handbook for Psychiatric Trainees*. London: Royal College of Psychiatrists, pp. 157–68.

14. **BMA** (2008). *Women in Academic Medicine: Developing Equality in Governance and Management for Career Progression: Executive Summary and Recommendations*. London: BMA.

15. **Thomas JM** (2014). Why having so many women doctors is hurting the NHS. *Mail Online.* 2 January 2014. <http://www.dailymail.co.uk/debate/article-2532461/Why-having-women-doctors-hurting-NHS-A-provovcative-powerful-argument-leading-surgeon.html>.

16. **Hawton K, Clements A, Sakarovitch C, Simkin S,** and **Deeks JJ** (2001). Suicide in Doctors: A Study of Risk Accoridng to Gender, Seniority and Specialty in Medical Practitioners in England and Wales, 1979–1995. *Journal of Academiology and Community Health* **55**:296–300. See also **Schernhammer ES** and **Colditz GA** (2004). Suicide Rates among Physicians: A Quantitative and Gender Assessment (Meta-analysis). *American Journal of Psychiatry* **161**(12):2295–302.

17. The Psychiatrists' Support Service (PSS) of the Royal College of Psychiatrists is a free, confidential support and advice service for psychiatrists at all stages of their career who find themselves in difficulty or in need of support. The service is available during office hours from Monday to Friday

18. **Department of Health** (2002). *Women's Mental Health: Into the Mainstream––Strategic Development of Mental Health Care for Women.* London: DoH. See also **Department of Health** (2003). *Mainstreaming Gender and Women's Mental Health: Implementation Guidance.* London: Department of Health.

19. **Simply Psychiatry** (2003). UK Maternal Deaths Enquiry (North East London Strategic Health Authority 2003). Report of An Independent Inquiry into the Care and Treatment of Daksha Emson MBBS, MRCPsych, MSc and her Daughter Freya. <http://www.simplypsychiatry.co.uk/sitebuildercontent/sitebuilderfiles/deinquiryreport.pdf>.

20. **Department of Health** (2005). Domestic Violence: A National Report.

21. **Care services Improvement Partnership and National Institute for Mental Health in England** 2006:10 High Impact Changes foe Mental Health Services.

22. **Council of Europe Convention on Action against Trafficking in Human Beings**. Warsaw, 16 May 2005. Treaty Series No 37 (2012). The Convention entered into force in respect of the United Kingdom on 1 April 2009. <https://www.gov.uk/government/uploads/system/uploads/attachment_data/file/236093/8414.pdf>.

23. **Ramsay R** and **Hollins S** (2011). Women in medicine. In: Brown T and Eagles J (eds). *Teaching Psychiatry to Undergraduates.* London: Royal College of Psychiatrists, pp. 301–13.

24. **Moody O** (2016). Women suffer as medical research focuses on men. *The Times,* 10 August 2016. <http://www.thetimes.co.uk/article/women-suffer-as-medical-research-focuses-on-men-8cnvfj6pb>.

25. **Psych Central**. A Challenge to 'Bashing the Borderline'. Psych Central Professional: 2016. <http://pro.psychcentral.com/a-challenge-to-bashing-the-borderline/0011086.html>.

26. **Kohen D** and **Arnold E** (2002). The female psychiatrist: professional, personal and social issues. *Advances in Psychiatric Treatment* **8**(2):81–8. DOI: 10.1192/apt.8.2.81.

27. **Dutta R, Hawkes SL, Iverson AC,** and **Howard L**. Women in academic psychiatry. *Psychiatric Bulletin* **27**(9):321–2. DOI: 10.1192/problem.27.9.321.

28. **Mason F**. Making a difference. Invited commentary on … Effects of domestic violence and sexual abuse on mental health. *Psychiatric Bulletin* **32**:450–1. DOI: 10.1192/pb.bp.108.022319.

29. **Lawn T** and **McDonald E**. Developing a policy to deal with sexual assault on psychiatric in-patient wards. *The Psychiatrist* **33**:108–11.

30. **Dutta R, Hawkes Sarah L, Iverson AC,** and **Howard L** (2010). Women in academic psychiatry. *The Psychiatrist* **34**:313–17.

31. **Henshaw C** and **Protti O** (2010). Addressing the sexual and reproductive health needs of women who use mental health services. *Advances in Psychiatric Treatment* **16**:272–8. DOI: 10.1192/apt.bp.107.004648.

32. **Howard L** (2012). Domestic violence: its relevance to psychiatry. *Advances in Psychiatric Treatment* **18**:129–36. DOI: 10.1192/apt.bp.110.008110

33. **Jenkinson J**, **Oakley C**, and **Mason F** (2013). Teamwork: the art of being a leader and a team player. *Advances in Psychiatric Treatment* **19**:221–8. DOI: 10.1192/apt.bp.111.009639.

34. **NHS Employers**. Consultant Contract. Terms and Conditions of Service—Consultants (England) 2003. Version 9, March 2013. <http://www.nhsemployers.org/~/media/Employers/Documents/Pay%20and%20reward/Consultant_Contract_V9_Revised_Terms_and_Conditions_300813_bt.pdf>.

35. McNally noted changes in working patterns with a move to shorter working weeks in **Eccles S** and **Sanders S** (2008). *So You Want to Be a Brain Surgeon*, 3rd edn. Oxford: Oxford University Press, pp. 86–8.

Chapter 5

Psychiatry and Patienthood

Rosemary Lethem

Introduction

For many years I described myself as having a double life: patient and psychiatrist.

When I retired early on health grounds in 2008 I gave a little talk to those who gathered for that last National Health Service (NHS) sandwich lunch. I said it was an opportunity for a few words of explanation, reflection, and justification. 'Explanation', because I thought my colleagues didn't know enough about me; 'reflection', to try to make sense of it all; 'justification', by way of apology for my perceived shortcomings.

I have been a psychiatrist since 1985 and was a consultant general adult psychiatrist for 12 years, working progressively more part-time until, when I decided it would be better for everyone if I stopped, I was working only three mornings per week. I have been a patient much longer than a psychiatrist, having suffered from affective disorder from the age of 12, virtually all of it depression. My final diagnosis, in 2001, was bipolar 2 disorder. I calculated that I had spent 11 years of my life being depressed (at least 12 now) and had had over 20 episodes.

This chapter uses my experiences as patient and psychiatrist and their interplay to explore themes relating to doctors' mental ill health and recovery. I prefer to use the term 'patient', which has been approved again by the Royal College of Psychiatrists (RCPsych), to alternatives such as 'mental health service user' or 'client'. Information about various topics can be found in the boxes.

Becoming a Psychiatrist

When Professor Robin Murray (Institute of Psychiatry, Psychology, and Neuroscience, King's College, London) was asked what he wished he had known as a junior doctor, his reply was: 'As we learn more and more about neuroscience and social science, psychiatry is poised to become by far the most interesting specialty open to young doctors. So my advice is: don't bury yourself in understanding the heart or kidneys, instead, step up to the exciting challenge of understanding how the brain processes the social environment.'[1]

Max Pemberton, author and psychiatrist, wrote: 'Psychiatry encompasses medical, social, psychological, legal and philosophical issues—I can't think of another specialty that is so intellectually stimulating. You develop strong, enduring relationships with patients, which makes it extraordinarily rewarding.[2]

What does a psychiatrist actually do? When I saw a new patient, I would try to work out why this particular person had come to see me, in this place, at this time. This requires facts but also interpretation, and the result is called a formulation—an attempt to make sense of the presentation, considering relevant biological, psychological, and social factors. There are various ways of doing this, but a good basic way of organizing information is shown in Table 5.1. I have created the example of a 22-year-old girl who has developed a psychosis (distortion of reality by hallucinations and/or delusions).

My path to psychiatry was long and unfocused. I was a clever but socially isolated girl, relying on my intellect and going to Cambridge University at the age of 17 to read Natural Sciences. Once there, I became seriously depressed, ended up in hospital, and returned home, where I had almost no treatment. However, I learned as much as I did at Cambridge by working as a lab technician locally. I returned for three depressive undergraduate years, emerging with a first-class degree in zoology.

I stayed on to do a doctorate. My subjects (snails) had no economic, agricultural, or medical significance whatsoever and the future was problematic until a friend suggested I think about medicine. This was the answer I craved, but instead, to avoid being a student even longer, I became a management trainee in a manufacturing industry, loathed it, got depressed, didn't recognize that I was not well, didn't even register with a general practitioner (GP), and finally embarked on medical studies only one year later than originally envisaged. My vocational confusion can probably be attributed to delayed maturation mainly due to illness.

I became a Senior House Officer (SHO) in psychiatry in 1985. I thought very carefully about choosing a career in psychiatry in view of my student depressive illness, but being motivated by fascination with the subject, as opposed to looking after myself or from some projected need to care for others, was acceptable. In reality, probably all those factors were relevant. My advice? Then, would have been the same: try it. Now, cautiously yes, try it, with information and support.

Table 5.1 An example of factors contributing to a formulation

	Biological	**Psychological**	**Social**
Predisposing	Uncle has schizophrenia	Sexually abused as a child	Smokes cannabis
Precipitating	Smokes cannabis	Assaulted three weeks ago	Smokes cannabis
Perpetuating	Acquired sexually transmitted disease Non-compliant with medication	Poor relationship with parents	Unemployed
Protective	Stopped smoking	Relationship with boyfriend	Lives in commune Stopped smoking

Being a Psychiatrist

For the first ten years, being a psychiatrist was like a background theme to the rest of my life. Being a patient was a much more prominent role. Life was an endless series of getting through things.

When I started my first job I was soon depressed. I did not realize I needed help and was entitled to it but rather I felt intensely guilty that I had been recruited to my job under false pretences, and kept my head down. 1987 was, in some ways, my *annus horribilis*, crowded with life events: we moved to London, where I became a registrar, started revising for Membership of the Royal College of Psychiatry (MRCPsych) Part 2 exam, coincidentally unintentionally got pregnant with twins, passed the exam, and got depressed. My condition was detected by Professor Anthony Clare, my head of department, (literally 'in the psychiatrist's chair'), saw a psychiatrist, and had the twins in November. Two years later I had another baby (despite contraception), and ante- and postnatal depressive illnesses, resulting in hospital admission for almost six months and my first electroconvulsive therapy (ECT) treatments (see Box 5.1).

Box 5.1 Electroconvulsive Therapy (ECT)

ECT was developed in 1938. It involves the passage of a small electric current across the hemispheres of the brain to induce an epileptic fit. It has had bad press in recent years: 'barbaric' and 'inhumane' are words commonly associated with it, probably because many people think of it as memorably portrayed in the film *One Flew over the Cuckoo's Nest* (1975). Contemporary ECT is nothing like this. It is a humane treatment, usually given for severe depression. It is not frightening for the patient. There are no absolute contraindications. Nothing better has replaced it so far.

ECT is given in hospital in a designated ECT suite, partly because it is used in severe illness and partly because it requires an anaesthetist to give a short-lived general anaesthetic so the patient is unaware during the treatment. A short-acting muscle relaxant is also administered to paralyse voluntary muscles as an unmodified fit can be a violent affair and in the past often led to broken bones. Usually only small twitching movements in the toes are visible. The electrodes, between which the current flows, are small pads on sticks. They are applied either to each temple (bilateral ECT) or to one temple and the top of the head (unilateral ECT). It has now been established that bilateral placement is more effective. The amount of current used is now titrated up during the first treatment to induce a fit of optimal length (around 30 seconds).

The other reason ECT gets a bad press is because of its potential side effects. The main ones described by patients are confusion and memory loss, particularly autobiographical memory. These are roughly in proportion to the amount of current used. There is no evidence that cognitive change is cumulative.

Source: data from Waite J, Easton E (eds) (2013), *The ECT Handbook*, 3rd edn. London: Royal College of Psychiatrists[3]

As a junior doctor in the 1980s I had to administer ECT. Prophetically, I could see myself on the bed. Between 1990 and 2011 I had over 70 treatments. The final time, I didn't notice any side effects. When I first had it, my memory was severely affected. For example, at home on leave I did not know whether I had shoes other than sandals or walking boots, or if we had any sellotape: these were complete blanks. I had absolutely no idea of the route to work. I talked to my neighbour at dinner thinking he was somebody completely different with a similar name. These acute events resolved over a few weeks; however, I think many memories are lost insidiously, such as memories of my children growing up. But how do you prove this? Are the memories still in my head or have they been permanently erased? The answer is still not known. Nevertheless, ECT is my treatment of choice for severe depression. It works and it is relatively quick.

In hospital, at last I recognized all the other illnesses for what they were. My diagnosis was recurrent unipolar depression (meaning mood change in one direction only) (see Box 5.2).

In 1996 I became a consultant. Being a psychiatrist was one of the balls I was keeping in the air, along with motherhood, domesticity, and being a patient, the last as inconspicuously as possible, yet much of my identity was bound up in it. My illnesses continued (see Box 5.3).

How did all this relate to me? For most of my professional career I maintained two identities: that of patient being much more prominent than my being a psychiatrist. In the early days I kept the fact of my illness well hidden because I was ashamed of my weakness. I was always adamant that being a psychiatrist did not cause or contribute to it. I over-identified with patients, particularly the ones with depression, usually noting that my illness was worse than theirs. However, I denied my need for care, twice ignoring the advice of GPs who wanted to sign me off from work. I was probably guilty of too much presenteeism but not enough absenteeism.

As a consultant, I certainly maintained a feeling of 'we're all in this together' with both patients and staff. By this time I was comfortable with other people knowing about my illness; in fact, I wanted them to know as a means of some sort of self-justification. I have always been sensitive about talking and listening respectfully to patients and offering explanations to orientate and include them. Even when someone is too disturbed to communicate conventionally, I believe they can still appreciate the effort, which may lead to a better therapeutic relationship. Other colleagues could plan projects, conduct research, teach, shape services, or dream dreams. My focus was clinical care, which I did well, and staying well enough myself.

Other psychiatrists have not always been comfortable with my status. I remember asking a question which revealed my history after a lecture at the RCPsych in the 1990s, and was disconcerted to receive a round of applause. My consultant colleagues must have been known that I was sometimes off work for long periods but, with a couple of exceptions, never acknowledged it. The medical director of the Trust reassured me that I was not considered a risk to patients (so that was all right!). The Trust got in locums and waited for me to return, for which I am grateful, until my decision to retire. It is likely to be different these days.

Box 5.2 Classification of Mood (Affective) Disorders

A classification is a way of seeing the world at a point in time (Sartorius).[4] Since the early 1960s, the Mental Health Programme of the World Health Organization (WHO) has been engaged in a programme designed to improve the diagnosis and classification of mental disorders. A glossary defining each category was also developed. There have been several revisions or updates of this work; the version in use at the time of writing is the Tenth Revision of the International Classification of Diseases (ICD-10) (1992).[4]

Mood disorders are classified using various specifiers, such as direction of change (towards mania/depression/both directions), severity (mild, moderate, or severe), presence or absence of psychotic or somatic symptoms, and frequency. Psychotic symptoms are delusions and/or hallucinations and somatic symptoms refer to a collection of characteristic disturbances in biological functions (sleep, appetite, activity, sexual desire, ability to feel pleasure, diurnal variation in mood) which may occur with depressed mood.

Categories

F06 Organic

F30 Manic episode

F31 Bipolar affective disorder

F32 Depressive episode

F33 Recurrent depressive disorder (includes seasonal affective disorder)

F34 Persistent mood disorders; e.g. dysthymia, cyclothymia

F38 Other; e.g. recurrent brief depressive disorder

F39 Unspecified

In the United States, the Diagnostic and Statistical Manual 5th revision (2013)[5] is used, designed to harmonize with ICD 11, which will be published soon. Although the categories of disorder and specifiers are based on those of the ICD, it uses a multiaxial system which involves assessment on five axes, each of which refers to a different domain of information.

Axis I Clinical disorders (illnesses)

Axis II Personality disorders, learning disability, other developmental disorders

Axis III Medical conditions

Axis IV Psychosocial and environmental problems

Axis V Global Assessment of Functioning (using GAF scale in the manual)

The axes reflect the bio-psycho-social model at the heart of modern psychiatry. It is good practice in the United Kingdom to consider them even though they are not formalized in ICD 10.

Box 5.3 Doctors' Mental Health

Mental health problems in doctors are common. Surveys continue to reveal high rates of depression, anxiety, and addictions.[6,7] Drug misuse is increasing. The risk of completed suicide is several times greater than the population average, particularly in female doctors. In 2005–13, 28 doctors being investigated under the General Medical Council (GMC)'s Fitness to Practice procedures killed themselves.[8] Sick doctors are becoming younger. Reasons are not hard to find. Take this fake advertisement:[9]

Wanted—medical Staff

High academic achievers only, with strong perfectionist and self-critical traits preferred.

Successful candidates will have had: 5+ years training in party-fuelled student culture followed by sleep deprivation and long hours in their twenties; regular exposure to death, loss and human misfortune; never-ending exams and lifelong study; constant onerous responsibility for other people's health and wellbeing; strict, hierarchical, conservative training with a hint of bullying and intimidation.

Easy access to Pharmaceuticals.

Doctors are competitive, perfectionist loners working in stressful environments with frequent changes of job, colleagues, and location, and difficulty in synchronizing employment with family commitments. There is an attenuated sense of 'belonging' since teamwork gave way to shift working. Add in hours, bureaucracy, constant scrutiny and assessment, and it is only too easy to let a healthy balance between work, family, and interests slip.[10]

Doctors are regarded as supermen/women by the general public and find it difficult to recognize or admit vulnerability, considering it weakness. There is still tremendous stigma around mental ill health. Doctors may not recognize their difficulties, deny them, or refuse to talk about them, fearing career suicide.[11] In a survey conducted by the Medical Protection Society in 2015 of members of all grades and specialties ($n = 631$) to explore their personal experiences of mental health issues, 41 per cent of respondents who had suffered psychological symptoms had not confided in anybody. Fifty-eight per cent of them said they did not need support.[6] They may stay at work when they are not fit (presenteeism): they do not want to 'let down' their patients, are fearful of being identified, and need 'permission to be unwell'.[12] This leads to a culture of 'named, shamed and blamed'. Dr Clare Gerada, who founded the Practitioner Health Programme, says that doctors need a healthcare system of their own.[13]

However, nearly all doctors who acknowledge their mental ill health either remain at work or soon return to it. It is highly cost-effective to treat them. The cloud of adversity may reveal a silver lining in terms of personal growth and resilience.

Box 5.3 Continued

There may be a move from independence towards interdependence and connectedness, and a clearer sense of what is important in career and life.[10]

Being a Doctor After Being a Patient

After being ill, the ways doctors relate to patients and think about themselves are likely to change.[14] Symptoms may be denied under the guise of 'coping' or intellectualization. Boundaries may shift: there may be over-identification with patients and excessive emotional involvement, or a sense of 'we're all in this together', and greater empathy. Behaviour towards patients can become more sensitive: listening, asking, explaining, forgiving. Doctors can inspire and teach.

Some doctors retire. This raises fundamental existential questions because doctors integrate their professional identities into a profound sense of themselves and their lives. Maintaining one identity is generally easier than having two. Medicine is much more than a job.

A recent study reported that over a third of clinicians and team leaders working in English community mental health teams had personal experience of mental issues, although less than half had disclosed this to colleagues. The merits of using this 'untapped resource' of 'dual identity' were discussed.[15]

Do Doctors Get Special Treatment?

The answer is yes, but not invariably, and it can be for better or for worse. The most extreme example of this for me was, more than once, having ECT as a day patient. The advantages of this arrangement with a young family are obvious, but I so longed for the burden of having to care for them or indeed to do anything to be lifted, but it rarely was. From 1991 until 2011 I was never an in-patient, despite having around 40 ECT treatments. I think people that ill should be in hospital. On the positive side, I was fully informed and decisions were discussed with me (only), but I wanted to be managed and treated like other patients. In this respect, I had several long spells at day hospitals which I found therapeutic and beneficial. However, these have been replaced by crisis care and home treatment teams, which cater for a different client group. Tacitly, in the twentieth century, home and work were not directly involved in my treatment. I was grateful for this as I didn't want my 'weakness' to be exposed, and certainly I did not consider myself an 'untapped resource' at work. There are now a number of organizations offering help for doctors with mental health problems (including stress) which were not available when I was a trainee (see Table 5.2).

Coping

For decades I coped as best I could (see Box 5.4). In the early days I was isolated and ignorant. In my acknowledged illness when I was aged 17 it was as though the sky fell

Table 5.2 Getting help

Organizations offering support to sick doctors	
BMA Counselling and Doctor Advisor Service	Professional telephone counselling Call 0330 123 1245 24hr/7day
Psychiatrists Support Service pss@rcpsych.ac.uk	Free, confidential telephone support and advice service on dedicated line Call 020 7245 0412 9 a.m. to 5 p.m., Mon–Fri
NHS Practitioner Health Programme <http://www.php.nhs.uk>	Free confidential service based in London for mental/physical health concerns and addictions Call 0203 049 4505
Health for Health Professionals (HHP) Wales	New face-to-face counselling service for all doctors in Wales. Free Call 0800 058 2738 9 a.m. to 5 p.m., Mon–Fri
Sick Doctors Trust <http://www.sick-doctors-trust.co.uk>	Independent, confidential help offered to doctors and medical students dependent on alcohol or drugs Call 0370 444 5163 24hr/7day
DocHealth enquiries@dochealth.org.uk	New psychotherapy service for all UK doctors, supported by BMA and RMBF. Self referral, not for profit Call 020 7383 6533
Royal Medical Benevolent Fund (RMBF) <http://www.rmbf.org>	Financial support and advice to doctors, medical students, and their families Call 020 8540 9194 9 a.m. to 5 p.m., Mon–Fri
Doctors Support Network (DSN) <http://www.dsn.org.uk>	Independent medical charity providing information and support for doctors and medical students through online forum and regional support groups

in. I went from having it all (Cambridge) to having nothing (return to parental home). After that I forced myself to continue studying and working for fear of disclosure and because I must not 'give in', aided by personality traits and plenty of denial. Privately I embraced my suffering. It was exclusive and often felt like all I had. I reached breaking point more than once. Other people helped, of course. Several women nurtured me and have enabled me to do the same for others.

Mood Charts, Moodscope, Life Line, and Writing.

These are all ways of charting or keeping abreast of what is happening. I have charted my mood and kept a life line for almost 20 years. As well as being interesting, it has many other uses, for example, demonstrating the effect of medication changes or life events. Since 2010 I have also used the online facility Moodscope[16] for mood charting. This has options including notifying 'buddies' of scores if wished. The basic version of Moodscope is free. I have always written privately about my life, infrequently until 1997, when I started keeping a diary, a book I write in when I make time. These days it's not very often. Rereading what

Box 5.4 Tips for Coping With Depression

I drew this up in 2008. It is what worked best for me.

1. Acknowledge it
2. Accept it
3. Deal with it

Don't put dealing with depression off. Life's too short. There is a lot you and others can do to help.

- Prioritize. What must you do? Then put the rest aside
- Structure time. Have something you can be doing; not too much, not too little
- Try to keep to a routine
- Stay neutral. Suspend judgement (especially negative)
- Don't shut yourself away
- Share it—with friends/family/colleagues/support group. Don't endure it alone
- Be kind to yourself. Have reasonable expectations. No self criticism
- Allow yourself to be (relatively) weak at this time
- Treat yourself. Any little thing which gives you pleasure (smelling the flowers in the garden, etc.)
- What are the special things about *you*?
- Remember that 'this too shall pass'

4. Get some help
   - GP
   - Psychiatrist
   - Helpline
   - Organization
5. Decide (with a helper or friend) who needs to know you are suffering

I wrote when I was 18, it is obvious I was depressed, though I didn't know it at the time.

Management of Depression

I have experienced many kinds of management of depression, some of which I shall describe, along with my (personal) evaluation.

Medical Model

Until 2001 I was treated in accordance with 'the medical model'. It fits poorly with many mental health problems, which can be chronic, with incomplete symptom resolution—as are, increasingly frequently, many physical conditions. Thus: I acquired an illness, which was something bad that happened to me and I needed treatment to get rid of it, by doctors, in hospital if necessary, primarily with medication. Less attention was paid to psycho-social factors. These days, in my experience, the term is often used dismissively by non-psychiatrists about psychiatrists, although the reality is that now most psychiatrists and professionals working in mental health services understand and treat mental illnesses in a multifaceted way.

Admission

The prospect of admission, for me, was as a haven where the burden of having to do things would be lifted and I would be taken out of the bruising flood of daily life. Other than two nights in Cambridge, this has only happened twice. I met remarkable people in hospital and several became friends. Some have died prematurely. I mention two because they were women without voices. One killed herself on leave. Nobody seemed to know her. I was given her photograph by the mother of another friend after he jumped in front of a train. The other person was a talented pianist and teacher who had a long history of paranoid schizophrenia and type 2 diabetes, which she could not manage properly. She was found dead in her fortress of a flat. I'd like to think things are different now.

Medication

I was first prescribed psychotropic medication in 1971 and have taken it continuously since 1992 (see Box 5.5). At the time of my retirement in 2008 I estimated I had consumed 39,000 pills. I have had my share of side effects, including tremor, clinical hypothyroidism, weight gain, reduced libido, abnormal movements, and dry mouth, the last being the most bothersome from day to day. However, overall medication has been necessary, and I have responded well to it.

Psychotherapy

During the 1990s I had experiences with psychotherapies (see Box 5.6) but did not find them particularly helpful. The personality of the therapist seemed to be the key variable. Cognitive Behavioural Therapy (CBT) struck me as common sense, but I appreciated its value more with the passage of time. The hope that it might act prophylactically to short-circuit or prevent future depressive episodes was soon dashed. So-called psychodynamic therapy (CBT had been requested) was much worse (for me) and, I think, harmful: it precipitated one of my breakdowns. I felt no rapport with the therapist and never emotionally engaged with the process. What I shall always appreciate are the many psychiatrists, nurses, occupational therapists (OTs), and social workers who possessed the 'core conditions' of unconditional positive regard and empathy, and engaged with me on a personal level in sickness and in health (see Figure 5.1).

Box 5.5 Medication Used in Treating Depression

Medication is the mainstay of treatment for moderate to severe depression (see Table 5.3), although not the only relevant treatment modality. It is not recommended for mild depression and it works best when there are somatic symptoms. There are several different classes of drugs which are all thought to exert a therapeutic effect by altering levels of the neurotransmitters noradrenaline and serotonin in the midbrain. How they do this is still not understood. There are many different receptor sub-types, other neurotransmitters may additionally be involved, and the drugs act at different points in the neural pathways. With the exception of agomelatine, they have no direct effect on the cerebral cortex, in which the experience of depression is located. The choice is individual and should be made by patient and doctor together, balancing potential benefit against tolerability of likely side effects.

For severe or recurrent depression, and for prophylaxis, antidepressants are often combined with other types of medication, particularly mood stabilizers such as lithium or sodium valproate, and atypical antipsychotics such as quetiapine and olanzapine.

About half the people prescribed an antidepressant will find about half of their symptoms resolved. Any benefit is not usually felt until two to four weeks after beginning treatment. Treatment should be continued for several months after recovery to reduce the otherwise high chance of relapse, and for longer with recurrent illnesses.

Table 5.3 Antidepressant medications

	Name of group	Examples	Main side effects
SSRI	Selective Serotonin Reuptake Inhibitors	Fluoxetine Citalopram Sertraline	Nausea, agitation, insomnia, shakiness, diarrhoea
SNRI	Serotonin and Noradrenaline Reuptake Inhibitors	Venlafaxine Duloxetine	Nausea, vomiting, agitation, anxiety, headache, dizziness
NaSSA	Noradrenergic and Specific Serotonergic Antidepressant	Mirtazapine	Increased appetite, weight gain, sedation, fluid retention
TCA	Tricyclic Antidepressants	Amitriptyline Clomipramine Lofepramine	Sedation, dry mouth, blurred vision, constipation, dizziness on standing
MAOI and RIMA	Monoamine Oxidase Inhibitors and Reversible Monoamine Oxidase Inhibitors	Phenelzine Moclobemide	Dizziness, insomnia, headache, drowsiness, nausea, bowel disturbance
Melatonergic	Acts on melatonin receptors	Agomelatine	Dizziness, abnormal liver function tests, abdominal pain

Box 5.6 Psychotherapies

Psychotherapy is the use of psychological methods to help a person change or overcome problems in desired ways. It has been practised for centuries by medicine men, prophets, philosophers, and ordinary people, but modern psychotherapy had its origins in the moral treatment movement of the nineteenth century. Now, over a thousand different named therapies have been described. It is usually practised as a one-to-one verbal exchange between a client and a therapist. The therapeutic alliance established between client and therapist is regarded as crucial to effective psychotherapy. Person-centred psychotherapy, developed in the 1950s, required the therapist to possess three 'core conditions': unconditional positive regard, genuineness, and empathic understanding. These non-specific factors are probably integral to the success of any course of therapy.

Some of the main types are:

Psychodynamic or insight orientated therapy, such as **psychoanalysis,** focuses on symptoms or character problems by revealing unconscious processes. This is done by using the therapeutic relationship to illuminate past experiences, typically over a long period of time.

Cognitive behavioural therapy (CBT) is widely used, including in primary care, because it is effective, brief, and therefore inexpensive, and therapists can easily be trained. It is focused in the present, and relates thoughts to feelings and behaviour. **Interpersonal therapy (IPT)** and **dialectical behaviour therapy (DBT)** are other variants, dealing with human relationships.

Humanistic therapies emerged in reaction to behaviouralism and psychoanalysis and are concerned with human development and needs of the individual. Examples are **person-centred therapy** and **compassion-focused therapy**.

Systemic therapies deal with the patterns and dynamics of groups of people, such as families.

Expressive therapies utilize primarily non-verbal forms of communication such as dance, drama, and art.

As with any treatment, some (10 to 15 per cent) of clients do not benefit or deteriorate further.

Psychotherapy is more effective than medication in mild depression and equally effective in moderate depression. In severe depression it is good practice to offer both physical and psychological treatment.

Support Groups

Since 2008 I have been a member of the Doctors Support Network[17] (see Box 5.7) and now facilitate one of the regional groups. These are supportive rather than psychotherapeutic; more like a gathering of friends, but we tackle big issues if necessary and ill people are welcome. It has certainly raised my self esteem. I would like to encourage all doctors who have or have had problems with their mental health to join.

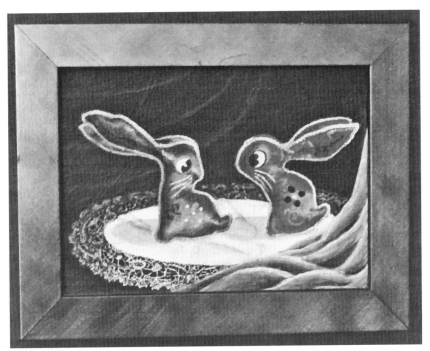

Figure 5.1 This shows one of my first paintings, which I have entitled 'It's good to talk'. I painted it for my mother-in-law, who had dementia, and she kept it on her bedside table.

My Recovery

My care in the twenty-first century became more holistic under the Care Programme Approach (CPA). This framework was introduced into the NHS in 1990 following several high-profile enquiries where individuals with psychosis had murdered professionals and others, including family members and strangers.[23] CPA requires that people with serious mental illness and living in the community should have a comprehensive assessment of their needs, allocated care coordinator, and regular review of their care plans. Accordingly, this century I have had not just a doctor to relate to but also a key worker: someone accessible who provides a gateway to other services.

I have had the good fortune to have the same person for the past 12 years. From her I have gained much insight. She is my first port of call in times of trouble. She instigated some compassion-focused psychotherapy sessions a few years ago to help balance out my well-developed threat and incentive systems (meaning competitive and self critical attitudes and behaviour) with some self care.[24] She says I have changed hugely in the past decade; I am kinder to myself and I do not always expect perfection. I have learned to be even more resilient (meaning I have become more flexible, strong, and tough).

Box 5.7 What is Recovery?

Contemporary ideas about recovery first surfaced in the United States in the civil rights movement about 40 years ago, when people who had experienced severe mental health problems declared that, nevertheless, their capacity to achieve life goals was not permanently impaired and their identity did not need to be defined by a disability. It challenged the traditional medical model, which placed little emphasis on the service user as a person. It became clear that stigma and exclusion were experienced by most people with mental health problems in most societies. There was thus a need for recovery-orientated mental health services, based on learning from service users themselves what worked for them.[18]

An internationally recognized definition states that recovery, as used in psychiatry, is 'a deeply personal, unique process of changing one's attitude, values, feelings, goals, skills and roles. It is a way of living a satisfying, hopeful and contributing life, even with the limitations caused by illness. Recovery involves the development of new meaning and purpose in one's life as one grows beyond the catastrophic effects of mental illness'.[19]

In the United Kingdom, the Royal College of Psychiatrists committed to developing and implementing the recovery approach in 2008.[20] The 'common principles' guiding the five year plan for mental health services in the United Kingdom (2016–21) include co-production with people with lived experience of services, their families, and carers; partnership working with public, private, and voluntary organizations; identifying needs and intervening as early as possible; and person-centred care, all underpinned by evidence.[21]

Co-production can be defined as 'a relationship where professionals and citizens share power to plan and deliver support together, recognising that both partners have vital contributions to make in order to improve quality of life for people and communities'.[21] It is based on principles including taking an assets-based (rather than deficits) approach; building on existing capabilities; reciprocity and mutuality; peer support networks; blurring distinctions; and facilitating rather than delivering care. It is the antithesis of 'the medical model'.

Considerable progress has been made.[21] A national survey recently reported that recovery orientation in English community mental health teams is high and there was some evidence that this was associated with personal recovery.[15] Many trusts have established recovery colleges which allow co-design and co-production by 'experts by lived experience' and 'experts by profession' of service user-led educational courses and activities. These challenge the conventional model of public services. Many now have websites devoted to recovery and wellbeing which can be accessed by the general public. Peer support workers are widely used, their work based on principles including mutuality, reciprocity, non-directive, strengths-based, and recovery-focused.

Psychiatry in the United Kingdom has always been practised with the needs of the individual uppermost, but changes to the curriculum for training junior psychiatrists to better develop person-centred care skills are planned.

Box 5.7 Continued

Dimensions of Recovery

There have been numerous attempts to measure recovery. This is difficult because it is subjective and both an outcome and a process. The following areas are typically covered: understanding mental health and how to manage it; physical health, activity and self care; addictive behaviours; life skills; social networks; relationships; work; responsibilities; identity; purpose and direction; self esteem, trust, and hope.

Five Ways to Wellbeing was designed to promote evidence based messages about good mental health directly to service users (and others).[22] It has been widely disseminated as a booklet and online. Wellbeing means having good relationships and being valued and respected. The five ways are: Connect; Keep learning; Be active; Take notice; Give.

key worker and my psychiatrist treated me primarily as a person who had an illness. I have seen psychiatrists who treated me as an illness, which is dispiriting. I continue to take large amounts of medication.

The chief therapeutic agents in my recovery have been people. I suggest this is usually so, and it is one of the reasons why psychiatry is such a rewarding discipline and career.

Retirement

Retirement has been surprising in the right sort of way: less patienthood and more psychiatry than I anticipated (see Figure 5.2).

On my formal retirement date in 2008 I had not actually been working for months. Nothing was planned. I was not ready to give up the identity of being a doctor so started being a Mental Health Assessor under Deprivation of Liberty Safeguarding (DOLS)[25] when it came into practice in 2009 (this authorizes detention in hospital or a care home of non-capacitous persons provided it can be shown to be in their best interests). Since the legal definition of deprivation changed in 2014, the volume of work undertaken by mental health assessors and the number of referrals everywhere has increased tenfold and the pioneering spirit is long gone. I decided to surrender my licence to practise in August 2017, rather than face more NHS bureaucracy and Section 12 renewal, not to mention CPD and appraisal. I have no regrets.

I could now be said to have a portfolio career. My latest venture is to establish a charitable fund to help individuals with their recoveries (work in progress), which I am starting with compensation money paid after I received a faulty hip prosthesis. This year I became a public governor of a mental health trust. I am involved in examining and teaching (including doctors' mental health to medical undergraduates). I facilitate a regional support group for the Doctors Support Network. In 2014 I became a

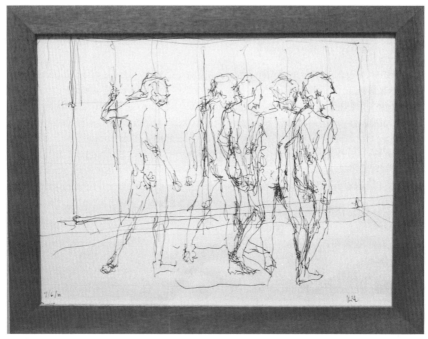

Figure 5.2 This shows an image made at a life-drawing class which was designed to show movement. Each figure was drawn in three minutes using my left (non-preferred) hand (which is less 'automatic' and a new challenge). I have called it 'Progression', and it could be seen as a metaphorical depiction of life after medicine.

member of an RCPsych's group considering ways to promote person-centred care in psychiatric training. (I have dual expertise—by profession and by lived experience).

I draw, paint, sing, write, and cycle (even in Sheffield).

I have enjoyed Mindfulness for Doctors[26] weekends and use mindfulness meditation at home. I have done some epic travelling. I am connected: a wife, mother, sibling, daughter, and friend. My children are affectionate and autonomous, despite everything. It gives me not a little satisfaction that I became a Fellow of the RCPsych in 2016.

I have learned that I can ask for help rather than wait until I'm so ill that other people notice, and that my illness is part of me, not something which happened to me.

Double life no more.

References

1. **Allen V** and **Hussain O** (2016). What I wish I'd known as a junior doctor. London: British Medical Association Publishing Group. BMJ Careers.
2. This quotation was on the RCPsych website but no longer appears. Other persuasive views on choosing psychiatry as a profession can be found at the site: <http://www.rcpsych.ac.uk/discoverpsychiatry/acareerinpsychiatry/choosepsychiatry.aspx>.

3. **Waite J** and **Easton E** (eds) (2013). *The ECT Handbook*, 3rd edn. London: Royal College of Psychiatrists, pp. 1–272

4. **World Health Organization** (2016). ICD-10 Classification of Mental and Behavioural Disorders, 10th revision. Geneva: World Health Organization.

5. **American Psychiatric Association** (2013). Diagnostic and Statistical Manual V. Lake St Louis, MO: American Psychiatric Association.

6. **Medical Protection Society** (2015). *Medical Protection Society Casebook* November 23:15–16.

7. **Royal Medical Benevolent Fund** (2016). Newsletter, Spring issue:4–5.

8. **Horsfall S** (2014). Doctors who commit suicide while under GMC fitness to practise investigations. London: General Medical Council,

9. **Stevens R** (2016). The Vital Signs. Our guides for doctors and medical students seeking help and advice. <http://www.rmbf.org>.

10. **Duggins R** (2016). The Rewards of Keeping Doctors Healthy. Doctors Support Network. <http://www.dsn.org.uk>.

11. **Grote H**, **Raouf M**, and **Elton C** (2012). Developing career resilience in medicine. London: British Medical Association Publishing Group. BMJ Careers.

12. **Oxtoby K** (2016). Tackling the stigma around mental health. London: British Medical Association Publishing Group. BMJ Careers.

13. **Gerada C** (2015). The wounded healer: Why we need to rethink how we support doctors. London: British Medical Association Publishing Group. BMJ Careers.

14. **Klitzman R** (2018). *When Doctors Become Patients*. Oxford: Oxford University Press.

15. **Leamy M**, **Clarke E**, **Le Boutillier C**, **Bird V**, **Choudhury R**, **MacPherson R**, **Pesola F**, **Sabas K**, **Williams J**, **Williams P**, and **Slade M** (2016). Recovery practice in community mental health teams: national survey. *British Journal of Psychiatry* **209**(4):340–6.

16. Moodscope. <http://www.moodscope.com>.

17. Doctors Support Network. <http://www.dsn.org.uk>.

18. **Roberts G** and **Boardman J** (2013). Understanding 'recovery'. *Advances in Psychiatric Treatment* **19**:400–9.

19. **Anthony W** (1993). Recovery from mental illness: the guiding vision of the mental health service system in the 1990's. *Psychosocial Rehabilitation Journal* **16**:11–23

20. **Royal College of Psychiatrists** (2008). Fair Deal for Mental Health: Our Manifesto for a 3-Year Campaign Dedicated to Tackling Inequality in Mental Healthcare. London: Royal College of Psychiatrists.

21. **Department of Health** (2016). Implementing the Five Year Forward View for Mental Health. London: NHS England.

22. The '5 ways to wellbeing' were developed as evidence-based mental health promotion messages at the request of the Government's Department of Science for the Foresight Mental Capital and Wellbeing Project 2008.

23. **Simpson A**, **Bowers L**, and **Miller C** (2003). The History of the Care Programme Approach in England. London: University of London Institutional Repository. <http://openaccess.city.ac.uk/8075/1/>.

24. **Gilbert P** (2009). *The Compassionate Mind*. London: Constable.

25. Mental Capacity Act 2005: Deprivation of Liberty Safeguards—Code of Practice. London: Ministry of Justice. <https://www.legislation.gov.uk/ukpga/2005/9/contents>.

26. Mindfulness for Doctors. <http://www.mindfulnessfordoctors.co.uk>.

Chapter 6

Perinatal Psychiatry: Motherhood in Mental Health Services

Jacqueline Humphreys

Perinatal psychiatry is the practice of caring for women with mental illness during pregnancy and the postpartum period (the year after giving birth). It is a relatively new subspecialty that only became a Faculty of the Royal College of Psychiatrists in June 2014. However, documented cases of women suffering from mental illness within the perinatal period stretch back over 200 years.

Historical Cases of Maternal Mental Illness

In 1858 Louis Victor Marcé, a French psychiatrist, published his treatise on maternal mental illness which described clinical syndromes with 79 case examples, and summarized the treatments of his era.[1] This anticipated much of what is now commonly known about mental illness in the perinatal period, such as the high risk of perinatal depression and postpartum psychosis.[2] Case notes from the 1800s refer to 'puerperal insanity', which often led to the patient's incarceration in a sanatorium or asylum (see Figure 6.1). One case involved Frances Sophia Davey, a former governess from Plymouth, who was admitted to Holloway Sanatorium in 1890 with a condition thought to be caused by premature confinement. Medical records describe her as a tall, delicate woman with light hair and a pale, freckled face. Although she was listless and rarely replied to questions, she believed her husband was not really her husband; she claimed he was, in fact, in heaven, as was she. A diagnosis of puerperal insanity led to her admission to the hospital for a little over a year, with no improvement. She was then 'relieved' to Camberwell Asylum under the authority of her husband.[3]

Similar cases can be found throughout the Victorian era and the first half of the twentieth century. During this time, women with serious mental illness such as postpartum psychosis were routinely separated from their babies, and there was an absence of women carers in positions of power within the asylums.[4] It was also a time when maternal death rates were high, and sepsis and haemorrhage were common complications of childbirth. A mother's mental state may have seemed secondary to these life-threatening conditions and may have been complicated by delirium. Figure 6.1 image shows a woman at four stages of 'puerperal mania', as it was then called.

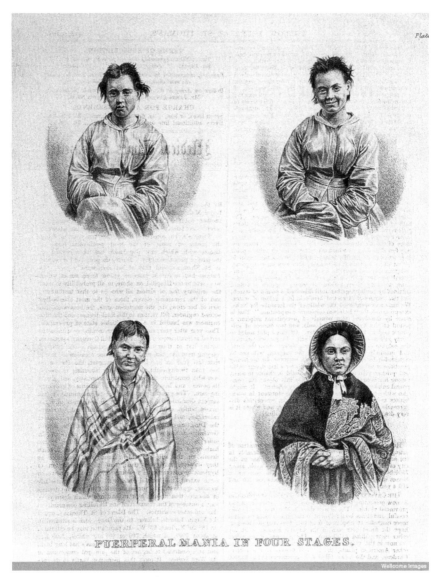

Figure 6.1 Puerperal mania in four stages, *The Medical Times and Gazette*, John Churchill and Sons London 1858.

Psychiatric Mother and Baby Units

The specific mental health of women during pregnancy and the postpartum period began to receive serious attention after the Second World War. The importance of the mother–infant bond and the impact of separation of children from their mothers was first discussed in the 1940s and 1950s. In 1951 John Bowlby wrote a report for the World Health Organisation which described the impact of maternal deprivation. Young children separated from their primary caregiver, generally the mother, developed long-lasting emotional and interpersonal difficulties.[5] This arose after studying the effect of the evacuation of children from London in the Second World War, and was further discussed by Bowlby in 1956.[6] In the same year Winnicott described the concept of primary maternal preoccupation—a period of heightened sensitivity of a woman towards her new baby which is almost like an illness, albeit one that is a normal and temporary state for mothers.[7]

As there became increasing recognition of the mental health consequences that separation from their mothers could have upon children, the practice of allowing them to stay together on paediatric wards also became more common.[8] Then, in 1948, a mother with non-psychotic depression was admitted with her toddler to the Cassel Hospital at her request. From 1955 the medical director of the Cassel Hospital started to admit other women suffering from puerperal episodes with their children, noting that it promoted positive elements of the mother–child relationship,[9] although this practice did not extend to women suffering from severe psychotic episodes. Other hospitals admitted women with psychosis to hospitals and doctors described how this practice was beneficial and hastened the recovery of the mother.[10]

In 1974 Dr Margaret Oates, psychiatrist, opened a two-bedded Mother and Baby Inpatient Unit (MBU) in Nottingham. Although not the first unit of its kind, its integration with a community perinatal service was an innovative approach to caring for women. Her analysis of the literature provided persuasive argument for the expansion of mother and baby units and specialist community services.[11]

Cultural Perceptions of Motherhood

Although the causes of mental health issues during pregnancy and the postpartum period vary, the assumption that pregnancy and child-rearing is always a joyful experience can exacerbate the feelings of failure, inadequacy, and anxiety some mothers experience. Women can be reluctant to admit they are struggling for fear of being labelled a 'bad mother'. From an early age they are told, often by their own mothers, that the day they have a child of their own will be the happiest of their life. It is implied that they will instinctively know what their baby needs, and that giving birth is 'the most natural thing in the world'.

The image of the perfect mother is strewn throughout art, culture, and religion (see Figure 6.2). Christianity, particularly Catholicism, is imbued with images of the Virgin Mary smiling serenely at the infant Jesus. Within Hinduism is Devi, another benevolent mother goddess. Greek mythology features Gaia, the original earth mother—a concept that has recently been adopted in the Western world to symbolize the woman

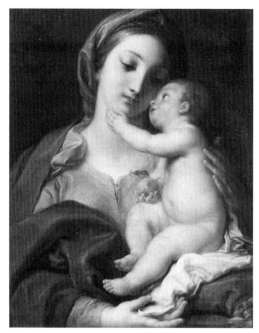

Figure 6.2 *Madonna and Child* by Pomeo Batoni.

who ensures everything she does is 'natural', from giving birth without pain control to feeding exclusively by breast and attachment parenting. Versions of the ideal mother and family are also prominent within Western literature,[12] such as in classic American novels like *Little House on The Prairie* and *Little Women*, in which tension exists between the women pushing against patriarchal oppression while at the same time colluding with it through domestic bondage and self-sacrifice.[13]

Although it is easier for women to speak out today, coupled with a growing acknowledgement that the 'perfect' mother is an insidious myth, modern women are not immune from social pressure once they become parents. One recent best-selling book, *Battle Hymn of the Tiger Mother*,[14] implied that mothers who are strict disciplinarians raise the highest-achieving children. Even when women don't subscribe to specific motherhood ideologies, they can still internalize the pressure to be a perfect mother and suffer from poorer mental health as a result of not meeting parenting expectations.[18]

Social media has added another layer of complexity to pregnancy and parenthood, allowing new mothers to share photos and videos of their children with a potentially vast audience of friends, acquaintances, and even strangers. The evidence about whether this is a help or hindrance to new mothers is contradictory. On the one hand, these communication systems offer a valuable form of peer support and information, and a way to reach more people than many traditional groups.[15] On the other, if all you see on social media are the days when someone's child is beaming and well behaved you may come to feel that your own parenting skills simply aren't good enough. In one study that examined Facebook use among new mothers, those who were more preoccupied with external validation of their own parenting experienced an increase in depressive symptoms in correlation with increased Facebook activity.[16] Another study found that people who stopped using Facebook for just one week reported increased life satisfaction and positive emotions.[17]

The Challenges of Motherhood

For women in many developed countries, having a baby can mean a sudden change from working full-time to staying at home, often with only your new baby for company. Erik Erikson, a German-born American developmental psychologist and psychoanalyst known for his theory on psychosocial development of human beings, claimed that this type of large role transition will normally result in a transitional crisis.[19] This is often complicated by sleep deprivation. For some women, a sense that they may not enjoy motherhood can also add feelings of guilt, shame, and regret to the slew of emotions they experience after giving birth.

In Western culture increasing atomization and isolation from the family unit has also reduced new mothers' contact with older women whom they trust enough to share their feelings of loneliness or anxiety. This may be less of a problem in some non-Western cultures. In Newham in London, the borough in which I work, there is a large migrant population from the Indian subcontinent. When women give birth, older women from their family often come to live with them for several months, taking over many of the responsibilities of looking after the new baby, any other children, and running the home so that the mother can rest and focus on establishing a breast-feeding regime (Figure 6.3).

The onset of motherhood can also bring about financial constraints due to the cost of providing for a new baby and the temporary or permanent cessation of employment. This has been speculated as one of the mechanisms behind the gender pay gap, which the UK government has attempted to tackle through introduction of the Shared Parental Leave (SPL) scheme. Unfortunately, a survey conducted one year after the scheme's launch showed that only 1 per cent of all men had taken up the opportunity to share their partner's parental leave to date. This may be due to multiple factors including a company's reluctance to allow men to take this leave and women's reluctance to share their maternity leave. It is hoped that there will be more uptake with time, with 87 per cent of men surveyed saying they would like to have longer leave to be fully involved in the care of their child.[20]

Single mothers often face the greatest financial difficulties and social isolation, factors associated with their higher risk of depression.[21] Nevertheless, having a partner doesn't always equate to emotional or financial support. In some cases it can actually put women at physical and emotional risk: the incidence of domestic violence against women is higher during pregnancy[22] and is associated with increased rates of depression, anxiety, and post-traumatic stress disorder.[23]

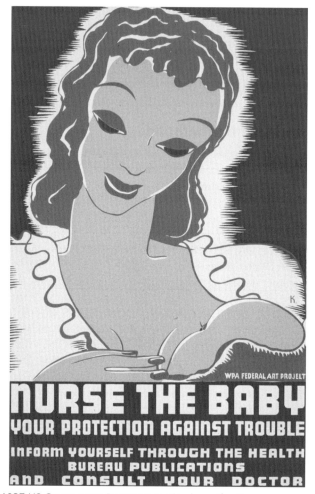

Figure 6.3 1937 US Government Poster promoting breastfeeding.

Detection of Maternal Mental Illness

When taking all these factors into account, it is not surprising that pregnancy and the postpartum period is the highest risk period of a woman's life for developing mental illness.[24] This can range from mild depression or anxiety to severe manifestations of these illnesses, or the most severe manifestation of maternal mental illness, postpartum psychosis.

While the stigma of mental illness has been much discussed in recent years, within perinatal psychiatry the added pressure of having to conform to societal ideals of motherhood can lead women to conceal or minimize their illness. One study reported in 2006 found that out of 1250 mothers half of those who had completed the Edinburgh Postnatal Depression Scale (EPDS) had given false information to conceal their symptoms.[25] A 1998 study identified that the fear that social services would remove their child if mental illness was identified was also common.[26] This still applies for many women that I see today. Thus, while there are reports that one in ten mothers experience mental illness at some point during the perinatal period, many others may not come forward, and the actual figure could be much higher.

Increased training and the use of standardized screening tools such as the EPDS means that midwives, obstetricians, general practitioners (GPs), and health visitors are getting better at detecting the presence of mental illness in women during pregnancy and the postpartum period, but no specialist services to refer patients on to exist. Maps showing the distribution of perinatal mental health teams and Mother and Baby Psychiatric Inpatient Units across the United Kingdom and Northern Ireland, produced by the Maternal Mental Health Alliance as part of the Everyone's Business Campaign launched in July 2014,[27] show large areas without any specialist services.

The Need for Specialist Services

Nevertheless, at a time of reduced resources for mental health services, some might argue that we cannot afford to allocate funds to specialist perinatal services. After all, the case for specialist funding rests on a limited body of evidence that proves dedicated perinatal services or mother and baby units lead to improved outcomes for patients. However, given that relatively few services exist; the accumulation of evidence proving their effectiveness will take time. Several large-scale studies are underway, including Effectiveness of Services for Mothers with Mental Illness (ESMI), a programme of research examining the clinical effectiveness and cost-effectiveness of perinatal psychiatry services.[28]

The answer to the question of whether to prescribe medication to pregnant and breastfeeding women, and if so which medication, is rarely a simple one. For example, it is important to consider the woman's past psychiatric history and her preferences, and combine this information with the most up-to-date evidence on certain medications. Yet these medications may be inconsistent with multiple other confounding factors; the most often-used ones are of little use if the patient finds the side effects intolerable, or if the medications are ineffective for her. The latest National Institute for Health and Care Excellence (NICE) guidelines recognize the complex nature of prescribing psychiatric medication for pregnant and postnatal women, and recommend that doctors take a more pragmatic view,[29] while emphasizing the importance of seeking up-to-date advice from a perinatal specialist.

To ensure women receive the best care, numerous professionals need to communicate effectively. A woman referred to a perinatal mental health service may encounter professionals from each of the following categories: midwives, obstetricians, psychiatrists, psychologists, parent–infant psychotherapists, mental health nurses, and health visitors. If safeguarding concerns are raised, this list can include social workers, and yet more professionals if a mother needs help from her local home treatment team or admission to a mother and baby unit. As such, women can feel that they have too many visits and appointments from professionals. Multi-professional team members therefore need to remain mindful that the woman and child are at the heart of their service and are watchful for psychological dynamics attributable to adverse circumstances and maladaptive relationships from the woman's childhood.

The Impact of Maternal Mental Illness

Undertreating mental illness can have serious repercussions for both mother and child. Without the appropriate treatment a mother's condition can deteriorate, and as a result they may struggle to care for their baby properly. This is not only the case for those women with psychosis; for example, a woman with obsessive compulsive disorder (OCD) might struggle with changing nappies due to fears about contamination.[30] Even if mothers can meet the child's physical needs, difficulty meeting its emotional ones can quickly lead to infant distress and ultimately attachment problems.[31] Consequently, medical professionals should always be mindful of the important relationship between mother and baby and be able to discuss any identified difficulties in the relationship in a sensitive manner; if the mother is already depressed it is important to avoid increasing her feelings of guilt.

Economic analysis published in 2014 estimated the financial cost of not treating maternal mental illness to be £8.1 billion per year.[32] This is largely due to the impact that untreated maternal mental illness has upon the woman's children. They often suffer much higher levels of mental illness than their peers, particularly depression by the age of 16, and behavioural problems such as conduct disorder. This has a knock-on effect upon social care and schooling budgets and adds to financial pressure within the NHS.

From 1997, Margaret Oates contributed to the UK's Confidential Enquiries into Maternal Deaths (CEMD).[33] These reports examine all maternal deaths in pregnancy and the postpartum period, both those directly attributed to pregnancy and those indirectly attributed. Deaths due to mental illness—which include suicide and drug abuse—were found to be the leading indirect cause of maternal deaths in the postpartum period, and has remained one of the leading causes of death in subsequent years. This evidence dispelled the commonly held view that pregnancy and the postpartum period were protective against suicide. Since 2012 the CEMD has been carried out by the MBRRACE-UK (Mothers and Babies: Reducing Risk through Audits and Confidential Enquiries) collaboration and reports are now issued annually.

The onset of postpartum illness—particularly postpartum psychosis—can be extremely sudden. The speed at which the mother's health can deteriorate has been underestimated in the past, as highlighted in the 2015 MBRRACE-UK report.[34] In the 2016 MBRRACE-UK report suicide was reclassified as a direct cause of maternal deaths, making it the leading cause of direct maternal deaths occurring up to one year after the end of pregnancy (111 recorded between 2009 and 2014).[35]

In rare but severe cases of mental distress there is a risk that the mother may not only harm or kill herself but may also kill her baby. Behind the development of perinatal services in Newham was the tragic death of a trainee psychiatrist, Dr Daksha Emson, and her baby daughter Freya. Daksha was a talented woman with a promising career ahead of her. She also had a diagnosis of bipolar affective disorder which she did not disclose to her employers due to the realistic fear that she would experience stigma. While she saw psychiatrists she was never formally under treatment by a community mental health team, again because of the fear of stigma that she would experience as a psychiatrist with a diagnosis of bipolar affective disorder.

In 2000 she gave birth to Freya, having come off her medication prior to conceiving. She then suffered a postpartum relapse but did not go back on her lithium medication as she was breastfeeding. Tragically, three months after giving birth, she killed herself and her daughter, stabbing them both several times before setting them both on fire. The independent enquiry into her death, which includes her life story and suicide note, is a sobering and heartbreaking read.[36] It concluded that the fear that she would be stigmatized was a significant factor in the failings of her care, and meant that she was treated as a doctor rather than as a patient. Several recommendations for developing perinatal mental health services were made, including producing guidance for commissioning these services, and additional training on perinatal mental illness for all psychiatrists.

However, the provision of perinatal services remain patchy in the United Kingdom. In December 2014, Charlotte Bevan, who had been diagnosed with schizophrenia and had been sectioned four times, walked out of St Michael's hospital in Bristol with her four-day-old daughter, Zaani Tiana, wrapped in a blanket. She walked to the clifftop at Avon Gorge and leapt to her death. It is unknown what her intention was at that time. Zaani was found dead in some shrubbery near the bottom on the gorge.

Charlotte had stopped taking her medication because she wanted to breastfeed. During the inquest into her death, Zaani's father and Charlotte's partner, Pascal Malbrouck, claimed she had been given contradictory advice about stopping her medication. At the time she left the hospital it was likely she was unwell from a psychotic relapse. The coroner, Maria Voisin, found there were a 'chain of failures' in Charlotte's care which ultimately led to the death of both her and Zaani. She wrote to NHS England about the provision of mental health services for pregnant women.[37] After the inquest, Charlotte's family urged the Bristol Clinical Commissioning Group to set up a dedicated perinatal unit for mothers with mental health issues.

The Rise of Modern Perinatal Psychiatry

In 1980, psychiatrists Channi Kumar, Ian Brockington, and James Hamilton helped to found the Marcé Society, an international society for the understanding, prevention, and treatment of mental illness related to childrearing[38] named after Louis Victor Marcé. The primary focus is to promote and communicate research into the mental health of women, their partners, and children. The society continues to hold a biennial scientific conference.

In recent years there has been a large influx of women into this specialty, and the majority of those practising within the United Kingdom are now women. Dr Oates deserves special mention for her outstanding and pioneering early work, for which she was awarded an Order of the British Empire for services to mental healthcare in 2009,[39] and a Royal College of Psychiatry Lifetime Achievement Award in 2013. Internationally, many other women have carried out high-profile research, such as Professor Louise Howard in the United Kingdom, Katherine Wisner in the United States, and Nine Glaungeaud-Freudenthal in France. A former chair of perinatal

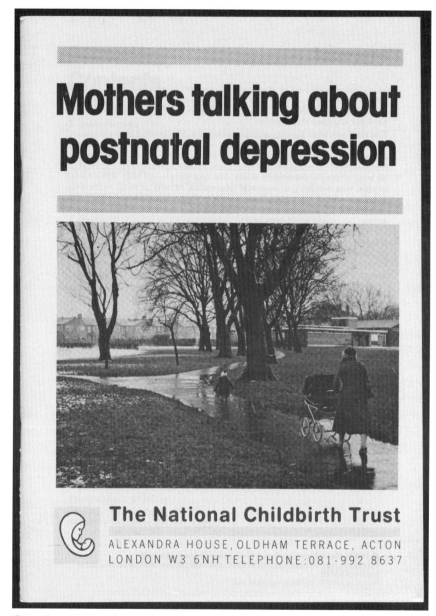

Figure 6.4. NCT Booklet: Mothers talking about postnatal depression.
© NCT/Wellcome Library, London, Wellcome Images. Reproduced under the Creative
Commons Attribution Licence CC BY 4.0

psychiatry, Dr Liz McDonald, also set up the excellent MBU within my own Trust in
East London. She has worked tirelessly to raise awareness of the specialty, to push the
agenda for increased training in perinatal psychiatry and more services, and is an inspiration to myself and others.

In addition, there is now a vocal group of people with lived experience of maternal mental illness, sharing their experiences through the media, and advocating for improved services and better recognition of women's mental health needs during and after birth (Figure 6.4).

The Maternal Mental Health Alliance (MMHA), is a coalition of national professional and patients organizations that has also been very active in raising awareness of the prevalence of maternal mental illness and the need for more perinatal services. Numerous women have shared their stories with the organization which have been used to inform storylines in television and radio. For example, a recent EastEnders storyline saw the character Stacey suffering from an episode of postpartum psychosis, leading to her developing delusional beliefs that her child is the Son of God. In addition to advising the storyline, women who have suffered postpartum psychosis have written blogs about their experiences, and the difference specialist care in mother and baby units made to their recovery.

Epilogue

Throughout history, the social and cultural pressures of pregnancy and caring for children have contributed to the suffering many women experience before and after birth, as well the stigma attached to women who suffer from mental illness during pregnancy and the postnatal period. As we have seen, when things go wrong for women and their children at this crucial life stage it can result in heartbreaking tragedy. While it is clear that there is much still to be done to improve mental health care for women during pregnancy and the postpartum period, there is also growing awareness that these conditions are treatable, there is no such thing as the perfect mother, and there is increased acceptance of fathers taking a more active role in caring for their children.

On a personal note, I would not be able to do the work I do today without the efforts of pioneers within perinatal psychiatry who have fought hard for increased recognition and services. I am lucky to have entered the specialty at time when there is growing momentum within both psychiatry and wider society around increased support for mothers and their families during a challenging stage of a woman's life, and for additional money to commission for specialist services. In short, it is an exciting time for myself, many colleagues, and the specialty, and I look forward to being involved in its future development.

References

1. **Marcé LV** (1858). *Treatise on madness in pregnant women, in women who have recently given birth, and in wet nurses, and medical/legal considerations on this subject. [Traité de la folie des femmes enceintes des nouvelles accouchées et des nourrices et considérations médico-légales qui se rattachent à ce sujet.* Paris: JB Baillière et fils.

2. **Trede K**, **Baldessarini RJ**, **Viguera AC**, and **Bottéro A** (2009). Treatise on Insanity in Pregnant, Postpartum, and Lactating Women (1858) by Louis-Victor Marcé: A Commentary. *Harvard Review of Psychiatry*, **17**(2): 157–65.

3. Holloway Sanatorium Hospital for the Insane Archives. Females no. 4: Certified female patients admitted July 1890–June 1891. MS 5157/5158, p. 83.

4. **Howard, L** (2000). The separation of mothers and babies in the treatment of postpartum psychotic disorders in Britain 1900–1960. *Archives of Women's Mental Health* **3**:1.

5. **Bowlby J** (1951). *Maternal Care and Mental Health*. Geneva: World Health Organization.

6. **Bowlby J, Ainsworth M, Boston M,** and **Rosenbluth B** (1956). The effects of mother-child separation: A follow-up study. *British Journal of Medical Psychology*, **29**: 211–47.

7. **Winnicott DW** (2012). Primary maternal preoccupation. In: Mariotti P (ed.). *The Maternal Lineage: Identification, Desire, and Transgenerational Issues*. London: Routledge, pp. 59–66.

8. **Cazas O** and **Glaungeaud-Freudenthal NM-C** (2004). The history of Mother-Baby Units (MBUs) in France and Belgium and of the French version of the Marcé checklist. *Archives of Women's Mental Health* **7**(1):53–58.

9. **Main TF** (1858). Mothers with Children in a Psychiatric Hospital. *The Lancet* **272**(7051):845–57.

10. **Bardon D, Glaser YIM, Prothero D,** and **Weston DH** (1968). Mother and Baby Unit: Psychiatric Survey of 115 Cases. *British Medical Journal* **2**(5607):755–8.

11. **Oates M** (1998). Psychiatric services for women following childbirth. *International Review of Psychiatry* **8**(1):87–98. DOI:10.3109/09540269609037821.

12. **Bassin D, Honey M,** and **Mahrer-Kaplan M** (eds) (1994). *Representations of Motherhood*. New York, NY: Yale University Press.

13. **Pope D, Quinn N,** and **Wyer M** (1990). The ideology of mothering: Disruption and reproduction of the patriarchy. *Signs* **15**(3):441–6.

14. **Chua A** (2011). *Battle Hymn of the Tiger Mother*. London: Bloomsbury.

15. **Henderson A, Harmon S,** and **Newman H** (2016). The price mothers pay, even when they are not buying it: Mental health consequences of idealized motherhood. *Sex Roles* **74**:512. DOI:10.1007/s11199-015-0534-5.

16. **Holtz B, Smock A,** and **Reyes-Gastelum D** (2015). Connected motherhood: Social support for moms and moms-to-be on Facebook. *Telemedicine and e-Health* **21**(5):415–21.

17. **Schoppe-Sullivan SJ, Yavorsky JE, Bartholomew MK, Sullivan JM, Lee MA, Kamp Dush CM,** and **Glassman M**(2016). Doing gender online: New mothers' psychological characteristics, Facebook use, and depressive symptoms. *Sex Roles* 1–14. DOI:10.1007/s11199-016-0640-z.

18. **Tromholt M** (2016). The Facebook experiment: Quitting Facebook leads to higher levels of well-being. *Cyberpsychology, Behavior, and Social Networking* **19**(11):661–6. DOI:10.1089/cyber.2016.0259.

19. **Erikson EH** (ed.) (1963). *Youth: Change and Challenge*. New York, NY: Basic Books.

20. **My Family Care**. *Shared Parental Leave—One Year On—Where Are We Now?—UK—April 2016*. <https://www.myfamilycare.co.uk/news/update/shared-parental-leave-where-are-we-now.html>.

21. **Brown G** and **Moran P** (1997). Single mothers, poverty and depression. *Psychological Medicine* **27**:21–33.

22. **Jasinski JL** (2004). Pregnancy and domestic violence: a review of the literature. *Trauma, Violence & Abuse* **5**:47–64.

23. **Howard L, Oram S, Galley H, Trevillion K,** and **Feder G** (2013). Domestic violence and perinatal mental disorders: a systematic review and meta-analysis. *PLoS Medicine* **10**(5):e1001452.

24. **Terp IM** and **Mortensen PB** (1998). Post-partum psychoses. Clinical diagnoses and relative risk of admission after parturition. *British Journal of Psychiatry* **172**(6):521–6.

25. **Russell S** (2006). Barriers to care in postnatal depression. *Community Practitioner* **79**:110–11.

26. **Nicholson J**, **Sweeney EM**, and **Geller JL** (1998). Focus on Women: mothers with mental illness: I. The competing demands of parenting and living with mental illness. *Psychiatric Services* **49**:635–42.

27. **Everyone's Business** (2014). *UK Specialist Community Perinatal Mental Health Teams (current provision).* <http://everyonesbusiness.org.uk/wp-content/uploads/2014/07/UK-Specialist-Community-Perinatal-Mental-Health-Teams-current-provision.pdf>.

28. **King's College London**. *ESMI: Effectiveness of Services for Mothers with Mental Illness.*<http://www.kcl.ac.uk/ioppn/depts/hspr/research/CEPH/wmh/projects/A-Z/esmi.aspx>.

29. **National Institute for Health and Care Excellence** (2014). *Antenatal and Postnatal Mental Health: Clinical Management and Service Guidance* (Clinical Guidance CG192). London: NICE.

30. **Humphreys J**, **Obeney-Williams J**, **Cheung RW**, and **Shah N** (2016). Perinatal psychiatry: A new speciality or everyone's business? *British Journal of Psychiatric Advances* **22**(6):363–72. DOI: 10.1192/apt.bp.115.014548.

31. **Murray L**, **Fiori-Cowley A**, **Hooper R**, and **Cooper P** (1996). The impact of postnatal depression and associated adversity on early mother-infant interactions and later infant outcome. *Child Development* **67**(5):2512–26.

32. **Bauer A**, **Parsonage M**, **Knapp M**, **Iemmi V**, and **Adelaja B** (2014). *The Costs of Perinatal Mental Health Problems.* London: London School of Economics.

33. **Oates M** (2003). Perinatal psychiatric disorders: A leading cause of maternal morbidity and mortality. *British Medical Bulletin* **67**(1):219–29.

34. **Knight M**, **Tuffnell D**, **Kenyon S**, **Shakespeare J**, **Gray R**, and **Kurinczuk JJ** (eds) (2015). *Saving Lives, Improving Mothers' Care: Surveillance of Maternal Deaths in the UK 2011–13 and Lessons Learned to Inform Maternity Care from the UK and Ireland Confidential Enquiries in Maternal Deaths and Morbidity 2009–13.* Oxford: National Perinatal Epidemiology Unit, University of Oxford.

35. **Knight M**, **Nair M**, **Tuffnell D**, **Kenyon S**, **Shakespeare J**, **Brocklehurst P**, and **Kurinczuk JJ** (eds) (2016). *Saving Lives, Improving Mothers' Care: Surveillance of Maternal Deaths in the UK 2012–14 and Lessons Learned to Inform Maternity Care from the UK and Ireland Confidential Enquiries in Maternal Deaths and Morbidity 2009–14.* Oxford: National Perinatal Epidemiology Unit, University of Oxford.

36. **North East London Strategic Health Authority** (2003). *Report of an Independent Inquiry into the Care and Treatment of Daksha Emson M.B.B.S, MRCPsych, MSc. and her Daughter Freya.* North East London Strategic Health Authority. <http://www.simplypsychiatry.co.uk/sitebuildercontent/sitebuilderfiles/deinquiryreport.pdf>.

37. **Voisin ME** (2015). *Regulation 28: Report to Prevent Future Deaths, Charlotte Bevan 2015-0418.* Courts and Tribunals Judiciary 2015. <https://www.judiciary.gov.uk/wp-content/uploads/2016/01/Bevan-2015-0418.pdf>.

38. **Glaungeaud N**. *History of the Marcé Society (1980–2016).* Available from <https://marcesociety.com/wp-content/uploads/2013/11/Marce-Society-History-1980-2016_nine_1September2016.pdf>.

39. **Honours: Order of the British Empire, Civil—OBE.** *The Independent,* Friday 12 June 2009. <http://www.independent.co.uk/news/uk/home-news/honours-order-of-the-british-empire-civil-obe-1703795.html>.

Dora Black

Rashmi Verma

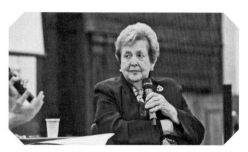

Figure P3.1 Dora's work as Vice Chair with Cruse national charity is one of her contributions of which she is most proud.

© Cruse Bereavement Care

Figure P3.3 Dora speaking at the Medical Women's Federation, Autumn Conference, November 2015.

© Medical Women's Federation

Prior to our several meetings, I had heard that Dora Black 'can be quite intimidating', as many successful, professional women are no doubt deemed to be. The Dora I met was warm, inspiring, and welcoming, proudly sharing her story. If ever there was a strong 'woman's voice' within the field of child and adolescent psychiatry, it surely belongs to Dora Black. Among her many achievements, she has been:

- NHS Consultant Child and Adolescent Psychiatrist, 1966–97

- Founder, Director and Child and Adolescent Psychiatry Consultant of the Traumatic Stress Clinic in London, the first of its kind for children in the United Kingdom
- Vice-Chairwoman of Cruse Bereavement Care
- A founder member and Chairwoman of the Institute of Family Therapy, 1989–92, the largest family therapy organization in the United Kingdom

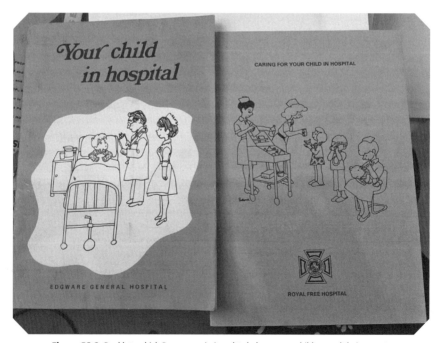

Figure P3.2 Booklets which Dora commissioned to help prepare children and their parents for hospital.

- Chief Psychiatric Consultant, Rhodes Farm Clinic, 1991–2001.
- Director of The Children's Trauma Service, Royal Free Hospital
- Consultant Child and Adolescent Psychiatrist, Royal Free Hospital

Life

Dora was born in 1932 in London. She describes a happy childhood but was only seven years old when she was evacuated at the start of the Second World War. Her mother took Dora and her younger sister to live in New York, and two years later they joined Dora's father, who was posted as a Royal Air Force liaison officer to the Royal Canadian Air Force. Consequently, Dora attended 16 different schools. She describes her mother as her constant support and perhaps her most significant female role model, encouraging her daughters to study and have careers.

Dora returned to England in 1945 and attended Hornsey High School, where she was able to catch up on her education, becoming 'more curious about the things we don't know rather than the things we do'. She then attended Hendon County Grammar School where she met her future husband.

Dora studied Medicine at the University of Birmingham, the first in her family to attend university, undeterred by the fact that very few women were accepted into medical schools at that time. She achieved distinctions in paediatrics, pathology, and neurology, and obtained her medical degree in 1955. Her further qualifications included: 1958–Diploma in Psychological Medicine (DPM), 1971–Member of the Royal College of Psychiatry (MRCPsych), 1979–Fellow of the RCPsych, and 1996–Fellow of the Royal College of Paediatrics and Child Health.

In 1955 Dora married Jack Black, a solicitor. They had three children and one grandchild together and celebrated their sixtieth diamond wedding anniversary in 2015. Dora has many non-professional interests including theatre, opera, concerts, art, travelling, and cooking; she began learning to play the piano from scratch in 2013.

Career

Despite being a trail-blazing pioneer, Dora describes herself as being 'accidentally ambitious', initially planning her career around her family commitments.

After her first house job in Birmingham, she moved to London due to her husband's job and did her second house job in Fulham Hospital. She wanted a specialty which would allow her to focus on being a wife and mother alongside being a doctor. There were few part-time posts available at the time in any specialty. Luckily for the field, the first job that came up was a full-time Senior House Officer in Psychiatry post at Napsbury Hospital, which established her career (Figure P3.4).

Dora trained in Psychiatry at the Maudsley and Bethlem Hospitals, working in the adolescent unit until she had her first child. She had her three children within the next three and a half years. In 1966 she became a part-time Consultant Child and Adolescent Psychiatrist at a Child Guidance Service in Hertfordshire. There she led a widowed mothers group as part of Cruse (Figure P3.1), the national charity for bereavement care and she 'started to have an ambition'. In this work she was particularly influenced by John Bowlby's ideas about separation and loss and Winnicott's notions of being a 'good enough mother'.

It was when she was attached to Great Ormond Street Hospital that she began her ground-breaking research into how to help bereaved children. Her work with Cruse is one of her contributions of which she is most proud.

Between 1968 and 1984, she set up a liaison service for paediatricians at Edgware Hospital. After her own experience of visiting her child in hospital, Dora introduced the practice of parents being able to stay with their children on the ward and she commissioned a leaflet to prepare them and their children for coming into hospital (Figure P3.2).

In 1974, she became a founder member of the Institute of Family Therapy and later became Chair of the Institute.

Dora's first full-time Consultant post, after her children had grown up, was at the Royal Free Hospital, leading a weekly session at the Tavistock Centre. She fought for and succeeded in getting medical student teaching time in child psychiatry and describes being 'ready for new challenges' at that stage. She founded a psychological trauma clinic for children and was the Co-Director of the Traumatic Stress Clinic between 1995 and 1997. She continued working as an Honorary Consultant until 2013. By the end of her career, Dora and her team had seen over 700 cases of children bereaved by one parent killing the other. It was at this time that she co-wrote the seminal text, 'When Father Kills Mother' (Figure P3.5).

In 1992, Dora was invited as a visiting professor at The University of Utah Medical School, Salt Lake City. In 1993, she was awarded the Winston Churchill Travelling Fellowship to study trauma services for children in the United States. In 1995, an invitation from UNICEF took her to Igalo, Montenegro to evaluate a respite care service for traumatized children from the war zones of Bosnia and Croatia. Her breathtaking CV displays a number of places that were keen to hear her expert

Continued on next page

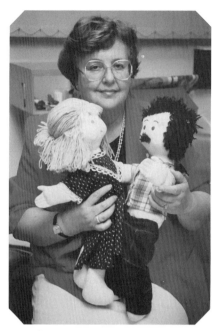

Figure P3.4 Dora's earlier clinical work.

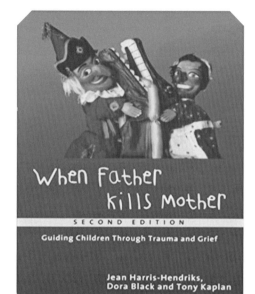

Figure P3.5 Dora's seminal textbook, *When Father Kills Mother*, 1993.

Reproduced from Harris-Hendriks J, Black D, Kaplan T, *When Father Kills Mother: Guiding Children Through Trauma and Grief*, Copyright (1993), with permission from Taylor & Francis

knowledge. Between 1983 and 2013, she gave over 60 main national and international lectures in 20 different countries, often being invited as a guest speaker. She travelled as far as China, Japan and South Africa to mention a few.

Dora was the Chief Psychiatric Consultant at Rhodes Farm Clinic for adolescent eating disorders between 1991 and 2001. She was Honorary Consultant Psychiatrist at Great Ormond Street between 1974 and 2007. Despite all these achievements, Dora describes herself as being foremost a woman with domestic responsibilities who was presented with opportunities ad hoc, grabbing chances where she could.

In 2009, Dora was the only female psychiatrist to be recorded for a Witness Seminar (oral history archive at the University of Glasgow) on the Development of Child and Adolescent Psychiatry between 1960 and 1990. Promoting 'the woman's voice', she spoke about the role of part-time female consultants, acknowledging that even when working 'part-time' herself, she was always at the end of a phone, balancing her family life, while trying to reach her academic potential and teach others.

Dora retired from the National Health Service in 1997 but continued to work as an expert witness for the courts. She fully retired in November 2014 at the age of 82 years. Despite laughing at descriptions of herself as "modest" and "unassuming," and instead describing herself as "quite bossy," Dora has undoubtedly been a formidable female force to be reckoned with…

Most Notable Works

Black D, Harris-Hendriks J, and Wolkind S (1998). *Child Psychiatry and the Law*, 3rd edn. London: Gaskell Press.

Black D, Harris-Hendriks J, and Kaplan T (1993). *When Father Kills Mother—Guiding Children through Trauma and Grief*. London: Routledge.

Black D and Cottrell D (eds) (1993). *Seminars in Child & Adolescent Psychiatry*. London: Gaskell.

Black D, Newman M, Harris-Hendriks J, and Mezey G (eds) (1997). *Psychological Trauma: A Developmental Approach*. Gaskell: London

She was a Home Office specialist adviser reviewing mother and baby units in prisons and made sixty-six recommendations promoting the welfare of children; all were implemented.

Dora has contributed to 45 books and 65 papers for well-known journals including the Lancet and the *British Journal of Psychiatry*, where she was Assistant Editor.

Favourite Quotations

'The apple doesn't fall far from the tree.' *American proverb*
'The most important thing that parents can do for their children is to survive their childhood.' Dr Kenneth Cameron, Consultant Child Psychiatrist at the Maudsley Hospital, London

Other Sources

Medical Womens' Federation. <https://youtu.be/XG5OFJ3qEws>. (Figure P3.3)

Channel 4 documentary: 'Killing in Mind', broadcast on Monday 25 September 1995 at 9 p.m. as part of the *Cutting Edge series*. Box Clever production. Produced and directed by Beth Holgate.

The Institute of Family Therapy. <http://www.ift.org.uk>.

Chapter 7

The Role of Women in Intellectual Disabilities: Clinicians, Scientists, Parents

Rupal Dave and Angela Hassiotis

My Path to Psychiatry (Rupal Dave)

As a 17-year-old schoolgirl applying to university, my understanding of medicine was based on a mixture of visits to a general practitioner (GP), voluntary work, Year Ten work experience in Hemel Hempstead Hospital, nosing through my big sister's lecture notes, and, crucially, watching TV medical dramas. The latter particularly fuelled my understanding that medicine was a fast-paced career that involved running down corridors, shouting instructions to all and no-one in particular. I confess that my understanding of psychiatry was more limited, and the psychiatry of intellectual disability (ID) was not a specialty I was familiar with at all. Psychiatry as a specialty certainly sounded different; more mysterious. It brought to mind an image of a homely doctor's office, complete with ubiquitous porcelain 'phrenology' bust (Figure 7.1), and a leather Chesterfield couch on which the patient would recline whilst being asked 'and how does that make you feel'? Perhaps, due to TV shows or films featuring psychiatrists (*Frasier* or *Good Will Hunting* spring to mind), I instinctively imagined that office, and that career, belonged to a male doctor. I am relieved, and proud, to have realized that I was incorrect and that women make up 59 per cent of those training in psychiatry.[1] The Faculty of the Psychiatry of ID has 430 members (full-time equivalent) with a high proportion being female. It is one of the smaller Faculties within the Royal College of Psychiatrists. In 2016, there were 44 female Specialist Registrars in the Psychiatry of Intellectual Disability in the United Kingdom, representing 64 per cent of the total number of Higher Trainees in the Psychiatry of ID (GMC Training Survey 2016, freedom of information request to GMC by RD; July 2016).

There is often a look of surprise, and a vague sense of confusion, when I tell friends, members of the public and even medical students about my occupation because it appears that the psychiatry of ID is a little-known specialty. Many questions regarding the role and daily job of a psychiatrist in ID follow including 'is that like a GP?', 'are you a psychologist?', and 'is there a crossover with the work of neurologists?' The answer to these questions is that the role is diverse and includes some aspects of all of these jobs.

Psychiatrists in ID diagnose and treat mental illnesses and behaviours that challenge in adults and older people with intellectual disability (ID). They also commonly play a

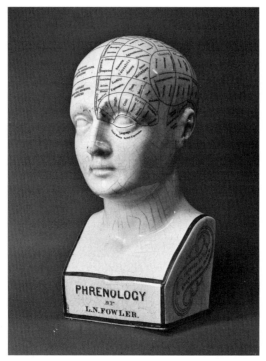

Figure 7.1. Phrenological Bust: 'Phrenology' was a theory introduced in the eighteenth century, popularized in the early nineteenth century and largely discredited in Britain by the middle of the nineteenth century. The theory proposed that specific regions of the brain were associated with emotions, behaviours, and personality traits, and that the size of these areas, described as 'mental organs', was proportional to the activity at this region of the brain. As such, assessment of the size and shape of the skull overlying the phrenological 'organs' of the brain would offer valuable insights into an individual's character. The organs were topographically mapped and publicized as images and later as engravings and phrenological busts.

© Wellcome Library, London. Reproduced under the Creative Commons Attribution Licence CC BY 4.0

role in managing physical and neurodevelopmental conditions frequently experienced by this group of patients, including epilepsy and autistic spectrum disorder. There are estimated to be 930,400 adults aged over 18 years with ID in England, comprising 2 per cent of the adult population. Perhaps this is an overestimate as the prevalence of ID is thought to be approximately 1 per cent globally.[2,3] However, only around 25 per cent of cases are known to healthcare services. Therefore, there is likely to be substantial underestimate of ID in the adult population as young people leave formal education. All mental illnesses may occur in patients with ID, and people with ID are more likely to experience mental ill health than those without ID.

Defining Intellectual Disability

Intelligence is commonly measured numerically as a full-scale 'intelligence quotient' (IQ). A full-scale IQ of 100 is the 'average' IQ in the general population. An IQ score of at least two standard deviations below the population mean represents a significant impairment of intellectual functioning. ID, commonly referred to as 'learning disability' in the United Kingdom, is defined as 'a condition of arrested or incomplete development of the mind, which is especially characterized by impairment of skills manifested during the developmental period, skills which contribute to the overall level of intelligence'.[4] The *Diagnostic and Statistical Manual* (DSM) 5th Edition has revised the term 'mental retardation' to 'ID', and the definition includes impairments in three domains: conceptual, social, and practical.[5] A further condition is that the disability must have manifested during the developmental period and must be associated with significant impairments in daily function, some aspects of which can be measured by psychometric testing. In clinical terms, ID may be described as mild (the person may not be easily identified as having an ID, may be a parent, maintain employment, and have good verbal skills); moderate (the person has higher level of need but may still be able to manage a few tasks independently such as dressing, snack preparation); severe (significantly impaired function and need for daily support, limited or no verbal ability), and profound (usually thought to perform below the age of a 12-month-old child). ID may occur secondary to a known cause, for example a genetic condition, perinatal difficulties or be due to socioeconomic adversity.[6] Recent research suggests that at least 11 per cent of cases with ID may be explained by genetic abnormalities.[7]

Mental and Physical Health in Intellectual Disability

The reported prevalence of mental ill health in persons with ID varies widely but it is found to be significantly higher when compared to the general population. Lower IQ score has been associated with increased risk for schizophrenia, severe depression, and other non-affective psychoses. In particular, poor mental health in persons with ID has been associated with female gender, more traumatic life events, the presence of severe physical disabilities or immobility, low education attainment, low social class, low income, and poor quality of relationships.[8,9] Physical illness and financial difficulty are also factors associated with lower IQ.[10] Finally, adults with ID of all causes, including Down syndrome, are at higher risk of developing dementia than the general population. The relative risk of having a diagnosis of dementia is between four to five times higher in people with ID.[11] Adults with ID have a reduced life expectancy and are more likely to die from preventable causes such as aspiration pneumonia or uncontrolled epilepsy.[12] The findings of the Confidential Inquiry into Premature Deaths of People with Learning Disabilities[13] showed that the average age of death of men with ID was 65 years and of women with ID was 63 years. This is 13 years younger than the figure for men in the general population and 20 years younger than women in the general population. There is a higher prevalence of physical health illnesses such as respiratory disease and epilepsy; increased rates of diabetes, osteoporosis, and chronic pain have also been reported.[14]

What Does a Psychiatrist in Intellectual Disability Do?

The key role of a psychiatrist in ID is to assess a person's mental state to diagnose mental ill health or review a change in mental state. We must consider all factors precipitating and maintaining change in mental health. This includes asking questions about physical health and enquiring specifically about vision, hearing, infections, presence of seizures, memory and movement disorders, all of which may affect mental state. Psychiatrists in ID work closely with GPs and may liaise with many other medical specialists when considering potential alternative or co-morbid diagnoses in their day-to-day clinical work.

It is important to consider psychological factors that might affect the patient such as recent life changes, trauma, and bereavement. A sound understanding of the patient's developmental trajectory, social circumstances, and environment are also important so home visits are common in our specialty.

In exploring treatment options, psychiatrists in ID, perhaps more than any other specialty, emphasize the importance of a 'bio-psycho-social' model. This considers biological, psychological, and social factors in mental ill health, and treatment approaches address all these factors. A role specific to the psychiatrist is to consider the need for pharmacological treatments for mental disorder, such as psychosis and depression. Regular reviews of the use of medication are conducted, noting side effects and interactions with other medications, monitoring therapeutic effects, and regularly considering risks and benefits of such treatment. The psychiatrist often works together with other professionals and treatments should be discussed and agreed with the patient and their family and paid carers.

Patients are most commonly supported with treatment in the community although at times a hospital admission may be needed. A community ID service may include community nurses, psychologists, occupational therapists, speech and language therapists, physiotherapists, dieticians, art, drama, or music therapists, as well as social workers. Health services may be integrated with social care services allowing the opportunity to work closely with social workers who provide input for decisions around access to daytime activities, skills training, accommodation, and finances. The psychiatrist formulates a broad management plan which involves a number of these other professionals.

All psychiatrists, but perhaps even more so psychiatrists in ID, must promote autonomy and patient-led decision making. This requires frequent assessments of the patient's 'mental capacity'. 'Mental capacity' is the ability to make decisions about aspects of care based on understanding information pertaining to that decision. If a patient is unable to demonstrate capacity to understand the relevant information on which to base specific decisions, the Mental Capacity Act 2005 requires that decisions are made on the basis of that person's best interests. A psychiatrist in ID also contributes to patient advocacy by promoting equal care, social inclusion, and equal access to resources such as universal physical and mental health services.

What Roles are There for Women in the Psychiatry of Intellectual Disability?

Clinical Leadership and Management

Psychiatrists in ID may develop specialist skills in clinical areas such as forensic psychiatry or management of epilepsy. Female doctors in all specialties commonly hold roles other than that as a clinician, and ID psychiatry is no exception. As a trainee, development of leadership and management skills is encouraged and doctors in training often undertake quality improvement projects in which they take initiative to identify and change specific aspects of a service, or of a patient's experience of the service, so that the service is improved. The consultant psychiatrist, who is an expert and has received certification of specialism, may also lead on service development. Consultants should work to involve service users and members of the wider multi-disciplinary team in service design and accessibility. Doctors engage in clinical audit to measure current standards of care and highlight areas for service improvement. Conducting an audit of current practice and performance allows for the development of mental and physical health services, and contributes to safe and high-quality care. One such recent audit evaluated the performance of 15 acute general health and mental health services in the United Kingdom delivering in-patient care to people with ID, and it identified multiple areas of in-patient care that could be improved to provide a safer, higher quality health service to patients with Learning Disability admitted to hospital.[15]

Research

Female researchers have been historically significant in the study of ID. For example, in the early 1900s, thousands of American women were employed as field workers to undertake 'family pedigree studies' and gather knowledge on the hereditary patterns of intelligence.[16]

There are several notable researchers in the field of ID but two in particular merit attention due to their important achievements in developing the field of the psychiatry of ID in the United Kingdom and internationally. Their work has also had tangible impact on the lives and care of people with ID. Professor Joan Bicknell (Figure 7.2), the United Kingdom's first Professor of the Psychiatry of Mental Handicap, as it was then known, was an early pioneer in the exploration of psychopathology in patients and families with ID and in the development of psychodynamic psychotherapy for those patients. Her paper 'The Psychopathology of Handicap', first published in 1983,[17] described the impact of ID upon the individual, their parents, and siblings. She noted that a catastrophic response to the diagnosis, and subsequent life events, may disrupt family cohesion and further impact upon the disabled family member. Professor Bicknell launched the first academic unit in the psychiatry of ID at St George's Hospital, in South London. A medical student essay competition is awarded in her honour by the Faculty of the Psychiatry of ID.

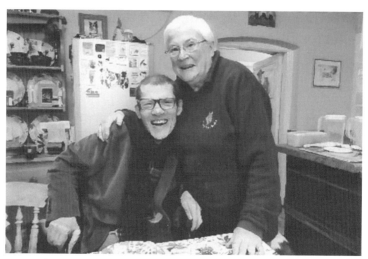

Figure 7.2 Professsor Bicknell at her home.
Reproduced with Permission from Joan Bicknell

Baroness Sheila Hollins (Figure 7.3), Emeritus Professor of Psychiatry of ID at St George's Medical School and cross-bench life peer of the House of Lords, is another formidable influence on the current generation of senior female psychiatrists (and several male ones who trained under her supervision) in ID. Baroness Professor Hollins

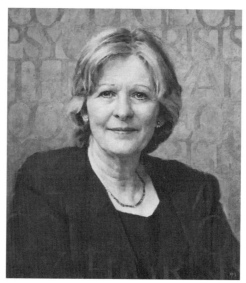

Figure 7.3 Professor Hollins' portrait, Royal College of Psychiatry.
© Keith Breeden

was President of the Royal College of Psychiatrists from 2005 to 2008 and previously Chair of the Faculty of the Psychiatry of ID at the Royal College of Psychiatrists. She is the creator and chair of *Books Beyond Words* (Figure 7.4), a series of picture books aimed at facilitating communication between patients with ID and their carers or professionals. Baroness Hollins considered her major achievements as Faculty Chair to have been elevating the 'section of Psychiatry of ID' to 'Faculty' and the change of its name and function from 'mental handicap' to 'Psychiatry of Learning Disability', emphasizing the mental health aspects of learning disability and also adopting a term which is accepted by users, carers, and other professional groups. She said: 'I guess I was seen as a modernizer'.[18]

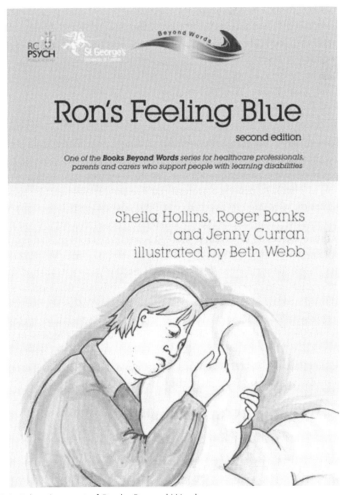

Figure 7.4 Advertisement of Books Beyond Words.
Reproduced from Hollins S, Banks R, Curran J [Authors], Webb B [Illustrator], Ron's Feeling Blue, Second Edition, Copyright (2011), with permission from *Books Beyond Words*.

Human Rights

The World Health Organization has identified disability to be a human rights issue due to the inequalities attributable to disabilities, including reduced access to healthcare. Psychiatrists in ID, alongside other professionals, often advocate on behalf of their patients and seek to address barriers to healthcare including *reasonable adjustments* to reduce discrimination faced in accessing services. Reasonable adjustments may include booking appointments of longer duration and offering 'easy-to-read' information that is presented in an accessible format.

Teaching and Training

The role of a doctor comes with an expectation that one will also engage in teaching duties, most commonly in education for medical students and junior medical colleagues. Additionally, psychiatrists in ID may lead in designing and implementing educational sessions to paid carers and family members. Several psychiatrists in ID choose to take on educator roles in shaping training curricula, managing changes in workforce, and building the skills of the doctors in training as supervisors and examiners.

Academic Careers

A survey by Killaspy and colleagues based on academic and NHS psychiatry posts of all specialties in 2001[19] demonstrated, disappointingly, that males were significantly more likely than females to have an academic rather than NHS post in psychiatry. Men occupied 80 per cent of all academic psychiatry posts, and within those posts women were less likely to occupy a professorial position. It was heartening to see that the representation of women in psychiatry of ID academic posts in London was more equal to that of men. However, due to the small numbers of this survey it is difficult to generalize this occurrence to psychiatry of ID academia across the United Kingdom or indeed globally.

The Equality Challenge Unit's Athena Swan Charter[20] was established in 2005 to address difficulties in the recruitment and retention of female academics, and to encourage commitment to advancing the careers of women in areas such as science and medicine, employment in higher education, and research. Members of the Charter commit to gender equality within their institution and the advancement of gender equality in academia, including the promotion of equal gender representation across academic disciplines and leadership positions, tackling the gender pay gap, and provision of a non-discriminatory working environment for all staff.

Future Developments in the Psychiatry of Intellectual Disability

The psychiatry of ID is a dynamic field populated by determined practitioners who are committed to enhancing research, improving teaching and training experience, and bringing high-quality care to ordinary practice. There are many areas of promising research within biomedicine, health services, and social care. In the last three years, two National Institute for Health and Care Excellence (NICE) guidelines have been developed to close the variation in service provision across England. One of these guidelines focuses on behaviour that challenges, a significant issue in the field of ID that has adverse consequences for the person and their families;[21] the second addresses mental health issues.[22]

Studies are not limited to researching new treatments for mental ill health but can also include assessing existing prescribing patterns, such as the review of the efficacy and safety of current clinical practice such as the prescription of antipsychotic medication for the management of behaviour that challenges.[23]

Caring for a Person with Intellectual Disability

A UK census has established that there are approximately 6.5 million carers of people with a variety of chronic and terminal conditions in the United Kingdom. It is estimated that the unpaid care they provide is worth £119 billion each year.[24] The Survey of Adult Carers in England (NHS Digital, 2012–13) found that 48 per cent of carers of an adult with ID spend 100 or more hours a week caring for that person, and 29 per cent of adult carers were not in paid employment because of their caring responsibilities. It is important to recognize the contribution of women, especially mothers, in this area. Women are more likely to be carers; 58 per cent of carers are female, and women are more likely to leave paid employment to provide care.[25,26]

Case Study

Sue is a mother of an adult with ID. Neil was born at full-term following a normal pregnancy. It became apparent that his development, including speech, language, and walking skills, was delayed from the age of six months. Sue attends to all household tasks and helps Neil with his self-care. Neil has epilepsy and diabetes, and Sue supports him to take his medication and attend medical and dental appointments.

Eighty-two per cent of carers who responded to the 2015 State of Caring Survey by Carers UK reported that caring had a negative impact on their health. Sue has severe osteoarthritis in her hips, hands, and knees.

Neil does not have the mental capacity to make choices and to communicate these choices. As such, Sue is his advocate and his voice. She has no immediate family nearby and only a small circle of neighbours and friends. Without this network she is especially isolated; she informs me 'people are nice, but they keep their distance'. Sue worked as a clinical psychologist and initially reduced her working hours before leaving her career altogether to care for Neil following the death of Neil's grandfather, who previously undertook a caring role. She noted that as a child Neil had many assessments and more support. He enjoyed attending a school for children with special educational needs, and later a college course. It is a shame that the service cuts and closures that Neil has experienced as an adult seem to be so common. The closure of Neil's day centre has resulted in loss of contact with his social group and loss of a safe, appropriate space to join in indoor leisure activities and develop new skills. Neil now goes out in the day with a single support worker and there has been a noticeable change in his everyday social interactions. He is more reserved, and at home is more restless and difficult to engage in activities. Sadly, a 2016 Mencap survey of young adults with ID revealed that

44.6 per cent of those surveyed do not think they spend enough time with friends and 17.8 per cent feel alone and cut off from other people.

Day services also provide a vital form of daily respite for carers. Mencap's Breaking Point Survey of families caring for persons with ID found 70 per cent of families reported reaching or coming close to 'breaking point' due to lack of respite services. Sue has not had a carer's break for over two years but has used local respite services when attending her own hospital appointments. The planned closure of this local short-stay service, an essential resource for carers and patients for many years, will undoubtedly affect the well-being of both Sue and Neil; with the support of Mencap she spends her few moments of free time writing letters and campaigning to prevent such closures.

> *I enjoyed my job as a Psychologist but I couldn't continue in employment whilst also acting as a carer. Caring for Neil is a full-time job, which I largely had to learn through trial and error. Being a full-time carer has certainly affected my own physical health and I rarely have any time to myself. But he is my son of course and he deserves the same life, love, support and rights as my other son who doesn't have learning disabilities. And I will continue to fight for his access to day services and respite services, even though I often feel I am fighting alone.*

Being a Mother with Intellectual Disability

There are approximately 375,000 adult women with ID in the UK[27] and it is important to highlight the challenges they face. Employment of people with ID is very low nationally with approximately 6 per cent in paid employment.[3] Men with ID were more likely to be in paid employment or self-employment than women with ID, and were more likely to be working over 30 hours per week than women.

Fortunately, it is increasingly recognized that women with ID have the same right to engage in relationships and be mothers as women without ID. The exact number of parents with intellectual disability is unknown, however it is estimated to be 1 in 15 adults with ID.[28] Approximately 40 per cent of parents in the National Survey of Adults with Learning Disabilities in England were not living with their children; some of these may reflect cases where the child has grown up and left home, however more commonly this is a result of the child being removed from the care of their parent. 'Valuing People Now'[29] highlighted the need to better support parents with ID so that they might benefit from the same mainstream information and initiatives available to parents without ID. Like many other mothers with ID, Jackie and Jill, report negative experiences with health and social care services.

> *I knew that you had to get pregnant but I didn't really know/understand what pregnancy involved. It was scary not knowing what was going to happen, I was in pain. I never really said much to them that I had a real learning disability because I was frightened what they might do*
>
> Jackie, mother of two

> *They said 'do you have someone that can come along with you, so we can talk to them and not talk to you?' We had to go to lots of meetings because they didn't think we understood how to bring the children up ... society thinks we can't cope. They were trying to teach us like children, as children having children rather than adults having children.*
>
> Jill, mother of four

Guidance for good practice when working with parents with ID[30] states that the specific needs of this group require particular knowledge and skills from professionals working with them so that an equitable service can be provided to parents with ID and their children. The aim should be to improve the well-being of the child and to provide the support required to enable children to live with their parents as long as this is consistent with the child's welfare.

Psychiatry of ID as a Career

Core psychiatry training is at least three years in duration and this training may include six months' experience with an intellectual disability service. Trainees must pass clinical examinations to become a Member of the Royal College of Psychiatrists (MRCPsych) and to enter higher training in the psychiatry of ID. The duration of higher training is at least three years and involves practice in community and in-patient settings. With respect to the quality of training in the specialty, the higher training scheme is noted to be well-managed and well-delivered, according to the General Medical Council (GMC).[31] There are many opportunities for gaining additional expertise and obtaining specific skills through competitive application to out-of-programme experience (OOPE). Trainees interested in research may also apply for PhD fellowships funded by either the National Institute for Health Research or Research Councils and/or charities.

As a woman, it would be wrong to shy away from discussing the chance offered by this career to maintain flexible working hours on completion of training. The Royal College of Psychiatrists supports flexible working arrangements for carers during training.

Like many aspiring doctors, I applied to medical school with a passion 'to help people and make a difference'. I was fortunate to volunteer with a befriending service for young persons with physical and intellectual disabilities, and this improved my confidence and understanding of the skills required to work in medicine. As a core psychiatry trainee, my six-month placement with a London psychiatry of intellectual disability team allowed me to realize that even within a busy inner-city NHS service, the specialty is one in which lasting relationships are made with patients and carers. The psychiatry of ID offers a holistic care plan and the opportunity to work with a skilled multi-disciplinary team to facilitate improvements in both mental and physical health.

The psychiatry of ID is a fascinating specialty in which women hold a number of rewarding roles as clinicians, leaders, educators, and researchers. In addition to sharing the notable achievements that can be held by female doctors specializing in the field, this chapter has also highlighted the incredibly important role of the women that we meet and work in partnership with every day; female carers striving to meet the challenges in caring for persons with ID and mothers with ID who face stigma and disparity of care in the service they receive.

Further information about the specialty, and useful resources for professionals, carers and patients, can be found on the Royal College of Psychiatrists website:

<http://www.rcpsych.ac.uk/workinpsychiatry/faculties/intellectualdisability.aspx>.

References

1. **NHS Digital** (2016). NHS Hospital & Community Health Service (HCHS) monthly workforce statistics—Provisional Statistics: HCHS Doctors by Grade and Specialty—Full Time Equivalent. <https://data.gov.uk/dataset/nhs-hospital-and-community-health-doctors-by-grade-and-specialty>.

2. **Maulik PK1, Mascarenhas MN, Mathers CD, Dua T,** and **Saxena S** (2011). Prevalence of intellectual disability: a meta-analysis of population-based studies. *Research in Developmental Disabilities* **32**:419–36.

3. **Public Health England** (2015). People with Learning Disabilities in England 2015: Main report. <https://www.gov.uk/government/publications/people-with-learning-disabilities-in-england-2015>.

4. **World Health Organization** (1996). The ICD–10 Classification of Mental and Behavioural Disorders: Diagnostic Criteria for Research. Geneva: World Health Organization.

5. **American Psychiatric Association** (2014). *Diagnostic and Statistical Manual*, 5th edn. <https://www.psychiatry.org/psychiatrists/practice/dsm>.

6. **Emerson E** and **Hatton C** (2007). Mental health of children and adolescents with intellectual disabilities in Britain. *British Journal of Psychiatry* **191**:493–9.

7. **Wolfe K, Strydom A, Morrogh D, Carter J, Cutajar P, Eyeoyibo M, Hassiotis A, McCarthy J, Mukherjee R, Paschos D, Perumal N, Read S, Shankar R, Sharif S, Thirulokachandran S, Thygesen JH, Patch C, Ogilvie C, Flinter F, McQuillin A,** and **Bass N** (2016). Chromosomal microarray testing in adults with ID presenting with comorbid psychiatric disorders. *European Journal of Human Genetics* (advance online publication). DOI:10.1038/ejhg.2016.107

8. **Cooper S-A, Smiley E, Finlayson J, Jackson A, Allan L, Williamson A, Mantry D,** and **Morrison J** (2007). The prevalence, incidence, and factors predictive of mental ill-health in adults with profound intellectual disabilities. *Journal of Applied Research on Intellectual Disabilities* DOI:10.1111/j.1468-3148.2007.00401.x.

9. **Rajput S, Hassiotis A, Richards M, Hatcha SL,** and **Stewart R** (2011). Associations between IQ and common mental disorders: The 2000 British National Survey of Psychiatric Morbidity. *European Psychiatry* **26**, 390–5.

10. **Meltzer H, Brugha T, Dennis MS, Hassiotis A, Jenkins R, McManus S, Rai D,** and **Bebbington P** (2012). The influence of disability on suicidal behaviour. *Alter European Journal of Disability Research* **6**:1–12.

11. **Strydom A, Shooshtari S, Lee L, Raykar V, Torr J, Tsiouris J, Jokinen N, Courtenay K, Bass N, Sinnema M,** and **Maaskant M** (2010). Dementia in older adults with intellectual disabilities—epidemiology, presentation, and diagnosis. *Journal of Policy and Practice in Intellectual Disabilities* **7**(2):96–110.

12. **Glover G** and **Ayub M** (2010). How People with Learning Disabilities Die. Durham: Improving Health and Lives: Learning Disabilities Observatory, England. <http://webarchive.nationalarchives.gov.uk/20160704181356/https://www.improvinghealthandlives.org.uk/uploads/doc/vid_9033_IHAL2010-06%20Mortality.pdf>.

13. **CIPOLD (Confidential Inquiry into Premature Deaths of People with Learning Disabilities)** (2013). <http://www.bristol.ac.uk/media-library/sites/cipold/migrated/documents/fullfinalreport.pdf>.

14. **Emerson E, Baines S, Allerton L,** and **Welch V** (2012). Health inequalities and people with learning disability in the UK. Durham: Improving Health and Lives: Learning Disability Observatory. <http://www.complexneeds.org.uk/modules/Module-4.1-Working-with-other-professionals/All/downloads/m13p020c/emerson_baines_health_inequalities.pdf>.

15. **Sheehan R, Gandesha A, Hassiotis A, Gallagher P, Burnell M, Jones G, Kerr M, Hall I, Chaplin R, Crawford MJ** (2016). An audit of the quality of inpatient care for adults with learning disability in the UK. *British Medical Journal Open* 6. DOI:10.1136/bmjopen-2015-010480.

16. **Carlson L** (2009). *The Faces of ID: Philosophical Reflections*. Bloomington, IN: Indiana University Press.

17. **Bicknell J** (1983). The psychopathology of handicap. *British Journal of Medical Psychology* **56**:167–78.

18. Faculty of the Psychiatry of ID (2011). Newsletter. <http://www.rcpsych.ac.uk/pdf/LDNewsletterMarch%202011_forwebsite.pdf>.

19. **Killaspy H, Johnson S, Livingston, G, Hassiotis A,** and **Robertson M** (2003). Women in academic psychiatry in the United Kingdom. *Psychiatric Bulletin* **27**:323–6.

20. **Athena Swan**. <http://www.ecu.ac.uk/equality-charters/athena-swan/>.

21. **National Institute of Health and Care Excellence** (2015). Challenging behaviour and learning disabilities: prevention and interventions for people with learning disabilities whose behaviour challenges. London: NICE.

22. **National Institute of Health and Care Excellence** (2016). Mental health problems in people with learning disabilities: prevention, assessment and management. London: NICE. <https://www.nice.org.uk/guidance/ng54>.

23. **Sheehan R, Hassiotis A, Walters K, Osborn D, Strydom A,** and **Horsfall L** (2015). Mental illness, challenging behaviour, and psychotropic drug prescribing in people with ID: UK population-based cohort study. *British Medical Journal* **351**:h4326.

24. **CIRCLE (Centre for International Research on Care, Labour and Equalities)** (2011). Valuing Carers 2011: Calculating the value of carers' support. <https://www.carersuk.org/about-us/36-for-professionals/policy-eng/report/5021-valuing-carers-2011-calculating-the-value-of-carers-support>.

25. **Carers UK** (2014). <https://www.carersuk.org/for-professionals/policy/policy-library/facts-about-carers-2014>.

26. **Carers UK** (2014). <https://www.carersuk.org/for-professionals/policy/policy-library/caring-family-finances-inquiry>.

27. Improving Health and Lives. <https://www.ndti.org.uk/our-work/our-projects/peoples-health/improving-health-and-lives-ihal>.

28. **Department of Health** (2005). Survey of adults with learning difficulties in England 2003/4: Final and summary reports. <http://webarchive.nationalarchives.gov.uk/20130107105354/ http://www.dh.gov.uk/en/Publicationsandstatistics/PublishedSurvey/ListOfSurveySince1990/Generalsurveys/DH_4081207>.

29. **Department of Health** (2009). Valuing People Now: A new three-year strategy for people with learning disabilities. <http://webarchive.nationalarchives.gov.uk/20130107105354/http://www.dh.gov.uk/prod_consum_dh/groups/dh_digitalassets/documents/digitalasset/dh_093375.pdf>.

30. **Department of Education and Skills and Department of Health** (2007). Good practice guidance on working with parents with a learning disability. <https://www.bristol.ac.uk/media-library/sites/sps/documents/wtpn/2016%20WTPN%20UPDATE%20OF%20THE%20GPG%20-%20finalised%20with%20cover.pdf>.

31. **GMC** (2014). GMC 2014 Report. <http://www.gmc-uk.org/PLD_report_FINAL.pdf_62652898.pdf>.

Helen Green Allison (1923–2011)
A Story of Hope, Faith, and Charity
Jane Mounty

Life

Helen Green was born in Princeton, New Jersey, on 7 February 1923. Her father was Joseph Coy Green and mother Susannah Miles Kinsey Green. Unfortunately, her mother died six days after the birth from puerperal sepsis. Joseph had served in the US State Department for many years. He remarried in 1927 and later became US Ambassador to Jordan between 1952 and 1953. It was during this sojourn in Amman that Helen married Tony Allison, a medical graduate from Oxford.

Earlier, at Vassar, an Ivy League College at that time admitting only women, Helen majored in history and was invited to become a member of the Phi-Beta-Kappa Society (an academic honour society) in her junior year, a rare distinction. As a young graduate Helen served in the Overseas Special Service (OSS, predecessor of the CIA), attached to the US Embassy in Cairo in Egypt, and Athens in Greece. She then attended the School for Advanced International Studies (SAIS), a branch of Johns Hopkins University, in Washington DC. She learned that the near-Eastern oil-producing countries were strategically important so she decided to study Arabic and Persian. In 1950 Helen obtained a Fulbright Fellowship to read Arabic and Persian languages, literature, and history for three years at Oxford University. For the first year she lived in college, Lady Margaret Hall (LMH), and then moved into a small apartment in north Oxford, where she met her future husband, Tony, when passing on the stairs. Helen was the only candidate to obtain a First-Class Honours degree in these subjects.

In 1958, while living in the London Borough of Mill Hill, Helen realized that her son Joe was not achieving developmental milestones (Figure P4.1).

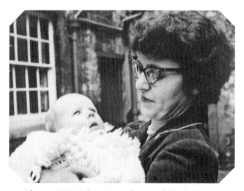

Figure P4.1 Helen Green Allison with her baby Joe.

He was agitated and avoided eye contact. Child psychiatrists deemed him 'mute and hyperactive' and thus not capable of being educated. She suspected autism and an American friend gave her an article describing a group of parents of autistic children who had bought a house in Long Island in New York. Together the parents renovated the house, decorating it, making curtains, and buying second-hand furniture. They hired teachers and soon after many autistic children 'came out of their attics' and went to school for the very first time.

Career

Hope: This spawned the idea of setting up a Society for Autistic Children (SAC) in the United Kingdom. The first step was to get national recognition for the plight of autistic children and their families. Helen lobbied the BBC and eventually appeared on Woman's Hour, on the then Home Service radio in November 1961. This broadcast led to a flood of letters from parents. She kept a record of all correspondence with a view to the later establishment of local branches and schools.

The next step was the meeting of a group of parents in north London. Initially, the group was set up in 1962 under the auspices of the National Society for Mentally Handicapped Children. Eventually a constitution was established with a number of officers elected. Helen was initially Honorary Secretary and later General Secretary when the premises for SAC was established in the garden room of 100 Wise Lane, Mill Hill, where Helen, Tony, and their two boys lived. The SAC phone used to ring day and night.

Also in 1962, a parent introduced her to Sybil Elgar, a Montessori-trained teacher who was running a small nursery for 'maladjusted and backward' children in her basement in St John's Wood. By this time, the situation with Joe was desperate: he was causing havoc at home and the family lived with locked doors, stained walls and ceilings, broken windows and furniture, and interrupted nights and days. She said to Sybil: 'Please take Joe; if you can handle him, you can handle anyone'.

Helen left the National Society for Autistic Children (renamed in 1962)[1] in 1968, and took up a part-time role as an administrator at the head office of the UK Medical Research Council. There she learned how to cope with British bureaucracy, another valuable lesson. In that year Sybil Elgar established the first school for autistic children in north London, at which Joe was a weekly boarder. Helen knew Wendy Landman from her days in Oxford and persuaded Wendy to become the inaugural principal of the second school for autistic children in Gravesend in Kent (Figure P4.2).[2]

This school was later named the Helen Allison School, and was officially opened by Harold Wilson, then leader of the Labour opposition party at the time, in 1973. Similar societies and schools, mostly based on the British model, were established in France, the United States, and other countries.

Faced with bringing up an autistic child, Helen cherished Joe all the more and worked tirelessly with Sybil Elgar and others to improve his schooling and, later, his residential care. Helen, Sybil, and a group of parents of autistic children set up Somerset Court in 1974 as the first autistic young adult community in the United Kingdom. She continued to contribute to the work of the Society[3] and in retirement researched the effects of bereavement in autistic adults.[4] She was secretary to the Somerset Court parents group, minute-taker, and typist extraordinaire. Sybil and Helen both received MBEs (Member of the Order of the British Empire) for their achievements. (Figure P4.3).

In mid-life, Helen had been able to turn a personal tragedy into a career that was to influence the welfare of hundreds of thousands of children and their families in many countries.

Faith: Helen had been brought up in the Episcopalian faith, the US counterpart of the Church of England. Throughout her adult life she read and thought about religion deeply and was influenced by the books of the theologian Reinhold Niebuhr and others. Helen later recognized that meetings of the Society of Friends (Quakers) had

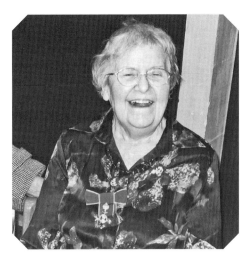

Figure P4.3 Helen Green Allison on the day she was awarded her MBE.

the combination of spiritual uplift and lack of ceremony that most appealed to her. She regularly attended Sunday meetings of the Society of Friends in Finchley, north-west London, with several members who had become friends and were so until the time of her death. Her religious faith sustained her while her bodily and mental functions were slowly declining.

Charity: With Joe at Somerset Court and brother Miles settled near Newport in Wales, Helen decided to move from London to an apartment in a Friends' Retirement community near Bath in Somerset. She had long since separated from her husband. Helen died aged 88 on 26 December 2011, just months before the National Autistic Society celebrated its 50th anniversary. By then the Charity had six schools across the country, managing well over 1,000 adults with autism through supported living and residential services and providing many more families, individuals, and professionals with support, information, and advice.

Favourite Quotations about Helen

- 'Helen could walk with aristocrats while retaining the common touch.' Tony Allison
- 'Helen fought bureaucracy strongly, like a tigress, and persistently, with a low profile that did not antagonize but eventually produced desired results.' Tony Allison
- 'Helen ... deserves enormous credit for her determination ... to obtain help, support, recognition of the existence of autism and understanding for

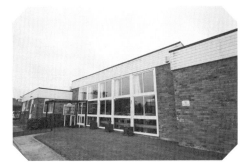

Figure P4.2 The Helen Allison School in Kent.
© The National Autistic Society

Continued on next page

the problems faced by those with autistic children. Autism was then a little known and misrepresented handicap. Many of us have benefited from her work. Helen should not be forgotten.' Lord Christopher Wakehurst

- 'Helen's initial aspirations of getting the right education for children with autism and securing an environment in which adults with autism can flourish and fulfil their potential, remains the vision of the NAS today.' Mark Lever, President NAS.

Acknowledgments

Dr Miles Allison, Consultant Gastroenterologist

Notes

1. For more information, see National Autistic Society (NAS) website: <http://www.autism.org.uk>.

2. Helen Allison School. See <http://www.autism.org.uk/>.

3. Allison, HG (1988). Perspectives on a puzzle piece. *Communication* 22:6–9. See also McGuire A (2012). The puzzle of autism. *Journal on Developmental Disabilities* 18(1): 96–100.

4. *Staff in Services for Adults on the Autism Spectrum*. London: The National Autistic Society, 2001. An updated version of Helen Green Allison's seminal book about how to deal with bereavement and grief for those with autism, including Asperger syndrome (2013) is available from the National Autistic Society website, <http://www.autism.org.uk>, NAS code 432.

Chapter 8

Are Women's Mental Health Units Needed?

Aoife Rajyaluxmi Singh

Introduction

In the United Kingdom, patients with psychiatric illness are admitted for acute in-patient care 'when a person's illness cannot be managed in the community, and where the situation is so severe that specialist care is required in a safe and therapeutic space'.[1] However this is different from the initial structure of psychiatric services in the nineteenth and early twentieth century where asylums provided the majority of care for all patients with psychiatric illness. Within the asylums, women and men patients were strictly segregated from one another and usually treated by nurses and attendants of the same sex. The 1970s heralded the start of significant changes in psychiatric care with a shift to treating more patients in the community. This was a response to various factors including the realization that patients should have the right to receive treatment in the least restrictive environment possible, advances in antipsychotic drugs, and the high costs associated with in-patient mental health care.[2] Subsequently, many asylums were closed, women and men began to be admitted to the same psychiatric wards,[3] and mixed-sex wards became part of normal practice and were generally viewed as therapeutic and progressive.[4] A national audit in 1995 of 263 adult acute admission wards and 33 adult intensive care wards in mental health units across England and Wales found that 94 per cent of the wards were mixed, 65 per cent of women patients did not have access to women-only sleeping areas, and 33 per cent had access only to bathrooms used by both male and female patients.[5]

It was not until the 1990s that changes in policy led once again to a move to segregating wards based on sex. In 1997 the government set the wider National Health Service (NHS) the goal of eliminating mixed-sex hospital accommodation, with a target of 95 per cent of Health Authority areas being compliant by the year 2002 in response to concerns about patient privacy, dignity, and safety.[6] Subsequently the Department of Health has set very clear guidelines regarding the provision of same-sex accommodation in both mental health hospitals and general hospitals, except under exceptional circumstances.[7] Breaches of this policy must be reported monthly by NHS Trusts and additionally these are also identified during routine Care Quality Commission (CQC) inspections. For mental health units, provision must include completely segregated sleeping and bathroom units and women's-only lounge areas. Trans people have equal rights to access single-sex wards and should be admitted to a ward in accordance with their preferred gender with the only exceptions in specific circumstances where there is genuine and necessary need. Professionals have a duty to ensure a trans person's dignity and privacy is maintained during their admission.[8]

A Community and a Hospital In-Patient Unit for Women

Here are descriptions of two very different Women's Mental Health Units (WMHUs): a community ward and a hospital ward both providing care for women only.

The community WMHU is an eight-bed crisis house which opened in 1999 aiming to provide holistic care to women requiring psychiatric admission. Early discussions involved service users and local organizations.[9] The aims were to provide women with mental illnesses a specific service in which therapeutic functions, policies, and day-to-day activities were designed and based on what women said worked and did not work for them.[10] This WMHU is set in a 1920s detached house in a residential area and from the outside it appears very much like any other house on the street. Inside it is designed to be homely, with patients having their own individual rooms, communal areas which are inviting and comfortable, a kitchen that is accessible to everyone, food cooked by staff daily and space for everyone to sit and eat together. There is a well-maintained garden with seating areas for quiet reflection. In response to women's feedback there is no clinic room and hence no queue of patients during dispensing times. This unit is staffed 24 hours a day by an all-female team of nurses and healthcare assistants. It is a nurse-led service with male and female doctors visiting twice per week. Women in need of psychiatric in-patient treatment but not in need of formal detention for assessment or treatment under the Mental Health Act 1983 (MHA) can be admitted directly from their homes or transferred from hospital wards. The majority of patients have diagnoses of mood and/or personality disorders which includes complex trauma. Available evidence suggests that this type of community WMHU may be as effective as a traditional psychiatric ward in treating women presenting with acute psychiatric problems and does not have an adverse impact on resource use.[11,12]

The hospital WMHU was established as a female-only ward in 2009. It has 20 beds, is a locked ward, and has male and female nursing and medical staff. Women have their own individual rooms but with peep holes in their doors so staff can observe and enter if clinically indicated. The multi-professional team includes sessions from an occupational therapist and a clinical psychologist. Garden space specifically for this unit is minimal but as patients recover they can use the extensive hospital gardens. The main reasons for admission are psychotic or manic illnesses.

Women's Experiences of Community and Hospital WMHUs

A key difference in the experience of women patients in these two units was with regards to consent. All women admitted to our community WMHU were able to grant consent and did so in order to be admitted and treated there. In contrast, most women admitted to the hospital unit were admitted formally under sections of the MHA, often against their expressed wishes, reflecting the degree and nature of their illnesses at the time of admission, and particularly the nature of risks to themselves or others. This meant that women on the hospital WMHU were usually very keen to be discharged

Box 8.1 Example Case History 1

A 40-year-old woman was admitted with a relapse in her schizo-affective illness. She was disinhibited towards male staff, particularly towards one male doctor to whom she presented love notes in the shape of roses, stating that they were married. She was overfamiliar in her body language and verbal communication. The staff team understood that this was a delusion and part of her mental illness. When she recovered and regained insight she was embarrassed about her behaviour. Staff reassured her that no-one had been offended, her presentation had been a symptom of her illness, and had resolved with appropriate treatment.

from the outset and often felt that their admission was unwarranted. Despite this, many women who had previously been admitted to the hospital WMHU under the MHA had a preference to be directly re-admitted there when they were again detained, instead of to a mixed triage ward as per the usual admission pathway. There was a sense from these women that sharing a therapeutic space with men who were unwell felt intimidating and frightening. The hospital WMHU is not a women-only environment and it was noticeable that for some women the presence of male staff could also be frightening. Sometimes women experiencing psychotic episodes developed beliefs that male staff were following them and entering their rooms with intention of harming or sexually assaulting them. Some patients were sexually disinhibited towards male staff; this behaviour would make them vulnerable on mixed wards (see Box 8.1).

In the community WMHU, the environment was largely experienced as a genuinely supportive place and the point of discharge could often be distressing (See Box 8.2). Women on this unit had made capacitous and informed choices to be admitted for treatment.

Box 8.2 Example Case History 2

A 42-year-old woman with a diagnosis of bipolar affective disorder was interviewed post-discharge from our community WMHU. Her admission was initially precipitated by the acute emotional reaction she experienced following the murder of a family member. She described how since discharge she often thought about the Unit and wished that it was in fact her home. It made her feel safe, cared for, and gave her the psychological space to reflect. She started to think about going back to college, something she had not thought about for many years. When she was discharged she went back to her own home setting where her mental state was stable, but she felt overwhelmed by difficulties with her family, finances, and housing. Our community WMHU was able to work with her community team to offer longer-term treatment.

Anecdotally, women in both these settings identified that they provided an important forum where they could discuss shared aspects of their lives with other women, such as poverty, racism, interpersonal violence, and their roles as mothers and partners. The need for female patients to share their experiences with other women has also been highlighted in the work by Cutting and Henderson[10] with one of the main themes identified in their qualitative work being 'a woman in a man's world'. However, particularly on the hospital WMHU, where most women were largely confined to the unit, interactions between women could also be a source of real difficulty. Evidence from non-clinical settings indicates that women may engage more often than men in relational aggression,[13,14] using relationships as the vehicle of harm, and at times women would form cliques, excluding or ignoring others, which would lead to emotionally charged interactions and sometimes violence.

Staff Experiences of Community and Hospital WMHUs

One of the most striking aspects of working in the hospital WMHU was the response of other mental health professionals. Many remarked sympathetically how difficult it must be to work in a WMHU and nursing staff who had previous experience of working on both female- and male-only wards highlighted that 'women are very difficult to manage when they are ill'.

Our experience is that there may be more challenges in interactions, particularly in the context of women who are acutely unwell and, as the evidence highlights, have experienced high rates of abuse and trauma compared to the general population.[15,16] These experiences may lead to interpersonal interactions in which women have intense feelings of abandonment and rejection, evoking primitive psychological defence mechanisms which can leave staff feeling attacked and vulnerable. The difficulty that the hospital WMHU staff expressed is that, given the pressures of managing acutely disturbed behaviour and staff shortages, it was difficult to provide the consistency that is often required to help these women feel contained and safe. This is ameliorated to a degree by the fact that some women have been admitted multiple times over the years or have lengthy admissions and therefore a trusting relationship with staff can develop (see Box 8.3). Given the high rates of abuse that women have experienced in the

---

Box 8.3 Example Case History 3

A 65-year-old woman with a diagnosis of paranoid schizophrenia and stable after a lengthy admission to our hospital WMHU was keen to be discharged. Despite complying well with her prescribed medications and follow-up care plan, she rapidly developed persecutory delusions about staff at her new residence. This culminated in her sleeping on the streets for a week. She was re-admitted to the hospital WMHU where these symptoms rapidly resolved and she felt safe again. This time a more gradual discharge to her new home was implemented, with time taken to introduce her to her new environment, neighbours, and residence staff.

general population[17,18,19] there must also be some consideration regarding women staff, what experiences they may have had, and how best they can be supported in providing this essential role in nursing women who are mentally unwell.

The staff in the community WMHU faced different challenges. Because all the patients are informally admitted, those with high levels of risk, usually in the form of suicidality and thoughts of self-harm, are managed in a non-coercive framework and staff tolerate higher levels of uncertainty compared to those faced in a locked in-patient unit. Staff in the community unit found that some stressful aspects of their roles were ameliorated by the clinical reflection and supervision built in to the culture of the unit, including weekly support group from a psychoanalytic therapist, debriefs at the end of shifts, and supervision by the team manager/senior nurses. Despite the fact that all the women had access to a kitchen and could come and go as they wished, the actual incidents of self-harm within the community WMHU were minimal. There was a view expressed by women that they did not feel impelled to self-harm whilst in the unit and that there was sense of mutual and genuine trust between both the women admitted there and the staff.

The Evidence for WMHUs

Although government policy has been explicit about the need for WMHUs, within the literature the evidence is not so clear.

First, the research into the preference of women patients for admission either to a mixed-sex or women-only unit has shown mixed results. Women's preferences for single-sex accommodation in acute psychiatry were shown by Leavey and colleagues,[20] and likewise in the study of Johnson and colleagues.[21] However, Cleary and Warren[22] found that although some women had experienced problems with safety in a mixed-sex psychiatric ward, the majority preferred this setting to a single-sex setting. Similarly Thomas and colleagues[23] and Mezey and co-workers[24] found that women overall would prefer to be on a mixed-sex ward. A key advantage of mixed-sex wards highlighted by women in these studies was that they felt the wards were more beneficial therapeutically, and they felt more balanced in them, that the wards were more social and were a truer representation of the outside world.[20,23]

Second, one of the main arguments for single-sex psychiatry wards was to protect women from harm from male patients. Although women may feel sexually threatened by male patients, they can still face physical and verbal violence from other women,[20,25] and a recent study highlighted that single-sex wards may not offer significant protection to potentially vulnerable victims.[26]

Finally, it has been highlighted that segregating wards based on sex is not enough in providing women-specific care. A report into Ashworth Hospital[27] highlighted major failings in the women-only in-patient personality disorder service. Concerns included women having accommodation considerably inferior to the accommodation for men, a considerable proportion of the nursing staff working on the women's wards not being trained specifically in mental illness nursing, and that medication was inappropriately used to sedate women. This is an extreme example in an organization that was failing in many areas but it highlights that women may receive sub-standard care in settings which nominally fit the notion of a WMHU.

The Challenges to Providing WMHUs

The question arises, therefore, whether women need specific mental health units and if so, what is essential to meet their needs? Finding answers to these questions is hampered by the fact that there is a lack of data comparing clinical outcomes, patient experiences, and cost effectiveness of mixed units to WMHU, and that generally most research within mental health largely ignores gender differences, potentially contributing to a failure to provide gender-sensitive mental health treatments and services.[28]

Safety was an important driving force in the policy shift to eliminate mixed-sex accommodation and provide WMHUs. However, physical aggression and violence are realities on both mixed-sex and WMHUs. The National Audit of Violence found that a third of in-patients had been threatened or made to feel unsafe while admitted.[29] Protecting women from violence and providing a therapeutic space therefore requires a consideration of the physical environment and staffing as overcrowding on wards,[30] increased use of bank staff, the ward layout, and lack of staff experience all contribute to this risk and it cannot be ameliorated just by segregating hospital wards by gender. Addressing these issues is complicated by the fact that most wards were commissioned and designed before current understanding of the impact of the physical environment on person-centred approaches to health, safety, privacy, and dignity,[31] and the considerable stress that in-patient psychiatric services in the United Kingdom are currently under. A recent report[32] on in-patient care highlighted that there has been a 39 per cent reduction in the number of in-patient psychiatric beds in England between 1998 and 2012, more than half of general adult in-patient wards are running at greater than 100 per cent occupancy, the number of patients in England travelling out of their local NHS Trust area for emergency mental health treatment has more than doubled in two years, and there are difficulties in recruiting and retaining permanent staff.

What is likely to be different in a true WMHU is the ability of professionals to provide an environment that is not experienced as disempowering and helps women understand and address underlying causes of their distress. Compared to men, women experience higher rates of poverty,[33] unemployment,[34] provide most childcare and other caring responsibilities,[35] and are more likely to be victims of domestic and sexual violence. The life-time rate of physical violence against women in the general community is reportedly between 21 per cent and 34 per cent[17,18,19] and the prevalence rate is increased for women in contact with psychiatric services with serious mental illnesses. A review of in-patient and out-patient studies of women with serious mental illness found that between 42 per cent and 64 per cent of women reported adult physical abuse.[36] A survey of mental healthcare service users in London reported that 70 per cent of women (and 50 per cent of men) had been victims of domestic violence as adults, with many (27 per cent of women, 10 per cent of men) experiencing recent and current domestic violence and abuse.[37] It has been suggested that acute in-patient care, by definition, is disempowering for many women, may unintentionally trigger feelings of powerlessness, and may cause them to feel re-traumatized, particularly when restraint and/or seclusion are used.[38]

Archer and colleagues[39] conducted a literature review to elucidate the needs of women in acute psychiatric units, and whilst they highlighted a lack of research into this area they were able to draw some conclusions for providing women-centred in-patient care. These included ensuring good interpersonal relationships with staff, a clear ward structure and routine, and the need for staff to have adequate support and training. They identified that women in-patients were more likely to have personality disorder diagnoses and histories of abuse/trauma with consequent complex and challenging interpersonal interactions. Unfortunately, the drive from higher management within NHS structures does not currently reflect the need to think about women's specific needs. When Agenda, an alliance of voluntary sector organizations, sent a freedom of information request to all the Mental Health Foundation Trusts in the United Kingdom, only one of the Trusts that responded had a strategy for providing gender-specific services for women.[40] Also highlighted within this report was that the majority of responding trusts had no policy of 'routine enquiry' about abuse, information that is one of the keys in providing gender-informed care, and only five services reported having a policy on actively offering female patients a choice of a female care worker.

The majority of acute in-patient services at present do not fit the criteria for a WMHU. Even if a unit is completely segregated by gender, it does not necessarily follow that it truly is a WMHU. The defining characteristic is neither one of safety (though this should be a given for all psychiatry wards) nor lack of contact with men, but that these units recognize the differential experiences of women that contribute to the development and perpetuation of their mental illnesses. Further research is needed to understand the core factors underlying women's mental illnesses and the specific skills and training that staff need to treat them.

Acknowledgements

I am sincerely grateful to Dr Koravangattu Valsraj, Consultant Psychiatrist and Associate Clinical Director, for his enthusiasm regarding women's mental health issues, his encouragement to write this chapter and for all of his contributions. He has been an immensely supportive trainer and colleague.

References

1. **Crisp N**, **Smith G**, and **Nicholson K** (eds) (2016). Improving acute inpatient psychiatric care for adults in England. Interim report. London: The Commission on Acute Adult Psychiatric Care. <http://www.rcpsych.ac.uk/pdf/0e662e_a93c62b2ba4449f48695ed36b3cb24ab.pdf>.

2. **Chow W** and **Priebe S** (2013). Understanding psychiatric institutionalization: a conceptual review. *BMC Psychiatry* **13**:169. <http://doi.org/10.1186/1471-244X-13-169>.

3. **Warner L** and **Ford R** (1998). Conditions for women in inpatient psychiatric units: The Mental Health Act Commission 1996 national visit. *Mental Health Care* **1**(7):225–28.

4. **Batcup D** (1994). Mixed sex wards: recognising and responding to gender issues in mental health settings and evaluating their safety for women. Interim report for the Bethlem and Maudsley NHS Trust. London: The Maudsley Audit Office.

5. **Warner L** and **Ford R** (1998). Conditions for women in inpatient psychiatric units: the Mental Health Act Commission 1996 national visit. *Mental Health Care* **1**(7):225–8.

6. **NHS Executive** (2000). *Safety, Privacy and Dignity in Mental Health Units.* London: Department of Health.

7. **Beasley C** and **Flory D** (2010). *Eliminating Mixed Sex Accommodation: From the Chief Nursing Officer and Deputy NHS Chief Executive.* London: Department of Health. <https://www.gov.uk/government/publications/eliminating-mixed-sex-accommodation>.

8. **Beasley C** and **Flory D** (2009). *Eliminating Mixed Sex Accommodation: From the Chief Nursing Officer and Director General of NHS Finance, Performance and Operations.* London: Department of Health. <https://www.gov.uk/government/publications/eliminating-mixed-sex-accommodation-in-hospitals>.

9. **Foxley Lane Women's Service staff** (2008). Radical ordinariness: the women's service in Purley. *Journal of Holistic Healthcare* **5**(4):13–18.

10. **Cutting P** and **Henderson C** (2002). Women's experiences of hospital admission. *Journal of Psychiatric Mental Health Nursing* **9**:705–9.

11. **Meiser-Stedman C, Howard L,** and **Cutting P** (2006). Evaluating the effectiveness of a women's crisis house: a prospective observational study. *Psychiatric Bulletin* **30**:324–6.

12. **Howard L, Flach C, Leese M, Byford S, Killaspy H, Cole L, Lawlor C, Betts J, Sharac J, Cutting P, McNicholas S,** and **Johnson S**(2010). Effectiveness and cost-effectiveness of admissions to women's crisis houses compared with traditional psychiatric wards: pilot patient-preference randomised controlled trial. *British Journal of Psychiatry* **197**:s32–s40. DOI:10.1192/bjp.bp.110.081083.

13. **Archer J** and **Coyne S** (2005). An integrated review of indirect, relational, and social aggression. *Personality and Social Psychology Review* **9**:212–30.

14. **Conway A** (2005). Girls, aggression and emotion regulation. *American Journal of Orthopsychiatry* **75**:334–9.

15. **Bengtsson-Tops A, Markstrom U,** and **Lewin B** (2005). The prevalence of abuse in Swedish female psychiatric users, the perpetrators and places where abuse occurred. *Nordic Journal of Psychiatry* **59**: 504–10.

16. **Sturup J, Sorman K, Lindqvist P,** and **Kristiansson M** (2011). Violent victimization of psychiatric in patients: A Swedish case–control study. *Social Psychiatry and Psychiatric Epidemiology* **46**:29–34. DOI:10.1007/s00127-009-0167-5.

17. **Bunch C** and **Carillo R** (1994). Global Violence Against Women: The challenge to human rights and development. In: Klare M and Thomas D (eds). *World Security: Challenges for a New Century.* New York, NY: St Martin's Press. pp. 256–73.

18. **Marshall P** and **Vaillancourt M** (1993). *Changing the Landscape: Ending Violence—Achieving Equality.* Ottawa: Canadian Panel on Violence against Women.

19. **Davies M** (1994). *Women and Violence: Realities and Responses Worldwide.* London: Zed Books.

20. **Leavey G, Papageorgiou A,** and **Papadopoulos C** (2006). Patient and staff perspectives on single-sex accommodation. *Journal of Health Management* **8**:79–90.

21. **Johnson S, Bingham C, Billings J, Pilling S, Morant N, Bebbington P, McNicholas S,** and **Dalton J** (2004). Women's experiences of admission to a crisis house and to acute hospital wards: A qualitative study. *Journal of Mental Health* **13**(3):247–62.

22. **Cleary M** and **Warren R** (1998). An exploratory investigation into women's experiences in a mixed sex psychiatric admission unit. *Australian and New Zealand Journal of Mental Health Nursing* **7**:33–40.

23. **Thomas B, Liness S, Vearnals S,** and **Griffin H** (1992). Involuntary cohabitees. *Nursing Times* **88**:58–60.

24. **Mezey G, Hassell Y**, and **Bartlett A** (2005). Safety of women in mixed-sex and single-sex medium secure units: Staff and patient perceptions. *British Journal of Psychiatry* **187**(6): 579–82. DOI: 10.1192/bjp.187.6.579.

25. **Henderson C** and **Reveley A** (1996). Is there a case for single sex wards? *The Psychiatrist* **20**(9):513–15. DOI:10.1192/pb.20.9.513.

26. **Bowers L, Ross J, Cutting P**, and **Stewart D** (2014). Sexual behaviours on acute inpatient psychiatric units. *Journal of Psychiatric and Mental Health Nursing* **21**:271–9. DOI:10.1111/jpm.12080.

27. **Fallon P, Bluglass R, Edwards B**, and **Daniels G** (1999). *Report of the Committee of Inquiry into the Personality Disorder Unit, Ashworth Special Hospital* (Vol. **1**). London: Her Majesty's Stationery Office.

28. **Howard L, Ehrlich A, Gamlen F**, and **Oram S** (2016). Gender-neutral mental health research is sex and gender biased. *Lancet Psychiatry* (4):9–11.

29. **McGeorge M, Shinkwin L**, and **Hinchcliffe G** (2007). *Healthcare Commission National Audit of Violence 2006–7*. London: Royal College of Psychiatrists.

30. **Lanza M, Kayne H, Hicks C**, and **Milner J** (1994). Environmental characteristics related to patient assault. *Issues in Mental Health Nursing* **15**:319–35.

31. **Williams J** and **Paul, J** (2008). *Informed Gender Practice; Mental health Acute Care that works for Women*. London: National Institute for Mental Health England. <http://webarchive.nationalarchives.gov.uk/20110512085708/http:/www.nmhdu.org.uk/silo/files/informedgenderpractice.pdf>.

32. **Crisp N, Smith G**, and **Nicholson K** (2016). *Old Problems, New Solutions—Improving Acute Psychiatric Care for Adults in England*. London: The Commission on Acute Adult Psychiatric Care. <https://www.caapc.info/publications>

33. **Oppenheim C** and **Harker L** (1996). *Poverty the Facts*. London: Child Poverty Action Group.

34. **Office for National Statistics** (1997). *Social Trends*. London: Her Majesty's Stationery Office.

35. **Montgomery, P** (1993). Paid and unpaid work. In: Kremer J and Montgomery P (eds). *Women's Working Lives*. Belfast: Her Majesty's Stationery Office, pp. 15–43.

36. **Goodman L, Rosenberg S, Mueser K**, and **Drake R** (1997). Physical and sexual assault history in women with serious mental illness: Prevalence, correlates, treatment, and future research directions. *Schizophrenia Bulletin* **23**:685–96.

37. **Khalifeh H, Moran P, Borschmann R, Dean K, Hart C, Hogg J, Osborn D, Johnson S,** and **Howard L** (2015). Domestic and sexual violence against patients with severe mental illness. *Psychological Medicine* **45**: 875–86. DOI: 10.1017/S0033291714001962.

38. **Judd F, Armstrong S**, and **Kulkarni J** (2009). Gender-sensitive mental health care. *Australasian Psychiatry* **17**(2):105–11. DOI:10.1080/10398560802596108.

39. **Archer M, Lau Y**, and **Sethi F** (2016). Women in acute psychiatric units, their characteristics and needs: A review. *British Journal of Psychiatry Bulletin* **40**(5):266–72. DOI:10.1192/pb.bp.115.051573.

40. **Agenda** (2016). *Agenda mental health gender responsiveness briefing*. London; Agenda. <http://weareagenda.org/wp-content/uploads/2016/11/Mental-health-briefing-FINAL.pdf>.

Chapter 9

Jail Birds: Challenges for Prisoners and Professionals

Annie Bartlett

Evil and Illness

There is a 'fine line between evil and illness' according to Joanne Taylor, the mother of one of the children who was a victim of the nurse, Beverley Allitt.[1] This conundrum is central to forensic practice, for clinicians, courts, victims, and perpetrators alike. Evil and illness as explanations for crime cannot overlap but they may still appear in the same paragraph of speech. How people and their criminal actions are understood is the stuff of forensic court reports and court proceedings. Court judgments tell us not only where people end up (i.e. in prison or in hospital) but also the tenor of the daily interactions of those who become prisoners with clinical and prison staff. The judgments will influence how both victims and perpetrators come to terms, or not, with what has happened. The mother in question was responding to the judge's comments on Allitt's possible sadism. This extreme behaviour is very rare in women offenders. Despite this, women who kill barbarically, who kill the very innocent, or who kill repeatedly tend to become far better known than their male counterparts.[2]

Clytemnestra would have understood the problem. She lost her daughter, Iphigenia, sacrificed to the war Agamemnon was keen to prosecute with the Trojans. Yet, when she in turn killed Agamemnon it ensured that she was established as the embodiment of female wickedness for centuries to come. Agamemnon returns from the Trojan wars with another wife, Cassandra, one of the spoils of war. Clytemnestra had to deal with two blows: the death of her daughter for the good of the state at the hands of her husband and then her abandonment and replacement by another woman as his wife. Life events, we might say now, are likely to have an effect on a woman's psyche. Her responsibility for the death of Agamemnon is not in doubt in the original plays by Aeschylus. Her action speaks for her, but today, personality is seen as underpinning behaviour and psychological understanding is privileged. Clytemnestra in the twenty-first century might be better understood as a mother responding to grief with rage, a possibly unbalanced, homicidal response to an unforgiveable injury rather than a politically ambitious, middle-aged woman with a new lover.

This potential for competing readings of Clytemnestra's actions is the starting point of this chapter. It considers the confusion of conceptual frameworks about women's crime. The primary focus is the nature and value of the various discourses on women who offend. This goes beyond the clinical and criminological. Historically, before criminology and psychiatry were born, women did bad things that were understood within moral and religious but also social codes. Social codes are gendered and tell us what constitutes normal behaviour for women and men, at a particular time. These earlier understandings have been elaborated and changed, in terms of formal discourse, by a combination of statute law, psychiatric and psychological models of mental disorder, tempered with the ideas of feminist criminology. The last body of writing has led both to rejection of early criminological theory and thus to the view that the way in which women offenders might be different from men offenders is different from the way that was previously believed to be true. The word 'belief' is, of course, key here as allegiance or adherence to all these modes of thought are ultimately a matter of personal preference and belief, even if they are underpinned by empirical evidence. Even the idea that women are different from men can be disputed. The recent government White Paper on prison reform[3] mentions women only twice in over 65 pages, not exactly a ringing endorsement of the need to have gender-specific interventions for women offenders.

The contested ground on which the contemporary female offender stands is challenging for women professionals who encounter her. This applies whether the woman in question is a minor offender (the vast majority) or amongst the handful of serious offenders. The particular current preoccupation with perpetrators and victims—women in prison and secure hospitals are usually both—is part of that challenge, encouraging professionals to imagine in two directions at once, to grasp the idea that a woman has been victimised but to hold in mind that she has also committed a crime. With an additional awareness of the representation of women and their adherence or deviation from what is perceived as normal (think of Lucrezia Borgia, Lady Macbeth, Medea), most obviously but not exclusively rehearsed in psychodynamic thinking on women and their disorders,[4] the professional can feel as if the ground is very wobbly. This can be exacerbated by working in high-profile prison settings. It becomes painfully apparent that there are significant differences between what professionals can as well as actually do compared with external perceptions of the nature of their work and the nature of the client group.

Old Ideas About Wicked Women

To Return to the Greeks

When Clytemnestra is in turn killed by Orestes, her son, who kills her to avenge his father, the reasonableness of his action is called into question. Put another way, should Orestes be arrested, or to be more psychodynamic about it, is he already arrested, at least developmentally? He is certainly haunted by the Furies who taunt him about his mother's killing. He is, in fact, or as close to fact as Greek theatre gets, acquitted of murder by the goddess Athene in the play that is the final play of Aeschylus' *Oresteia*. This verdict is debated but upheld in a modern version seen in London in 2016.[5] The chief character witness for the prosecution, Electra, Clytemnestra's daughter, dwells on her view of her mother as an adulterous wife and ignores the grieving mother and the adandoned wife. Clytemnestra's own brothers absolve Orestes of any guilt for matricide. Thus, Clytemnestra becomes a person whom it is reasonable to kill because she has committed an evil deed herself. Killing war heroes went down badly amongst the Greeks but she has also offended against a social code as a woman who kills. Mary

Beard argues that in killing she is seen not as female but as male; indeed, Clytemnestra is not a popular children's name in contemporary Greece, whereas Orestes and Agamemnon apparently are.[6]

The plays which are based on this story and written by Aeschylus[7], Sophocles,[8] and Euripides[9] should be required reading for anyone who wants to work with women offenders. They equip us with the understanding that while the social world of the Greeks is not ours, ours is a social world in which the way in which women and their actions are understood has a context. As professionals working with women who offend, we share this context. In turn, it shapes our views on women. We will have professional and personal perspectives on women offenders and their actions. These professional views should not be assumed to be either objective or neutral, although they may be rational and supported by logic, experience, and evidence; they too must be informed by the social context in which we live. Our personal views may at times simply be moral judgements.

Wicked Witches

A different temptation, if that is not a loaded word in this context, is to see women as dangerous. This is seldom in the sense of being physically dangerous, except to children. The idea of dangerous women encompasses ideas of seduction, leading men astray, of deceit, and, of course, also of conjuration.

The history of witchcraft and, in particular, the uses to which accusations of witch-craft were put is salutary. Historically, to be a witch was not to be either Hermione Granger from *Harry Potter* or Samantha from the TV series 'Bewitched', with a twitchy nose and an uncanny ability to tidy the house by magic. Both these twentieth-century creations are winners. Their cleverness is praised, not punished. Hermione is cleverer than both Ron and Harry and often gets them out of scrapes by her mastery of magic.

Older witches were less lucky. Witch hunts were most common in the sixteenth and seventeenth centuries. Women were often accused of 'putting the evil eye' on someone and were thought to be more susceptible than men to the devil in all his forms. This idea seems to follow the ancient story of the Garden of Eden, where Eve was tempted by Lucifer and thus in turn tempted Adam into trouble he might otherwise have avoided. Older women, women who were skilled with herbs, women who were alone, and women who defied convention were, at particular times, at risk of the accusation of witchcraft and at risk of the severe punishment, usually hanging, that went with it. In the Essex Assizes, 92 per cent of those accused of witchcraft were women.[10] A highly gendered approach to religion and morality to enforce the social conventions of the day and, in the case of England, enshrined in the English Witchcraft statutes.

The true history of the witches of Salem exemplifies these ideas.[11] The community of Salem in New England was populated for the most part by white Anglo-Saxon settlers for whom Protestantism was a driving force in their lives. Religious observance was key to social cohesion. With it came a familiarity with and acceptance of the idea of spirit possession. A series of accusations arose within the community centred on the idea that witches were inflicting a range of physical symptoms on their neighbours. The first to be accused were women who were not well integrated into the community. The number of accusations grew in number and court hearings were held to try indi-viduals of whom this accusation had been made. Experts in witchcraft were consulted.

The result was that 18 people, mainly women, were executed, most by hanging, after the courts accepted that they were witches and guilty of malign behaviour. The symptoms of which the sufferers complained would now, in a more secular but perhaps no less credulous age, be seen either as feigned or perhaps as genuinely hysterical (in the sense that unconscious conflicts can be relieved by somatic symptoms). Neither of these modern interpretations would lead to wholesale execution.

The continuing salience of witchcraft and possession as ideas that can explain the cause of an injury is evident in the Victoria Climbié inquiry.[12] Victoria Climbié died at the age of eight, murdered by her aunt, Marie-Therese Kouao, and her aunt's boyfriend, Carl Manning. Kouao took the child to hospital on occasion and worried individuals alerted social services staff. However, Kouao also took Victoria to more than one church, where she claimed the child was possessed. One pastor considered this a plausible explanation for the already present, significant injuries the child displayed. He said prayers to cleanse her of the Devil. Carl Manning also believed that Victoria, a female child, was Satan. The formal inquiry focused on the failings of many statutory agencies and concluded that the child's death was avoidable principally because there were many opportunities for them to have intervened. Secular understandings of the patterns and origins of violence did not, in this case, trigger effective child protection against a violent step mother and her partner.

Criminal Women in Criminology

Criminological understandings of crime and violence in women have come a long way from the essentialist biological theories of Lombroso and Ferrero, via the idea that female criminality was an expression of abnormal female sexuality and a general tendency towards deceit and cunning.[13] These early figures were taken to task by feminist scholars[14,13] who concluded that there had a been a wholesale failure to distinguish between sex, a biological attribute, and gender, a social construct. This began investigation of the relationship between gender and crime, including the relevance of the ways in which boys and girls were differently socialized and what was considered normal for each. It followed that women and men occupied different social spaces with different opportunities for crime. Crime committed by men and women could also be differently received, including by the courts. This second wave of academic work put paid to the idea that women were neglected in social theories of crime but it offered little by way of solutions. Mercifully, it dispelled the idea that women's social and political emancipation led to crime. It also suggested that, by and large, women who entered crime did so from straitened social and economic circumstances, often including severe physical and sexual abuse.[15]

But What is the Matter with Her?

Even so, modern empirical feminist criminology left room for individual explanations of criminal action necessary to underpin the work of those involved in the supervision and care of criminal women. Psychiatric and psychological explanatory models have accordingly found a prominent place in contemporary understanding of criminality and violence in women. Nowhere is the psychologization of female crime better illus-trated than by the rebuild of Her Majesty's Prison/Youth Offenders Institution (HMP/YOI) Holloway in the 1970s. The old prison building was levelled to the ground, only the stone griffins survived from the old building. A new prison was designed and built on the debatable premise that what criminal women needed was therapy not rehabilitation.[16] Architecturally distinctive as a prison, with long corridors and poor sight lines for surveillance of prisoners, this version of HMP/YOI Holloway survived without much physical alteration until its closure in summer 2016. Initially, vocational training for prisoners of a kind designed to equip women for work on release was com-pletely lacking.[15] While ostensibly designed with therapy in mind, it conspicuously lacked interview and therapy spaces. Its physical limitations, regardless of intended function, were repeatedly criticized by prison inspectors.[17] However, the very lack of efficiency engendered by the building design meant that it needed a higher ratio of of-ficers to prisoners to maintain safety of both staff and inmates. So it was saved from the worst excesses of the now notorious benchmarking policy brought in by the Secretary of State, Chris Grayling, in 2010. This cost cutting exercise was ostensibly to stand-ardize staff to prisoner ratios across the prison estate but in fact led to the loss of a quarter of the national prison officer workforce by 2014.[18]

Both psychiatric and psychological models share several appealing characteristics. They may offer a kinder way of thinking about a woman than criminal justice super-vision, demanding a style of engagement with women in criminal justice settings that is person-centred and alert to personal and perhaps maladaptive styles of commu-nicating. In providing explanations that can go beyond symptoms, to encompass a narrative about unwanted or regretted actions or experiences, they can sometimes aid resolution and help even women who have committed serious crime to move on in their lives. They offer cure rather than moral judgement. They also rely on some degree of empirical certainty. The pills are not smarties. Cognitive behaviour therapy has an evidence base.

In truth, however, the majority of therapeutic work in women's prisons is little to do with understanding crime and much more to do with dealing with incidental mental health problems.

Women in Prison: Numbers and Problems

Today, women constitute about 5 per cent of the total daily population of 85,000 pris-oners in England and Wales. However, the population of women in prison has varied dramatically since 1900. Between 1915 and 1917 the proportion of women in the total prison population reached a maximum of 18 per cent. However, since the 1950s, women have constituted 3 to 5 per cent of the total prison population. Rates of impris-onment, per capita of the general population, have also varied enormously over time. While the population of male prisoners was 152 per 100,000 of the male population in 1901 and dropped in the first half of the twentieth century, it rose to more than double that, 356 per 100,000 in 2015. In contrast, the number of women imprisoned in 1901 was 27 per 100,000 of the female population and was much lower during most of the next 100 years, rising recently so that in 2015 it was 16 per 100,000.[19]

The background to these wild fluctuations is beyond the scope of this chapter but acknowledgement of past and probably future variations is important. It should make us wary of out-of-date estimates of health problems in a women's prison estate of varying size and criminological composition. It should encourage us to be clear about the current situation.

It has become a commonplace of prison healthcare that the women who find their way into custody are multiply morbid. In truth, there is little up-to-date mental health epidemiology based on this population; the most recent major study was published almost 20 years ago.[20,21] This reported high rates of psychiatric disorder in women prisoners: personality disorder 50 per cent, functional psychosis 14 per cent, and neurotic disorders 66 per cent. Similarly high rates of alcohol and drug abuse and dependence were reported. Roughly half of all women entering custody had used crack cocaine, heroin, and cannabis in the 12 months prior to imprisonment, and half were assessed as drug dependent.[22,23] Thirty-four per cent were viewed as being harmful drinkers. Women frequently present with more than one psychiatric disorder, this being highest in the remand prison population (83 per cent), and slightly lower, though still relatively high, in sentenced prisoners (70 per cent).[20]

Plugge and colleagues[24] also noted high rates of psychiatric caseness on arrival in prison and there is some evidence that these levels of psychiatric caseness are likely to remain high in women as custody continues.[25]

Women contribute disproportionately to the total number of incidents of self-harm in prison, although recent figures suggest that self-harm in male prisoners is rising faster than in women prisoners.[26] A small proportion of women in prison account for most of the self-harm incidents.[27] Suicide rates in women dropped to an all-time low in 2012 but have risen subsequently, as have all causes of deaths in custody.

Women prisoners' social backgrounds have been well documented in recent years.[28] They can be seen to predispose them to physical and mental health problems and, to some extent, identify women prisoners as having gender-specific issues. They are more likely than their male counterparts to be victimized as children and adults[29] and are more likely to have been in care. They share poor education records, disrupted families, and poor social support. They are more likely than men to have significant childcare responsibilities; in turn there is concern about the effects of involvement in the criminal justice system on their children.

While women are commonly in prison for violence against the person, conviction statistics over many years show that they seldom commit serious violence compared to men and almost never commit sexual offences. Ninety per cent of principal suspects for homicide are men.[30] However, violence in women, whether fatal or not, has been more frequently linked to mental illness than in men.[31,32]

Within the terrain of psychiatric and psychological discourse, two points are clear: first, that diagnosis alone will not be enough to establish a meaningful hierarchy of need that matches a woman's sense of her own difficulties; second, that all psychiatric and psychological formulations have merit, but the presence of competing, emanating from the multi-disciplinary team, professional understandings including epidemiology, trauma-informed formulation, personality disorder, and complex needs[33] within the broad domain of mental health is complex for both the women themselves and for practitioners.

Professionals' Stories

The Nature of the Challenge

One challenge of providing services is how to deal both with the small number of women who are serving life or indefinite sentences for grave offences as well as the larger number of women whose lower-level offending is often linked to drug and alcohol dependence and ingrained interpersonal difficulties. While the focus of this chapter is mental health, in practice most services within women's prisons are not focused on mental health. Only a small proportion of the overall health budget is devoted to what would normally be considered secondary mental healthcare. Services are holistic and comprise primary care, substance misuse services (detoxification and psychosocial programmes), sexual health and maternity services. There is a need to work coherently with the other components of healthcare.

Another challenge of what is, in effect, a polyclinic is how all these services, including mental health, can conduct effective clinical work in an environment where the majority of custodial staff are primarily and properly concerned with custody, education, and vocational needs.

The intrinsic institutional challenges are compounded by the high churn rate of women's prisons; that is, the predominantly low level of offending results in brief remand periods and short sentences. For healthcare this means that thought needs to be given to both what can be achieved within the walls and what should and can be delivered on release. Much depends on the attitude of the woman towards continuing contact with health services. The lack of fixed accommodation (often lost on reception into prison) plus membership of a stigmatized group (former women prisoners are not necessarily welcomed onto general practitioner rolls) may contribute to effective exclusion from all but urgent care. External secondary mental health services can have restrictive policies, making it hard to find teams happy to work with them outside prison. The following case vignette illustrates this.

Helen was 23-years old and had been in prison on 4 occasions. On the most recent occasion, she arrived pregnant and did not want to keep the child. She was charged with actual bodily harm. When intoxicated, she had assaulted a market trader who had made suggestive comments to her. She had a documented history of drug-induced psychosis. Her periods in the community were made more difficult because she had not had stable accommodation since she was first in prison. She had been the subject of repeated referrals to learning disability and community mental health teams. Various reasons for not accepting her had been offered, including a history of non-engagement, her having too high an IQ, and her suffering from no major mental illness. The team in prison felt she could not cope with life in the community without greater support and that she was vulnerable to exploitation. She coped with distress by using street drugs.

While aspects of this case may be typical, there are different challenges in the nature of work with women who stay longer. The next case study attempts to bring these issues to life.

Sonia was 35-years old and had killed her male partner after a bout of drinking. She said he was the love of her life and that it was an accident. She was known to have called the police on repeated occasions as he was also violent. The killing was very brutal and she had been given a life sentence. She spent a year in prison before trial and had been distressed, self-harming on several occasions. After her sentencing, she became withdrawn and intermittently refused to see the psychotherapist who had been working with her prior to her trial. She had denied any history of victimization as an adult and was full of shame. She could not see how her sentence could be endured and felt she was unworthy of people's efforts to engage her.

The clinical staff who deliver mental health care to women's prisons are, in my experience, more often women than men. There are opportunities and risks for people of both genders but here the focus is on those issues that may emerge for female staff.

Working in prison is not a traditional route to career stardom. Women's prisons have routinely had a bad press, being variously described as holiday camps and environments characterized by difficult and boundary-violating staff groups, and having high rates of suicide and self-harm in the prisoner population. Women's prisons have been the graveyard of many medical and nursing careers. It is only since the advent of National Health Service (NHS) commissioning of services in 2006 that the situation has changed.[34] This connectivity with the NHS, even where the providers are private sector companies, has led to increases in funding, the introduction of NHS expectations of parity of service with those not in prison, and regular monitoring of services delivered. There is a consensus, even if it lacks hard evidence of efficacy, that much has improved.[35] Nonetheless, for staff there is a risk of shared stigma with the women prisoners and a lack of formal recognition of the clinical skills acquired and required to work successfully within prison settings.

4 Risks and Opportunities

For women professionals working within mental health, there are specific risks and opportunities. The first risk is that the sheer intensity of the work can be overwhelming. The extreme nature of many women prisoners' experiences can be very challenging and can result in clinical apathy. This becomes more likely when the number of clinicians is reduced by difficulties in recruiting and retaining staff. Equally, women staff working with women prisoners often invites both sympathy and empathy between the two. This can lead to better understanding of women prisoners but also perhaps to an overidentification with an prisoner's problems and/or overdisclosure of personal circumstance. The risk here is not simply that a clinical professional may stretch beyond boundaries which protect both staff members and patients but can also result in a professional working in a custodial setting becoming open to blackmail.

Opportunities exist in well-managed and well-resourced prison settings to offset potential risks. The key to this is the provision of reflective practice space. This kind of meeting offers both clinicians and officers a chance to mull over elements such as the use of restraint, the stress induced by very high and seemingly insurmountable levels of self-harm, injury to staff members and the prisoner patient who sabotages all the help that she is offered. These meetings can also be useful to spot the exhausted member of staff, the person whose professionalism might slip under pressure. Linked with this should be an insistence on close managerial contact, impromptu visits by management to parts of the prison seldom normally visited. An open-door drop-in policy in a locked setting is vital. Both formal supervision and informal conversations and cups of coffee with staff to see which prisoners are causing concern can go a long way towards anticipating problems prisoners and staff may have. It is desirable and possible to foster a richness of discussion of women's problems that allows for several simultaneous perspectives, be they within a clinical framework[36] or between clinicians and officers (such as multidisciplinary care planning meetings attended by safer custody officers, healthcare governors, and clinical staff) who jointly work to tackle serious issues, including those that might upset the prison regime. This move towards working with the multiple discourses of clinical care and custody includes the social in the limited sense of the Social Care Act but also, more meaningfully, an appreciation of the social roots of criminality and mental health difficulties.

Allen and colleagues[37] highlighted the benefits of open and multi-perspective discussion among all prison based staff including flexibility within necessarily rule-driven, rigid institutions. The possibility of clinical choice in institutions that reinforce, by their very nature, a lack of autonomy can similarly be promoted by clinicians working knowledgeably and who are aware of alternative approaches. The lack of autonomy is also gendered. Women who have been victimized, who have found it hard or impossible to escape brutal relationships, and who then find themselves in a regime offering little option for self-expression or personal preference may find that a women's prison resonates with unwanted parts of their personal histories. Gender awareness amongst prison staff is not a uniquely female attribute but being a woman may help staff empathize with female prisoners, so too will appropriate training.[38]

It is interesting to note that in 2015, of all nine London prisons, it was decided that the one women's prison, HMP/YOI Holloway, would close. There were many objections to the closure.[39,40] As a female institution, its rapid and unwanted closure symbolized how little power women can have over their lives when the imperative from a male justice minister is to raise financial capital for men.

This then is routine. Less routine is the need for explanations for horrific acts e.g. the killing of children and parents or homicides of particular barbarity or the failure to protect children from sexual invasion or even active participation in sexual acts with children. These types of crimes test the professionalism of most people. They defy the common perception of women's usual gender roles as care givers and protectors of children and pose distinct challenges for both the prison in which such women are incarcerated and, in particular, protection for the women who have commited such acts. The circumstances in which this kind of criminal act may have occurred may range from involvement of a vulnerable woman with a predatory and violent paedophile man to a first episode of psychosis. To have explanations of this type of crime is extremely important for everyone involved: for patients, for families and for professionals. However, explanations of such acts can take a long time to emerge and may never appear. It is no accident that there was a small library of detective fiction in the Forensic Psychiatry Department at St George's Hospital offering comfortingly, available explanations of serious crime, in contrast to the uncomfortable loose ends of real clinical work.

Strong feelings arise inevitably, particularly for staff with children. Hearing and reading about grave criminal acts are difficult and often not necessary for all members of the team. The production and maintenance of good case records will also protect the patient from overly intrusive, repetitive questioning by medical and other authorities.

But for someone to know the facts is important, not least because for the woman to get to a position of full acknowledgement may be impossible. Life sentence prisoners will become used to changes in the team but maintaining threads of understanding, a matrix of non-judgemental knowledge alive to the gravity of past action will serve them well. The secret shame will often translate into a reluctance to engage therapeutically. They may challenge the purpose and utility of anything mental health has to offer. Treating the person either psychodynamically or via the routine professionalism of a good prison officer will often be the start of a difficult and frequently never completed journey towards rehabilitation and release. Managing distress and creating an authentic narrative using words or art or any medium will most likely be necessary along a route to possible parole a journey which has multiple technical hurdles.

The Limitations of Psychiatry and Psychology

We might reasonably ask how robust these clinical formulations and options are for women who offend? What do they offer professionals and women professionals who work with them? Sometimes psychiatry and psychology may not seem enough.

We come full circle and return to the use of evil as an explanatory framework. It has no place in clinical treatment but it may have a common sense quality. A clinical diagnosis or a psychological formulation relies on. Other people having suffered the same symptoms for similar reasons. Occasional cases challenge the value of these frameworks, particularly when the criminal actions concerned are so far beyond the norm as to make the case virtually unique. The cases of Dennis Nielsen and Peter Sutcliffe are instructive. Nielsen was responsible for the deaths of many young men; his sexual interests appear to have been in the dead. Peter Sutcliffe was responsible for the deaths of many young women whose bodies were severely mutilated. In Nielsen' case a psychiatric understanding was rejected in court, perhaps because diagnosis applicable only to a single case was inconsistent with the commonly accepted basis of diagnosis i.e. problems shared by multiple individuals, creating a recognizable pattern.[41] In Sutcliffe's case psychiatric evidence of psychosis was ignored and he was sentenced to prison, probably because the crimes were so awful that schizophrenia, a common illness, did not seem sufficient explanation, and because he would be at risk of release if given a hospital order.[42]

Evil is a word that might not unreasonably be applied to these men's actions, perhaps also to them as individuals, at least by a public whose influence on their futures is minimal. The use of this explanation in the case of any woman and her acts, given the way in which wickedness in women has been constructed over the centuries, combined with the almost complete absence of comparable crimes in women in the United Kingdom, makes it seem less appealing. Perhaps even the consideration of using evil as a rationale for specific criminal acts is a mark of the gravity with which those acts, and that woman, is considered, even as it has no clinical place. It might appear in the mind of the professional even as it is rejected as a suitable mode of clinical conceptualization. There are a handful of women such as Rosemary West, Myra Hindley, and Beverley Allitt whose actions, like Clytemnestra's, have turned them into enduring, quasi-mythological figures, but they are few and far between over the past 40 years.

References

1. **Batty D** and **Agencies** (2007). Serial killer nurse Allitt must serve 30 years. *The Guardian*, 6 December 2007. <https://www.theguardian.com/uk/2007/dec/06/ukcrime.health>.

2. **Heidensohn F** (1985). *Women and Crime*. Basingstoke: MacMillan, pp 84–109.

3. **Ministry of Justice** (2016). Prison Safety and Reform White Paper <https://www.gov.uk/government/publications/prison-safety-and-reform>.

4. **Welldon E** (1988). *Mother, Madonna, Whore: The Idealization and Denigration of Motherhood*. London: Karnac.

5. **Icke R** (2015). *Aeschylus' Oresteia*. London: Oberon.

6. **Nixey C** (2017). Radio Choice Woman's Hour *The Times*, 25 February.

7. **Stanford W** (ed.) and **Fagles R** (trans.) (1977). *Aeschylus, The Oresteia: Agamemnon, The Libation Bearers, The Eumenides*. Harmondsworth: Penguin.

8. **Watling EF** (trans.) (1953). *Sophocles, Electra*. Harmondsworth: Penguin.

9. Grene D and Lattimore R (eds) and Townsend Vermeule E (trans) (1959). *Euripides, Electra*.Chicago, IL: University of Chicago Press.

10. **Macfarlane A** (1999). *Witchcraft in Tudor and Stuart England: A Regional and Comparative Study*, 2nd edn. Oxford: Routledge.

11. <https://en.wikipedia.org/wiki/Salem_witch_trials>.

12. **Lord Laming** (2003). Victoria Climbié Inquiry. Norwich: London: Her Majesty's Stationery Office. <https://www.gov.uk/government/uploads/system/uploads/attachment_data/file/273183/5730.pdf>.

13. **Heidensohn F** (1985). *Women and Crime*. Basingstoke: MacMillan.

14. **Smart C** (1977). *Women, Crime and Criminology*. London: Routledge.

15. **Downes D** and **Rock P** (1995). Feminist criminology. In: Downes and Rock (eds) *Understanding Deviance: A Guide to the Aociology of Crime and Rule Breaking* revised 2nd edn. Oxford: Clarendon Press, pp 304–27.

16. **Maden T** (1995). *Women, Prisons and Psychiatry: Mental Disorder Behind Bars*. London: Hodder Arnold.

17. **Her Majesty's Inspectorate of Prisons** (2016). Report on an unannounced inspection of HMP and YOI Holloway by HM Chief Inspector of Prisons. London: Her Majesty's Inspectorate of Prisons. <https://www.justiceinspectorates.gov.uk/hmiprisons/wp-content/uploads/sites/4/2016/02/Holloway-web-2015.pdf>.

18. **House of Commons Justice Committee** (2015). Prisons: planning and policies. Ninth Report of Session 2014–15. London: The Stationery Office.

19. **Allen G** and **Dempsey N** (2016). Prison Population Statistics Briefing Paper. SN/SG/04334 4 July, House of Commons Library. <http://researchbriefings.parliament.uk/ResearchBriefing/Summary/SN04334>.

20. **Office for National Statistics (ONS)**, **Singleton N**, **Meltzer H**, and **Gatward R** (1997). *Psychiatric Morbidity among Prisoners in England and Wales*. London: The Stationery Office.

21. O'Brien M, Mortimer L, Singleton N, Meltzer H, and Goodman R (2003). Psychiatric morbidity among women prisoners in England and Wales. *International Review of Psychiatry* **15**(1–2):153–7.

22. Light M, Grant E, and Hopkins K (2013). *Gender Differences in Substance Misuse and Mental Health Amongst Prisoners.* London: Ministry of Justice.

23. Borrill J, Maden A, Martin A, Weaver T, Stimson G, Farrell M, and Barnes T (2003). Differential substance misuse treatment needs of women, ethnic minorities and young offenders in prison: prevalence of substance misuse and treatment needs (Home Office Online Report 33/03). London: Home Office Research, Development and Statistics Directorate.

24. Plugge E, Douglas N, and Fitzpatrick R (2006). *The Health of Women in Prison Study Findings.* Department for Public Health, University of Oxford.

25. Hassan L, Birmingham L, Harty MA, Jarrett M, Jones P, King C, Lathlean J, Lowthian C, Mills A, Senior J, Thornicroft G, Webb R, and Shaw J (2011). Prospective cohort study of mental health during imprisonment. *British Journal of Psychiatry* **198**:37–42

26. Ministry of Justice (2016). Safety in Custody Statistics England and Wales; Deaths in prison custody to September 2016, Assaults and Self-harm to June 2016 Ministry of Justice Statistics Bulletin 27 October 2016.

27. Chris Kottler, Jared G. Smith & Annie Bartlett (2018). Patterns of violence and self-harm in women prisoners: characteristics, co-incidence and clinical significance. *The Journal of Forensic Psychiatry & Psychology*, DOI: 10.1080/14789949.2018.1425475.

28. Ministry of Justice (2012). *Prisoners' Childhood and Family Backgrounds.* Ministry of Justice Research Series 4/12 March 2012. London: Ministry of Justice.

29. McCellan DS, Farabee D, and Crouch BM (1997). Early victimisation, drug use and criminality: A comparison of male and female prisoners. *Criminal Justice and Behaviour* **24**(4):455–76.

30. Ministry of Justice (2016). Statistics on Women and the Criminal Justice System 2015. <https://www.gov.uk/government/uploads/system/uploads/attachment_data/file/572043/women-and-the-criminal-justice-system-statistics-2015.pdf>.

31. Wessely S (1997). The epidemiology of crime, violence and schizophrenia. *British Journal of Psychiatry* **170**(32):8–11.

32. Flynn S, Abel KM, While D, Mehta H, and Shaw J (2011). Mental illness, gender and homicide: a population-based descriptive study. *Psychiatric Research* **185**:368–75.

33. Flynn S, Humber N, Bartlett A, and Shaw J (2016). Women offenders and mental health. In: Abel K and Castle D (eds).*Comprehensive Women's Mental Health.* Cambridge: Cambridge University Press, pp 148–60 at p 152

34. HMPS and NHS Executive (1999). *The future organisation of prison healthcare. Report by the Joint Prison Service and National Health Service Executive London.* London: Department of Health.

35. Public Health England (2016). Rapid review of evidence of the impact on health outcomes of NHS commissioned health services for people in secure and detained settings to inform future health interventions and prioritisation in England. <https://www.gov.uk/government/publications/health-outcomes-in-prisons-in-england-a-rapid-review>.

37. Allen S, Sadie C, Lockwood R, Maclennan F, Probert R, and Stewart P (2016). Freedom to think—the value of multiple clinical narratives in women's prisons. *Journal of Forensic Psychiatry & Psychology* DOI:10.1080/14789949.2016.1244282.

38. **Bloom B**, **Owen B**, and, **Covington S** (2005). *A Summary of Research, Practice, and Guiding Principles for Women Offenders. The Gender-Responsive Strategies Project: Approach and Findings*. Washington, DC: National Institute of Corrections.

39. **Hyde S** (2015). Closing Holloway Prison to make room for luxury flats isn't a triumph, George Osborne—it's just cruelly ironic. *The Independent*, Thursday 26 November 2015. <http://www.independent.co.uk/voices/closing-holloway-prison-to-make-room-for-luxury-flats-isnt-a-triumph-george-osborne-its-just-cruelly-a6749891.html>.

40. **Mansfield M** and **Pittaway H** (2016). Closing Holloway Prison will leave vulnerable women out in the cold Left Foot Forward <https://leftfootforward.org/2016/04/closing-holloway-prison-will-leave-vulnerable-women-out-in-the-cold/>.

41. <http://www.crimeandinvestigation.co.uk/crime-files/dennis-nilsen/trial>.

42. **Smith J.** (1989) *Misogynies*. London: Faber and Faber.

Considering the Predictive Value of the Risk Assessment Score

While you pretend to be sleeping
I restore to clarity
an armsreach of kitchen.

While I pretend you are sleeping
I tally the foiled-again blisters of paracetamol
fingertip them onto the high shelf,
divert your tins of soup to the low one.

While we are both pretending, I arrange the knives
in size order – paring, slicing, carving –
but do not sharpen them.

Our ears edgy as blades,
our skins pieced and popping
like beautiful bubblewrap, we concede
only this small circumference of wipeclean,

these blocked knives,
this shelf unreachable –
we know you're sleeping.

Emily Wills

Chapter 10

The Maternal Lap and the Mental Health Trust

Jo O'Reilly

In this chapter I describe how psychoanalytic ideas about maternal function can deepen and enrich our understanding of patients who need care from staff within mental health trusts (MHTs). As Figure 10.1 shows beautifully, the deep level of emotional engagement between mother and baby involves physical and emotional holding. The infant needs to be securely held on the mother's lap but it also needs the mother's mind to be emotionally available to recognize fully the passion and intensity of early emotional life and to respond to her baby with interest, care, and understanding. I am suggesting that the function of the maternal lap as could be termed *concave*, illustrating its ability to receive and hold the infant both physically and psychologically. This receptive and understanding response from another forms the basis of emotional and psychological development in early life.

The psychiatric organization too needs to function as a concave receptacle that is able to observe, enquire into, and thoughtfully respond in order to optimally understand and treat our patients. This requires an emotional state of receptivity and careful response from the clinical staff. Just as the maternal lap allows the infant to be safely held and protected, providing a secure base from which to address the world, the MHT provides services to individuals requiring safety, holding and understanding. However, pressures from various sources can limit the capacity of services to fully take in our patients' experiences, increasing the risk of superficial attachments and the repetition of harmful experiences of misunderstanding and rejection.

A *convex* surface represents an insecure or rejecting lap that cannot fully absorb or process communications. Under situations of excess pressure or demand an MHT can operate in this more convex way. Services based on more convex model can lead to treatment being organized with overly rigid entry requirements for example, in which patients can experience multiple assessments and discharges whilst never being fully understood. An encounter with the convex rather than the concave can mean opportunities to recover, grow, and develop are denied.

From infancy onwards, the thoughtful attention of another is essential in developing a coherent sense of identity and emotional growth and this is also the case at times of crisis in adult life. When the mind's capacity to function is fragile, processes of fragmentation and confusion can take over, referred to accurately as a 'breakdown'. Intense

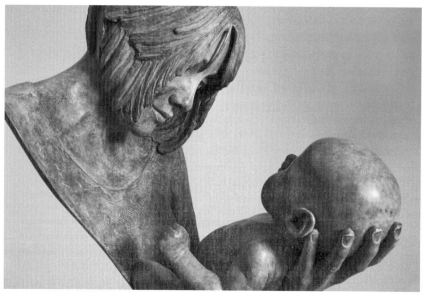

Figure 10.1 Sarah and Molly by Charles Westgarth
Charles Westgarth Sculpture. Reproduced with permission from Philippa Shimmin, the owner who originally commissioned the sculpture of Sarah and Molly.

emotional states that the individual cannot contain become dominant, and the mind is acutely sensitive to the responses it receives. The capacity to think becomes lost, along with any perspective other than complete identification with the prevailing emotional state. Psychiatric symptoms, including bizarre perceptual experiences and delusional beliefs, can loosen contact with reality. The past can flood the present with all the unmet need, traumas, and abusive relationships that this may contain.

The process by which we perceive and respond to others, both individuals and in groups, through the lens of our past experiences, is termed the transference (Table 10.1) in psychoanalytic terms. The transference can distort and disrupt our understanding of present situations and is acutely intensified in crisis—so much so that the present situation can be experienced concretely as the past. Witness the paranoid patient who responds to ordinary care with suspicion of attack or the borderline patient accusing caring teams of being neglectful and cruel. Staff working in the psychiatric hospitals and community teams that make up a modern MHT need to understand these processes and to be supported to do so in order to provide a receptive and sensitively attuned response to patients and to avoid repeating harmful patterns of relating.

In this chapter I describe clinical scenarios to illustrate some of these processes. All clinical cases are disguised and are condensed accounts of various cases gathered over many years of practice.

Although I write about maternal function I am not implying this relates to gender; men have laps as well and they can also provide this role, just as more paternal aspects of care can also be carried out by women.

Table 10.1 Definitions of terms used in Psychoanalysis

Transference	An unconscious process of the patient transferring or redirecting their feelings for a significant person from their past to the therapist. In psychoanalytic theory, this is ubiquitous and powerfully affects how we relate to others.
Counter-transference	When another's feelings are felt by the other person; such as when an infant's distress is felt by the mother. This is an unconscious process which can powerfully affect how we feel about others and respond to them.
Projection	Mechanism by which countertransference works. Aspects of emotional life and feelings that are too much to fully know are unconsciously transmitted to another. It can be a way to get rid of unbearable feelings but also to communicate and get these feelings understood by another.
Projective identification	A process by which unbearable feelings are split off and evacuated into the mind of another and have an impact when received by the other.
Splitting	The separation of feelings and experiences into categories of very good and very bad. In this way, they can feel more manageable.
Denial	An unconscious psychological defense mechanism that involves the obliteration of something that is known or seen.
Dissociation	A discontinuity of experience and memory
Containment	A response to another that recognises fully their emotional state without becoming overwhelmed. Allows an appropriate and attuned response based on emotional digestion rather than emotional reaction.
Psychotherapy	In psychotherapy a patient's emotional difficulties can be explored through the magnifying lens of transference/countertransference leading to increased recognition of unconscious feelings, fears and desires, making them more conscious and hence easier to understand and resolve.

The Medical Psychotherapist in the Mental Health Trust

As a medical psychotherapist I am trained as a medical doctor, a psychiatrist, and a psychoanalyst. Through my medical training I have learnt about biological aspects of illness while my psychiatric training taught me about the myriad presentations and managements of mental disturbance. My psychoanalytic training has allowed a deeper exploration of the mind, of the impact of the early nurturing environment and relationships on our adult functioning, and of the power of unconscious processes to inform how we perceive and relate to others.

Medical psychotherapists could be described as scientists with a wish to nurture and promote development; it is a popular career choice for women and for psychiatric trainees who are required to undertake training in psychotherapy early in their psychiatric careers.

In my National Health Service (NHS) role I work in a psychotherapy service to which patients are referred for therapy, usually with difficulties in emotional development, relationships, childhood trauma, and a wide range of symptoms suggesting psychological difficulties and suffering. Although they may attract a variety of diagnostic labels, patients referred to the service almost all describe difficulties in establishing and maintaining nurturing and secure intimate relationships and this is often the main cause of their isolation and distress. Not surprisingly these problematic relationship patterns are repeated in encounters with clinical staff and understanding this forms a key part of the therapeutic relationship.

My role within the MHT is wider than this, however, and the organization in which I work supports staff in their need to reflect about their work in order to improve patient care in a variety of creative settings. This means I also work with staff caring for patients with severe and enduring mental illness, psychotic conditions, and severe personality disorders. Psychiatric diagnosis often fails to capture the complexity of their presentations and how this relates to their early life experiences which are often characterized by abusive and neglectful experiences, traumas, and losses. Complex case discussions, a risk panel, supervision, and reflective practice groups provide essential opportunities to consider and understand some of the most violent, self-destructive, and disordered emotional states that staff encounter in their daily work. Often these cases need containment beyond what can be provided by the treating teams and the request to these panels is to process and consider what may be being communicated by some of these behaviours in order to best understand the patient as the basis for deciding clinical management.

Such work needs a theoretical model. These panels have learnt to formulate patients' difficulties from their earliest life experiences onward and how this can be key to understanding the presentation. We have also learnt that in addition to factual histories, the staff accounts of their emotional responses to the patient (the countertransference) can provide an essential tool to develop a deeper level of understanding of what the patient may be trying to communicate through unconscious processes. It can be fascinating to hear how similar stories of loss and adversity can elicit very different responses in team members, such as feeling overwhelmed, disbelieving, struggling to hold the history in mind, or deeply moved. This can be fundamental to learning about the patient's emotional experiences of early nurture and how this can be recreated in the present.

This work involves the application of psychoanalytic theory which itself has a fascinating history in discovering and describing the key role of maternal function in developing and maintaining psychological resilience.

Psychoanalytic Theory and Maternal Function

Sigmund Freud[1] described mental disorder as understandable in terms of development. He saw symptoms as having meaning for the individual, even if disguised as a psychotic or neurotic condition. Whilst he strongly emphasized the importance of early emotional development he wrote little about the importance of maternal functioning in shaping the early emotional world of the infant.

Subsequent psychoanalytic theorists have expanded on and explored the key importance of the mother–infant relationship in psychological development. These maternal aspects of relating have both physical and psychological components; just as the baby on the mother's lap needs to be physically held and supported, the developing infant's emotions need recognition and response. Whilst physical aspects of this care may include feeding, holding securely, clearing up dribbled milk, preventing falls, picking up, tucking in, and letting go, maternal function also includes responses to the emotional components and aspects of experience as they are expressed in early utterances, cries, gurgles, and bodily changes. The emotional correlate to this is the maternal mind, as concave as a lap in its capacity to capture and hold the baby's communications and to be able to express them back thoughtfully in more processed and digestible form.

The psychoanalyst Melanie Klein recognized how hungry from the start the young human is for relationships. Through her observations of infants, Klein described psychotic functioning as present in earliest emotional development.[2] She saw meaning in children's play and drawings and both early relationships and constitutional factors as being key to how we build up our own internal world and then perceive and respond to the external. Through transference mechanisms our formative early experiences continue to exert pressures in the present; we all perceive our environment and relate to others through early templates based on interactions between our infant selves and key caregivers.

These psychoanalytic ideas offer much to support psychiatric practice. The biology (constitutional factors) and role of early development and relationships combine to develop psychological resource and vulnerability, along with a sense of identity. Containment of intense emotional states in early life is seen as crucial in supporting psychological functioning and development and the same holds true in psychiatric breakdown. The ability to function in an integrated and healthy manner can be lost at times of increased stress and anxiety when we can all return to more fragmented functioning and lose a more robust and thoughtful perspective.

The following examples illustrate how important it is for staff working in mental health services to have the capacity to respond with some of the containing function of the maternal lap; we need to be able to absorb, understand, hold, and process our patient's experiences in order to help them to recover when their own capacity to manage emotional states has become overwhelmed.

MS V: Early Trauma and the Containing Mind

Ms V had a history of severe sexual and physical abuse throughout her childhood with little experience of safety and nurture. High levels of anxiety with panic attacks characterized her adult life and her relationships were chaotic and filled with conflict. Like many people who have been abused, she sought to hide her vulnerability behind an aggressive stance. She suffered severe nightmares and flashbacks about her abuse and had difficulty sustaining any employment due to her high levels of emotional arousal and agitation; it was as if the past was relentlessly flooding her present. Her emotional difficulties were played out in all her relationships, including with mental health services, meaning she had never engaged in any form of treatment.

Ms V did find, however, a way of starting to talk about her experiences to her general practitioner (GP), whom she consulted over many years about her daughter's asthma. This slowly evolving process required the sustained and patient approach of the GP in recognizing and sensitively responding to her high degree of anxiety and, at times, provocative behaviour; the GP managed not to fall out with her. After several years of attending appointments with her daughter Ms V started to refer to her own abuse. Eventually she agreed to a referral to an NHS psychotherapy service and was offered regular sessions, a few weeks apart, by a therapist. There was no agenda set by the therapist and sessions were consistently offered despite Ms V's initial erratic attendance.

From the start Ms V was forcefully dominating in these sessions, recounting how powerful she had been in situations of conflict with others, understood by the therapist as a defensive bluster against her terror of being vulnerable again. Her experiences of abuse were communicated in fragments of dissociative material in which she would abruptly communicate in the voice of a terrified child, or in written half-sentences on fragments of paper. After these disclosures she would abruptly leave the room.

The therapist initially felt bombarded by both terrified and terrifying emotions and struggled not to feel overwhelmed with anxiety and confusion. To think cohesively and hold a thread of understanding under the pressure of such high levels of agitation and fear in the sessions was a challenge and it could feel traumatizing to be with Ms V. On several occasions the Trust Crisis Team added additional support when suicidal thoughts become predominant. The therapist also felt contained by this external support.

Over time Ms V was able to establish a working relationship with the therapist which allowed more space for thought, discussion, and understanding to emerge about her distress and defensive behaviours. She started to settle to the extent that she was able to attend regularly and to engage in specific treatment for her arousal levels and flashbacks within a specialist trauma service. She continued to see the psychotherapist throughout this work and over a six-year period her quality of life improved and her relationship with psychiatric services became more consistent and less explosive. Her symptoms were less intrusive and she stopped having altercations with others; she became calmer but also sadder and seemed able to start mourning the childhood she never had. She had become able to listen herself and spoke of feeling listened to for the first time. She spoke of experiencing occasional feelings of happiness as a new experience and she started to write poetry.

Psychiatrists and mental health staff may all be familiar with similar cases where highly disturbed and symptomatic psychological states and behaviours can settle within the context of a containing relationship with staff. Ms V hadn't engaged in formal psychotherapy and at times was involved with several services simultaneously. The constant factor was the working relationship with the therapist, who had been consistent, reliable, and able to tolerate the ebbs and flows in Ms V's levels of fear and capacity to think

Klein described the process of containment of intense emotional states and recognized how the careful attention of the mother allows the infant to move from states of high arousal and anxiety to quieter states of mind. The infant depends upon the mother to take in his emotional state fully and communicates using all forms available to him or her; verbal, non-verbal, and unconscious processes. These include psychological mechanisms familiar to mental health teams such as projection, by which intense emotional states are felt powerfully by the other as a form of unconscious communication, and splitting, by which good and bad experiences are kept apart, thus preventing excessive anxiety from preventing a good attachment.

These ideas were elaborated further by the psychoanalyst Wilfred Bion who described how raw forms of unprocessed emotional experience are projected forcibly into the caregiver for emotional digestion.[4] If the care is sufficiently nurturing, the caregiver is able to process and return the emotional experience to the infant in a more manageable state. Under good enough conditions, the anguished screams of a baby in distress or pain are soothed by a mother who responds with a degree of urgency but not panic; this enables the baby to progress from a state of fragmentation and terror to a state of integration. A containing mother is not overwhelmed but is aware of the degree of distress and knows what to do. This is the bedrock of emotional development.

These processes persist in adult life. Under conditions of high anxiety, we too can fragment, lose the capacity to think, and become overwhelmed with emotion. At such times we need the attuned mind and empathic responses of another to bring us back to ourselves. The experience of being with Ms V seemed at times to be in contact with and share a state of terror beyond words in which it seemed that raw pieces of traumatic experience and emotion were forcibly projected into the therapist. The task of the therapist was to recognize the terror and confusion without being overwhelmed, while continuing to think: the process of containment. This process, repeated many times in the sessions, led eventually to a quieting of anxiety and integrated state of mind; Ms V's fragments of writing became poems.

Concave and the Convex: Rejection at the Lap

I have described how maternal function, like the physical lap, requires the maternal mind to work as a concave receptacle, able to gather a range of communications and signals, expressed physically, verbally, and through projective processes. The concave receptacle is able to recognize and absorb these signals and respond as needed by the infant so that raw distress, physical and emotional pain, confusion, states of anxiety and calm are given meaning and returned as identified and manageable states. These processes are observable in the ordinary interactions between mother and infant; the calm but timely response to cries, the enquiry into what the matter is, and conveying understanding through touch, words, tone of voice, and action. The response needs to reflect back what is being communicated, but not too quickly; to bounce back, for example, by reacting with excessive anger or anxiety can exacerbate a state of fear or distress. Similarly, responses such as an emotional blankness or being overwhelmed leaves the infant alone with all the confusion and intensity of their anxiety and distress. The mind of the other needs to neither under- or overreact, and the carer needs to be attuned to what the infant can manage and bear.

In contrast to the concave function of the maternal lap and mind, a convex surface cannot take in or make itself available to engage with the other. Its capacity to absorb signals is limited; it bounces back rather than absorbs. As mental health services function under situations of financial or other pressures, strict criteria and higher thresholds for accessing services can invite staff teams to function as convex rather than concave receptacles. This limits the capacity of the team to enquire into the underlying causes of the patient's disturbance and how to understand them. In a convex state of mind curiosity, receptivity, and kindness can be lost, and patients thus encounter both a symbolic and sometimes an actual closed door. The ward round which discusses only management, the locked door of the nurses' station, repeated assessments and re-ferrals on to yet another service are all ways in which services can function as convex surfaces, defending what is behind the boundary rather than being receptive to com-munications from the outside. These processes are heightened in situations of staff pressure, when teams may be organized along rigid diagnostic lines and when there is a lack of opportunity to reflect about the work.

Patients presenting to mental health services need their emotional states to be recog-nized, understood, and contained. Key to this is the development of a relationship with the staff team that seeks to make sense of some of their experiences and sees under-standing as the foundation of care and recovery. This work can be highly challenging. As with all forms of relating there are unconscious factors at play. Communication may be expressed verbally (although the contents of what is described can seem bizarre), non-verbally (such as odd behaviour, self-harm, or aggression), and/or projected through the emotional impact of the patient's disturbance on staff (the countertransference).

Many patients presenting to mental health services have experienced high degrees of disorganized, abusive, cruel, and neglectful early care; it is not surprising that this correlates with a higher susceptibility to psychological breakdown. Within mental health services we frequently see how early and problematic patterns of relating are re-enacted throughout adult life and we find that the feelings elicited in the staff team by the patient can be key to understanding how these unconscious pressures from the past can powerfully mold present experience. If the countertransference is seen as an attempt to communicate then it can be a rich source of material which can lead to a fuller understanding of harmful patterns of repetition in adult life while avoiding being drawn into further enactments of these patterns.

The Risk-Management Panel and the Maternal Lap

If mental health services provide opportunities for staff to reflect about their work, then the capacity of the teams to engage fully with their patients is enhanced. One such resource in my own organization is a Trust risk-management panel at which patients who present high levels of risk to themselves or others can be discussed. The panel is composed of senior managers from clinical backgrounds, a consultant medical psy-chotherapist, a consultant psychiatrist, and the Trust security officer, an ex-policeman. The process of curious enquiry into the patient's background and the feelings elicited in the team by the patient leads to a formulation of the case that can allow new ways of understanding how behaviours have developed as well as their function and meaning. This can help to relieve staff from situations of intense clinical anxiety and impasse; it could be said the panel acts as a maternal lap for the staff team, supporting them to think carefully about the case in order to work out what the underlying problem may be and what to do about it. Countertransference reactions in the team can be explored and this can reduce the likelihood of management decisions being based on an uncon-scious reaction to the patient's presentation, which may contain pressures to repeat what has previously occurred in the past as the following case illustrates.

Mr B was a 19-year-old man born to a drug-addicted mother who was reported to also have a psychotic mental illness. His father left when he was a baby and he was taken into care at two years of age due to neglect whilst in the care of his mother. Mr B's aggressive behaviour resulted in multiple failed placements with foster families and children's homes. He was deemed unmanageable and difficult to place by the age of eight, and was moved between different institutions including secure children's homes and residential psychiatric placements in adolescent units due to his violent and self-destructive behaviour; at times he seemed to be psychotic and substance misuse added to his problems. As soon as he turned 18 he was no longer eligible for children's services and was referred to adult services.

Mr B's relationships with psychiatric services were characterized by confusion and conflict. He did not meet the clear diagnostic categories or the typical behavioural patterns required by the current configuration of adult psychiatric services. He regularly used a wide range of drugs and at times drank heavily; he was self-destructive, impulsive, and chaotic, and spoke of hearing voices of abusive men and vulnerable children. At times, he seemed to identify with these abusive figures and he could be violent and abusive to both staff and other patients. It was unclear if he had a psychotic illness, whether drug addiction was his main problem, or if the fundamental problem was an underlying personality disorder.

Mr B's first referral into adult services resulted in a series of assessments with a psychiatrist working in a service for young adults with psychotic illnesses. He engaged well with the assessment and seemed to get on with the psychiatrist who was deeply puzzled by his escalating risky behaviour which culminated in a serious overdose at the end of the assessment process. The high level of risk and anxiety amongst staff lead to his being presented at the Trust risk-management panel, which allowed a full and detailed discussion of the case.

What emerged from this meeting was the discrepancy between the team's view that telling Mr B that he didn't, in their view, have a psychotic illness and therefore did not require ongoing care from their team, was good news, and their bewilderment at his subsequent suicidal reaction to this news. This in turn led to the breakdown of his relationship with members of the team who felt betrayed by his actions. The team felt they had fully explained the assessment process and possible outcomes to Mr B, who had seemed to accept their rational explanation of the service's referral criteria. As a result of this diagnosis-based decision, Mr B was not eligible for treatment in this team; he would instead be referred to another service deemed more suitable.

This is a clinical scenario that many of us will find familiar. Complex cases such as this young man are often difficult to place, leading to their being referred repeatedly between services organized along diagnostic and at times rigid guidelines, without quite meeting the criteria of any of them. The pull of the countertransference towards a patient who has experienced multiple rejections can amplify the process meaning that the MHT continues to re-enact this pattern of rejection and failed placements. This is an unconscious process which can be supported by rational-seeming arguments about diagnostic criteria or thresholds of entry which the patient must meet in order to receive care. The organization acts as a convex boundary and the rejected child becomes the unplaceable patient.

The risk-management panel provides an opportunity to reflect, away from the clinical pressures facing the clinical teams. In the view of the panel, Mr B 's response could be understood in terms of the relationship he had formed with the psychiatrist and team and the rejection he felt at this news; it could only be understood in relational terms. Given his early history of rejection by both parents, disrupted attachments, and repeatedly failed placements, it was of prime importance that psychiatric services recognized the pressures which could continue to re-enact these early relationships. After discussion with the team, the management was changed; it was agreed that the team needed to work with him over the longer term, avoiding as much as possible further failed placements and rejections. The underlying emotional and relational issues were paramount and the unclear diagnostic issues increased the risk of history repeating itself for this young man who could then continue to be deemed 'impossible to place' within the MHT. Thus, the pattern of harm would be re-enacted by well-meaning services who nevertheless were not addressing the deeper meaning these processes had for this patient.

In this instance, the organization risked behaving as a rejecting and unavailable maternal lap, unable to recognize either the nature of the distress or the need to hold such a disorganized and chaotic patient securely. The team's initial response was not sufficiently attuned to the underlying anxieties and experiences. Helpfully, the team also recognized their discomfort and brought the case to the risk panel to allow more reflection; all mothers need support and similarly so do mental health teams when pressures and anxieties become excessive and their own capacity to think under pressure is challenged.

Psychiatric Services, the Total Transference, and the Brick Mother

One strength of psychiatric training is the value placed on taking a detailed personal history from our patients and from other sources when available. However, there is a risk that the biographical information gathering leads to a belief that the past can be addressed adequately at a verbal and rational level. At the same time, we know as clinicians that our patients can present with a vast range of symptoms and behaviour that defies rational explanations or justifications. This can be most marked in how patients relate and respond to clinical staff and mental health services, and it is crucial we are able to tune into the unconscious processes in order to understand our patients' experiences.

Mrs M, aged 88, was admitted to a psychiatric ward for older adults for observation and investigation of memory problems. A previously mild-mannered woman, she became acutely distressed and aggressive on the ward; staff reported her responding to their approaches as if they were a threat to her, and at times she was violent towards them. Her family were shocked by this behaviour which was entirely new; they did report, however, that she had grown up in a children's home and had never spoken of her experiences there. Possible organic causes, such as dementia particularly affecting her frontal lobes, were considered but investigations were inconclusive and it seemed to make more sense to consider the meaning of this behaviour as a possible repetition in her mind of her earliest experiences in the care system in which perhaps she had been treated with violence or experienced abuse. The feelings she elicited in staff seemed most important in trying to understand her behaviour; they felt as if they represented danger to her and the intention to cause harm.

Discussion of this behaviour as having such a meaning enabled the team to think about addressing it differently, to provide concrete explanations about why they were approaching her with reassurances they would not harm her and were there to help. This seemed to settle the behaviour and she become very tearful on the ward, allowing staff to comfort her.

It seems in the cases described so far that a present situation was being responded to as if it were the actual past, be it abandoning, threatening, dangerous, and so on. The psychoanalyst Betty Joseph[5] wrote about how everything of importance in the patient's life will be lived out in some way in the transference relationships created in the present and saw transference as a ubiquitous, living, and shifting process that she termed the 'total transference'. This is not a conscious process but it powerfully shapes how all of us relate to events, people, and organizations in the present through the lens of earliest formative experiences. The psychiatrist and psychoanalyst Henri Rey coined the term 'the Brick Mother'[6] to describe the importance of the hospital building itself as representing safety and stability to patients frightened about mental fragility and breakdown; it is the nature of this mother which I am trying to explore in this chapter.

Behaviour, Symptoms, and Meaning

Psychiatry can be practised in such a way that prioritizes the eliciting of information for diagnostic purposes rather than considering the meaning of symptoms. This could be thought of as an emotionally detached mother able to tick off symptoms such as crying or screaming in her child and responding rather mechanically with food and shelter—essential to provide but in not seeking to understand why the distress has arisen at that point the meaning of the response and behaviour has been lost. In contrast, if we seek meaning in even the most bizarre seeming symptoms, we can more adequately understand the anxieties underlying the disorder as the following case illustrates.

Ms T was an in-patient on a psychiatric ward with a psychotic illness; both her parents had schizophrenia and her young sons had been taken into care two years previously as she was unable to look after them safely. On the ward she was preoccupied by how unjustified this was in her view, and frequently requested that the staff arrange for her to see her children. When a supervised access visit was arranged, however, she refused to go, saying she wasn't prepared to see her children until staff had arranged for their return to her care permanently, an unrealistic proposition which effectively meant not seeing her sons at all. She then took to her bed saying she had pain due to all the cracked eggs in her ovaries. Staff felt frustrated and helpless, but after discussing this new symptom in supervision, her key nurse was able to recognize it as a communication of her anxiety that her sons, like her, were 'cracked' and damaged by her, an anxiety she couldn't bear. The nurse was able to make sense of Ms T's feelings and was able to talk to the patient about how the children were doing in reality, directly addressing the anxieties that lay behind the psychotic belief. The rational explanations Ms T gave had disguised this anxiety which emerged in symbolic form as a psychotic symptom.

Ms T was visibly relieved and settled when she felt understood. The team arranged visits under more open conditions which were unlikely to be agreed to and equally likely to be cancelled again if Ms T's anxieties had remained unchanged.

In this chapter, I hope to have described how the MHT can act as a receptacle for patients' emotional states linked with their experiences of early nurture, intensified at times of crisis, and, through the transference directed to their clinical teams, to be understood and contained. These processes mirror the response needed by the infant on the maternal lap. This task requires staff to feel listened to and understood, and this chapter has described how this can be embedded in mental health work in order to provide services which are best able to promote recovery and psychological growth. Psychiatric training now recognizes the crucial role of careful reflection about our work which is now enshrined in our training and lead by medical psychotherapists.

References

1. **Freud S** (1911). Psychoanalytic notes on an autobiographical account of a case of paranoia (Dementia paranoides). In: *Standard Edition of the Complete Psychological Works of Sigmund Freud*, Vol **XII**. London: Vintage, pp. 3–79.
2. **Mitchell J** (ed.) (1998) Notes on some schizoid mechanisms. In: *The Selected Melanie Klein*. London: Vintage. pp. 1–24.
3. **Segal H** (1973). *Introduction to the Work of Melanie Klein*. London: Hogarth Press.
4. **Bion W** (1962). *Learning from Experience*. London: Heinemann.
5. **Joseph B** (1985). Transference the total situation. *International Journal of Psychoanalysis* **66**:447–54.
6. **Steiner J** and **Harland R** (2011) Experimenting with groups in a locked general psychiatric ward. *Psychoanalytic Psychotherapy* **25**(1):16–27.

Chapter 11

Historical Child Sexual Abuse

Joanne Stubley, Victoria Barker
and Maria Eyres

In this chapter we describe three aspects of Historical Child Sexual Abuse (HCSA):

◆ The historical perspective in relation to psychiatry/psychotherapy's response to the issue.
◆ The role of the mother in HCSA
◆ The aftermath of HCSA; the request by the patient for a gender-specific therapist

Historical Perspective

One may wonder why historical child sexual abuse HCSA is an issue that requires a chapter in its own right in a book entitled *Women's Voices*. Current evidence suggests that sexual abuse occurs much more frequently to girls than boys although there is considerable recognition of under-reporting for boys. The majority of the perpetrators are male.[1] These statistics suggest that this is predominantly a crime of men against women and often takes place within the family. It took the feminist political movement of the 1970s to give voice to the violence perpetrated by men within the setting of patriarchal dominance, and this allowed for a greater societal recognition of both domestic violence and child sexual abuse.

In this chapter we hope to demonstrate how the nature of this form of trauma impacts upon society in such a way that it has been repeatedly denied or disavowed. This in turn has influenced how psychiatry and psychoanalysis have responded to a history of childhood sexual abuse in their patients.[2,3] One may make use of a psychoanalytic understanding of trauma also to conceptualize the repeated instances where these professions have become embroiled in bitter, polarized debates and conflicts centred on child sexual abuse.

It is in the very nature of trauma that the capacity to symbolize or to use words to think about the traumatic event is impaired. The process of symbolization has been described by psychoanalysts as a capacity to be sufficiently separate from important others that one can use temporary replacements for the other. Thus, the symbol can truly represent the thing it symbolizes. Perhaps the most obvious symbols are words which stand for, represent, and describe the thing they symbolize. Trauma inevitability disrupts the capacity to use words in this way, rendering them instead as something more concrete and sometimes confused with what they are meant to describe.

As an example, a traumatized woman who had been assaulted with a knife could no longer use that word because when she did, she physically felt the knife once again on her neck.

Trauma overwhelms, fragments, and renders one helpless in the storm of powerful anxieties of annihilation, persecution, and dread. The psychological defences employed to attempt to survive the psychic threat will inevitably also be powerful. These include splitting, denial, projection, projective identification, and dissociation. We will describe these further.

In the normal course of development, the way in which an infant attempts to manage unbearable anxieties such as annihilation and disintegration is to employ the technique of 'splitting' to separate their feelings and experiences into categories of very good and very bad. In this way, feelings and experiences can feel more manageable and it is only gradually, as the mind develops, that it can begin to integrate its view of the world. As development continues, there is a gradual acceptance, all being well, that most feelings and experiences in life are mixed, which is a more mature and healthy way of perceiving oneself and others. The other major defence mechanism that holds sway in these early times is projective identification. What this essentially means is that what is unbearable is split off and evacuated into the mind of another. This has an impact on the other.

The polarized viewpoints representative of splitting are repeatedly found within the arena of childhood sexual abuse. They have been fought over in the clinical field and in the court room. One is invited to 'take a side'—external trauma versus internal conflicts or false versus recovered memory being two examples where choices become presented as either/or, with no room for a more integrated or nuanced approach.

The roots of such black-and-white thinking in relation to HCSA can be traced to Freud's initial conceptualization and his subsequent turning away from it. When Freud published 'The aetiology of hysteria' in 1897,[5] 18 cases of hysteria were described in detail, and in all cases he reported there was evidence of childhood sexual abuse. This led to Freud describing his seduction theory where he proposed that these cases of hysteria were aetiologically linked to previous experiences of childhood 'seduction'. This was a bold claim to make for a neurologist striving to establish his reputation and pursue a career in repressed Viennese society. Freud was already showing considerable daring in his 'talking cure', whereby he suggested that the doctor should listen to his hysterical patients—a novel and untried form of treatment in that era. Much has been written about Freud subsequently turning away from his seduction theory to his theory of infantile sexuality and the Oedipus complex with the psychoanalytic focus on psychic reality. Reports of child sexual abuse were therefore interpreted as fantasies driven by the adult's unconscious wishes.

The literature on this particular issue serves to demonstrate the marked polarities of opinion that repeatedly emerge on the topic of HCSA where one is asked to choose between extremes. Jeffrey Masson's book, *The Assault on Truth*,[6] suggests that Freud, through a form of moral cowardice, turned his back on the pervasive reality of child sexual abuse in Viennese society. Many psychoanalysts would vehemently refute this claim, emphasizing that Freud never wholly rejected the notion of the seduction theory; rather, he shifted focus, with his assertion that the neuroses were aetiologically embedded in unconscious fantasies.

Sandor Ferenczi, a prominent psychoanalyst close to Freud, provoked considerable consternation and debate when he presented his paper, 'Confusion of tongues between adults and the child', in 1932.[9] In this presentation he emphasized the pathological consequences of early sexual trauma, highlighting his belief in the greater frequency of these abuses than had been previously recognized and the profoundly disturbing consequences to the child who suffers such abuse. Many professionals working now within the field of HCSA would recognize a great deal of what Ferenczi described and yet this paper failed to reach publication in English until 1949, and he was personally ostracized by the psychoanalytic community.[9]

The repetition of these kinds of responses over the last 100 years may also be understood through the consideration of Freud's concept of the repetition compulsion. It is also important to note that these theoretical discoveries by Freud came out of an acknowledgement of external trauma in the form of the First World War. It highlights his capacity to hold both internal psychic life and external reality in mind when seeking to better understand the difficulties his patients described to him.

In 'Remembering, repeating and working through', published in 1914, Freud observed that some patients had an urge to repeat in action continuously, rather than consciously remember, difficult early experiences that had been forgotten and repressed.[11] Freud also saw the repetition compulsion as an attempt to gain mastery over the original trauma by turning previous passivity into activity. The unbearable nature of helplessness, a central feature in any traumatic experience, urges action, and one form of action is through the repetition compulsion. Through repetition of a traumatic experience, one can choose at an unconscious level to identify with different aspects of the traumatic scenario—victim, perpetrator, rescuer, and witness. Through the psychological defense of projective identification, relational events require taking up one of these positions unconsciously, endlessly repeating the essence of the trauma in action.

Messler, Davies, and Frawley suggest that in HCSA one can see, at a societal level, a repetition of the four positions of victim, perpetrator, saviour, and uninvolved/denying other which are also endlessly played out unconsciously.[8] This links with the nature of traumatic memory; the dissociation that occurs leads to the paradox of knowing and not knowing. The traumatized individual cannot remember in a truly symbolic, autobiographical manner and yet through the repetition of the re-experiencing symptoms—endless flashbacks and intrusions, traumatic nightmares—also cannot forget. Through the repetition compulsion, the traumatic scenario is unconsciously endlessly re-enacted within the various identifications. Within the professional working with the patient or the profession working in the field or society living with the issues, these repetitions evoke powerful feelings and responses, and inevitable actions and reactions are set in motion.

The paucity of publications on child sexual abuse within both psychiatry and psychoanalysis, alongside other mental health areas, for much of the first half of this century was reflected in the broader silence in society regarding the extent and the impact of sexual abuse. Moral welfare workers, working with vulnerable children largely in a voluntary capacity prior to the Second World War, emphasized maternal incompetence and 'mental deficiency' (of mother, victim, and abuser) in explaining cases of abuse. Abusers were termed 'deranged or unbalanced', with an increasing move towards viewing abusers as needing medical treatment rather than punishment.[10] Abused children were often seen as feeble-minded as well as sexually precocious.

A review in 1957 of child sexual assault in the magazine *Moral Welfare* described a forensic psychiatrist's opinion that in many cases there was de facto consent, and some children either did not realize the nature of the act or were indifferent to it. A 1963 study, 'Child victims of sex offence', asserted children's tendency to lie about abuse. It also suggested it was often a problem within the family, specifically mother's jealousy and envy of her daughter which caused the problem.[30] One may see this as a societal identification with the uninvolved, denying other where the child's experience is denied and invalidated.

The 1970s saw increasing media coverage of HCSA with a greater recognition of its reality in society. The reasons for this are multifaceted and may include a more sexualized culture, an increasingly child-centric view in education, justice, and leisure, and an increasingly outspoken press. However, Judith Herman,[12] a prominent psychiatrist in the United States working in the field of trauma, has suggested that it took feminism to allow these women's voices to be heard. It is her contention that the systematic study of trauma requires a political movement for support. With women's groups evolving and growing, the evidence regarding the existence of sexual and domestic violence became increasingly difficult to ignore. Herman was responsible for coining the term 'complex trauma' to describe a constellation of symptoms seen in repeated and sustained trauma due to captivity. She encompassed the experience of veterans alongside those women subjected to repeated domestic violence and adult survivors of childhood sexual abuse. With the link to the growing anti-war movement following the Vietnam War, the psychiatric diagnosis of post-traumatic stress disorder finally emerged in the 1980s in the *Diagnostic and Statistical Manual of Mental Disorders.*[13] This marked a new level of recognition and respectability for 'trauma' linked to an increasing acknowledgement of childhood sexual abuse.

The impulse to turn away from this reality remains very powerful, however. In 1980, the leading American textbook of psychiatry still claimed that incest occurred in less than 1 in 1 million women and that its impact was not particularly damaging.[14]

Research in this area only began in earnest in the mid-1980s and has been plagued by practical issues around data collection, prevalence rates, false positives or negatives, and barriers to disclosure. Nevertheless, large-scale population studies such as the Adverse Childhood Experiences Study[3] demonstrate a disclosure of 21 per cent of the general population for childhood sexual abuse. Alfred Kinsey's well-known study on female sexual behaviour in the United States in 1953 showed similar figures cited for HCSA experiences, and yet virtually no interest was shown in this statistic, although the figures for premarital sexual activity and adultery provoked public outcry.[4]

Perhaps one of the starkest examples of the polarized battles and the enactments of traumatic scenario is in the recovered/false memory debate that raged within the American psychiatric system and spilled over into vociferous legal battles in the 1990s. These centred on claims of women who, during psychotherapy, had apparently recovered memories of abuse which were usually familial in nature. In March 1992, the False Memory Syndrome Foundation (FMSF) was established in the United States by Ralph Underwager, Hollida Wakefield, Pamela Freyd, and Peter Freyd. The Freyds publicly alleged that their adult daughter had wrongly accused her father of sexual abuse. The daughter, Professor Jennifer Freyd, a cognitive psychology expert, then spoke publicly for the first time. She had consulted a mainstream clinical psychotherapist for problems including promiscuity, anorexia, drug abuse, and feelings of shame, guilt, and terror. Memories of abuse had apparently begun to emerge in the second session. In speaking out against her parents, Jennifer Freyd had not given details of these memories but had provided a graphic description of a family life dominated by intrusion, control, manipulation, and constant crossing of sexual boundaries. She subsequently published a book, *Betrayal Trauma: The Logic of Forgetting Childhood Sexual Abuse* (1996).[37] In this book, she described how amnesia for the abuse may serve as an adaptive response, allowing a dependent child to remain attached to her abusive caregiver.

Many repetitions of the scenario where a father is accused by his grown-up daughter of childhood sexual abuse ensued. The parents report a memory of a happy family life whilst the daughter describes an intrusive, boundary-less atmosphere. Therapy is sought for non-specific problems but memories of abuse begin to emerge. Through legal channels the battle takes place, increasingly in the public domain. Therapists are sued for the implantation of false memories whilst fathers are accused of abuse within the legal and public arena. The polarity of the battle is defined by the publication of 'The Memory Wars', by Frederick Crews,[7] where two essays, originally written for the *New York Review of Books* are reprinted with many powerful letters in response. Battle lines were drawn up and one was required to choose a side—real or imagined, false or recovered, father or daughter—who was to be believed?

The struggle to acknowledge the reality of abuse and the wish to turn away from something so infused with shame, guilt, and intrusive aggression continues to be played out in the present day. In the repeated delay, due to loss of several chairpeople, of the government's Independent Enquiry into Institutional Childhood Sexual Abuse the wish again to turn away, deny the reality, and return to societal amnesia as a means of maintaining attachment to institutions of authority.

The Children's Commissioner Report on Childhood Sexual Abuse published in 2015 estimates 450,000 cases of sexual abuse in children took place in England from 2014 to 2016.[1] In the same period, only 50,000 cases were known to statutory agencies. Whilst the figures are disturbing, particularly in relation to the estimation of cases where the abuse may be continuing, the existence of this report, with its clear agenda for action from the government, serves to demonstrate that child sexual abuse is currently increasingly visible within our society. Indeed, the media reporting of high-profile celebrities found guilty of HCSA in recent times, most notably Jimmy Saville, alongside investigations and enquiries into institutional abuse from within the church, social care, sports clubs, and private education serves to keep child sexual abuse to the forefront of our minds.

There is considerable evidence now that those with psychiatric illnesses experience a much higher incidence of HCSA.[15] It is seen in a wide variety of disorders including depression, anxiety, post-traumatic stress disorder, substance abuse and dependence, eating and personality disorders, particularly borderline personality disorder.[31]

The publication of the next edition of the European psychiatric classification—the *International Classification of Diseases* (ICD 11) —is imminent. It is said to contain the new diagnosis of complex post-traumatic stress disorder (PTSD) which will draw on Judith Herman's original description of complex trauma, based on survivors of sexual abuse. It is likely that this will lead to a further crisis point in the history so far described, a moment in which the acknowledgement of the reality of HCSA may be debated by the mental health system as a new perspective on diagnosis, based on the presence of traumatic events rather than symptoms alone, may be required.

The Role of the Mother and Child Sexual Abuse

It is the custom of every good mother after her children are asleep to rummage in their minds and put things straight for next morning, repacking into their proper places the many articles that have wandered during the day. If you could keep awake (but of course you can't) you would see your own mother doing this, and you would find it very interesting to watch her. It is quite like tidying up drawers. You would see her on her knees, I expect, lingering humorously over some of your contents, wondering where on earth you had picked this thing up, making discoveries sweet and not so sweet, pressing this to her cheek as if it were as nice as a kitten, and hurriedly stowing that out of sight. When you wake in the morning, the naughtinesses and evil passions with which you went to bed have been folded up small and placed at the bottom of your mind; and on the top, beautifully aired, are spread out prettier thoughts, ready for you to put on.
JM Barrie[36]

While stemming from a bygone era, the image that Barrie paints of a mother who knows her children so intimately that she can delve into their minds and tidy away anything unsavoury that she finds somehow still echoes in current views of motherhood. It suggests that any mother should be able to tell if her child is being abused, but also that she doesn't want to hear any unpleasantness that occurs in her children's lives and wants to pack it away with other 'evil passions'. Airing children's experiences is reserved for prettier thoughts and experiences. What is implicit here is that when a child has suffered from sexual abuse and the mother does not recognize what is going on, she is either a bad mother who can't see inside her child's mind or she knew about the abuse and was colluding with the abuser, not least in placing it at the bottom of her own mind. Indeed, the idea that the mother is somehow complicit in the abuse of her child goes back a long way.

After renouncing his seduction theory in 1897, Freud went on to develop his ideas on the Oedipus complex. The blame for seduction moved from the perpetrator to the child with the idea that scenes of infantile sexual trauma are derived from phantasy and not from actual events. In his later work, Freud came to see the mother as the instigator of sexual trauma through early genital contact in her ministrations to the child:

And now we find the phantasy of seduction once more in the pre-Oedipus prehistory of girls; but the seducer is regularly the mother. Here however, the phantasy touches the ground of reality, for it was really the mother who by her activities over the child's bodily hygiene inevitably stimulated, and perhaps even roused for the first time, pleasurable sensations in her genitals. Freud[16]

'By the care of the child's body, [the mother] becomes its first seducer.'[17]

Thus, the mother is accused of abusing her child even in the act of caring for her. However, most mothers are not involved in or complicit with the abuse and do not know that their child is being abused due to the abuser's high level of manipulation of both adults and children. The abuser grooms not only the child but also the non-abusing parent so as to minimize the risk of detection. The abuser may also insidiously drive a wedge between the non-abusing parent and the child in order to make the child more dependent on him and to limit the opportunity for disclosure.[18] In father–daughter incest, daughters feel emotionally abandoned by both parents and comply with their father's sexual demands out of dread of actual desertion; they view women's roles as depreciated and self-sacrificing.[19] Responsibility is removed from the abuser and placed on the mother when focus lands squarely on her shoulders. The consequence of this is that the mother is made to feel guilty for the sexual abuse of her child.

The theme of maternal absence is a common one in the context of childhood sexual abuse and the mother of the sexual abuse victim has, in the past, been represented as cold, deficient in maternal love, distracted, and unable to hear and respond to her child's distress. In his seminal work on the consequences of early sexual trauma, Ferenczi writes:

Usually the relation to a second adult ... the mother—is not intimate enough for the child to find help there, timid attempts towards this end are refused by her as nonsensical.[9]

This picture of the mother of the abused child as absent and uncaring, complicit in the abuse in order to avoid the intrusions of her partner or, frankly, abusive herself, has been widely accepted. There is a lack of recognition that this is not always the case, nor are attempts made to understand the circumstances which lead a mother to be unable to protect and prioritize her child, something that would seem to be natural under normal conditions.

It is important to understand why a mother might be absent, distant, or respond negatively to disclosure of child sexual abuse. It may be due to the grooming described earlier or to the common observation that the mothers in families where there is sexual abuse tend to be unwell mentally or physically and so are unable to be emotionally available. This may result in a 'role reversal', where the daughter takes on the obligations of the mother and the mother is then blamed for abdicating her responsibilities.[20] Whatever the cause of this distance, it is important to note as emotional alienation between mother and daughter increases the risk of sexual abuse to the girl.

The majority of children who experience sexual abuse will disclose it to their mothers if they disclose it at all,[21] and the majority of mothers (60 to 70 per cent) provide some level of support and/or protection to their child when abuse is disclosed.[22] A mother's belief that the abuse has occurred generally rests on the word of the child versus that of the abuser as there is rarely any other evidence of the abuse. Whether or not a mother believes her child is wrought with complexity and reflects the conflict between the mother's valence toward the child and the perpetrator. Although a mother may believe her child's allegation, she may also struggle to believe that her partner, whom she loves, is capable of sexually abusing her child. Ambivalence is normative when the costs of disclosure are high.[23] If she does believe her child she may feel unable to provide support or protection due to her own fear of or financial dependence on the abuser. Mothers who are being psychologically or emotionally abused are more ambivalent and less supportive when their children disclose sexual abuse.[24] Rather than a cold, distant, and uncaring mother, this gives us a picture of a woman who is herself oppressed and victimized and unable to cope with the emotional demands of the situation. It has been found that mothers were less likely to believe and take protective action when they were currently in a sexual relationship with the abuser, and this is particularly the case when her relationship to the abuser is more dependent or intimate.[24] Mothers were also less likely to support and protect their child when they had prior knowledge of the sexual abuse, the child victim exhibited sexualized behaviour, and when they had given birth to their first child before reaching adulthood.[25] Victims of incest consistently receive less support from family members than do victims of extra-familial abuse.

One thing that is clear from the literature is that mothers who have themselves experienced child sexual abuse do not respond more negatively to a child's disclosure of sexual abuse, but maternal substance abuse and social isolation appear to have a mediating effect in the negative responses to disclosure.[26] Other factors found in non-supportive mothers include criminal behaviours and problematic relationships with male partners.[27] A history of disrupted attachment relationships between grandmother and mother, and mother and child, characterize families in which sexually abused children do not receive maternal support, attesting to a trans-generational nature of the influences on maternal response to sexual abuse. Here then is a woman who is powerless, oppressed, abused, and struggling and who may have a difficult relationship with her own mother.

Ambivalence in a mother's response may also be either a defense against or an effect of the traumatic experience of the disclosure of abuse. Mothers of sexual abuse survivors show heightened levels of depression and anxiety and diminished maternal attachment behaviours.[28] All of this is likely to have an impact on the mother's capacity to respond in a supportive and caring manner to her sexually abused child. It does seem that when mothers are aware of sexual abuse and don't act, it is due to their being oppressed and powerless,[29] as stated by Yvonne Tormes of mothers in incestuous families:

> By brutality and by superior initiative, her husband has nullified her roles as wife and mother. Even prior to tolerating incest, she seems to have tolerated an increasing amount of deviant behavior, violent and non-violent from him.[30]

It would seem that one way to understand the turning away of the mother from the abuse of the child echoes something of society's turning away from revelations of child sexual abuse as previously discussed but on a much smaller, more intimate scale. In the face of something so unbearable, the mother and society identify with the helplessness that is central to the traumatic experience as described by Freud (1914)[11], and the intolerable nature of this leads them to take up the role of uninvolved and denying other. However, this is complicated because the mother in these cases is also often confronted with the reality of her own position as helpless victim.

The Request by the Patient for a Gender-Specific Therapist

Response to the adversity of HCSA plays out and can be explored on two main planes; the public one, including the societal, legal, and the political arenas, and a private one, where it can impact on the capacity to relate, which in turn can become apparent in the consulting room.

The societal aspect of HCSA is costly and includes poor relationships with others, domestic violence, marital breakdown, poor educational and employment records, forensic aspects including increased rates of crime and delinquency, as well as substance abuse. It can affect care-giving capacities, and as such lead to safeguarding procedures, including children being taken into care, temporarily as well as permanently.

The personal impact of HCSA can be enormous, on both physical and mental health. Patients have an increased risk of physical health problems such as somatization, chronic pain, and unexplained illness, hypochondriasis, body dysmorphic disorder, frequent or recurrent infections, severe eczema and other skin conditions, autoimmune disorders, increased risk of obesity, Type 2 diabetes, hypertension, heart disease, respiratory disease, and cancer.

It is vital that all health professionals working with those patients are aware of the HCSA potentially underlying those presentations, feel able and equipped to enquire about it, and aware where to refer, should this be a factor. There is a lot to be done to ensure that professionals are trained to the standard required to explore those issues with compassion and professionalism, without embarrassment, and without turning away from the patient.

In terms of mental health, personality disorders, and especially borderline personality disorder, are the most common sequela of child sexual abuse,[31,32] with antisocial and narcissistic personality disorders being less common, followed closely by depression, bipolar disorder, anxiety, social anxiety, obsessive–compulsive disorder (OCD), PTSD, dissociative disorders, eating disorders, substance misuse and addictions, sexual dysfunction, psychotic disorders; child sexual abuse involving penetration has, in particular been identified as a risk factor for developing psychotic and schizophrenic syndromes[33] and self-harm and suicide.

In the therapeutic encounter, individuals who have experienced child sexual abuse frequently present with these. What is often much subtler and more difficult to elucidate is the impact on relationships, including those with health professionals, that historical child sexual abuse may have. We want to explore one aspect of this in relation to an action that may occur before the therapeutic encounter has even begun.

There is anecdotal evidence that some women with a history of childhood sexual abuse prefer to be seen by female therapists and that requests of this nature are more common in this group of patients on the whole when compared to patients without a history of HCSA.

As mentioned in the opening lines of this chapter, research indicates that the majority of perpetrators are males, which might be a contributing factor in survivors of child sexual abuse requesting gender-specific therapists when seeking psychological help.

We conducted a brief survey in two adult psychological therapies services in two different London Trusts. We received 50 responses from experienced therapists, with a gender ratio of 40:60 male to female. Almost one-third of the therapists estimated that the requests for the gender specific therapist are as frequent as one in ten. The estimation of the whole group was that the female therapist is requested in 95 per cent, with 36 estimating that 85 per cent of the patients requesting a gender-specific therapist presented with HCSA, and 15 per cent with adult sexual assault.

The survey free comments are gathered in the following:

Free Comments

Female patients often claim to get on better with women when they had emotionally difficult relationship with their mothers. Same goes for male patients and their fathers although not as frequently.

Women presenting with a past history of sexual abuse feel more comfortable speaking about this with a female clinician, particularly within ongoing therapy. The issue can be referred to and acknowledged at assessment stage but not in-depth if the assessor is male. Females can often request female therapists in order to explore the impact and experience of sexual abuse in childhood.

I may be wrong; this may be because often the abusers tend to be male (I am aware they can be female also) People will often speak to a female therapist more freely then perhaps a male. But I do think its individual.

Sometimes we have not agreed in the first instance to offer the gender-specific request and with discussion the patient accepts that the gender is also a euphemism for a certain type of understanding that might not be the sole territory of a woman or man.

This is an interesting survey. As a male therapist, I have had referrals in which the female Service User has asked for a female therapist, which is absolutely fine. However, for some Service Users, it can be a really reparative experience to relate to and be helped by a gender linked to the gender of a past abuser. I have also had male Service Users referred who did not want to meet a male due to feeling ashamed disclosing to a male. Again it can be reparative for some to meet a male. It does seem in my experience that male therapists are more questioned than female. I understand that this will be to do with power and the constructions of gender in society. Ultimately I think gender is a basic and simplistic concept if only binary about humans and we are much more complex than the way we look. I look masculine, have a beard, can be strong and yet I have zero interest in football, I am creative and have an affinity with a more bi-gendered identity ... what really then is my gender? ... how can we manage the faulty assumptions of who we are just based on what we look like?

Sometimes it could be helpful to work with a therapist who is of the gender that someone has requested not to have. Though I think this would probably be more so the case in an ongoing piece of work, rather than time-limited.

I feel that we should always try and meet our clients' requests for gender-specific therapy if possible. However, this could reinforce unhelpful ideas about gender. I think it needs to be considered on a case-by-case basis.

Therapists should do their best to accommodate the client's best interest. I have never taken it personally and would not consider it an unreasonable request.

When I was taking patients on for therapy, the issue of therapist gender was not considered because of limited resources.

The results of this brief and limited survey suggest that the requests for gender-specific therapists are indeed more common with patients who have HCSA. Further exploration of what drives these requests as well as what the individual therapists' and the services' responses are to these requests is needed.

Clinical experience suggests that the requests for a female therapist from female patients with HCSA by a male perpetrator are not straightforward and can be made for a variety of reasons. These range from a more benign initial wish for a female figure who can protect and nourish to an attempt to avoid the repetition of the past. They may also be fuelled by unconscious attempts to assert different power dynamics, or be driven by the unconscious drives towards situations where patients feel they are not being protected, or feel aggrieved and in need of retribution.

Some patients may initially hold a very concrete belief that they can only see a female therapist which may suggest a powerful splitting in operation; mother or female being good, father/male bad. For others, the mother/female might be seen as a better or at least 'less bad' option; although the mother/female may have failed to protect her child from the abuse, she may also have been experienced as the only manifestly non-abusive relationship the patient has had.

It is a well-known fact that people relate to others following the patterns which are similar to those established in their early childhood relationships, especially towards their caregivers. In the context of therapy, this is understood as the unconscious phenomenon of transference which is the process of the patient transferring or redirecting their feelings for a significant person from their past to the therapist. In turn, the therapist's feelings towards the patient which emerge in response to transference are known as countertransference. Patient's emotional difficulties can be explored through the magnifying lens of transference/countertransference, leading to increased recognition of patient's unconscious feelings, fears, and desires, making them more conscious and therefore easier to understand and resolve. The past trauma can reveal itself in endless re-enactments when a patient might repeatedly take on any of the four basic positions associated with trauma described by Messler Davies (the abuser, the abused, rescuer, or the witness).[8] As the therapy unfolds, the patients may take on any and all of those positions, and the importance of anticipating these potential re-enactments of the abuse right from the beginning is vital and may require adaptation of the therapeutic technique. The therapist has to be constantly aware of the pulls in these different directions and to monitor their countertransference carefully—not to act out the abuser, but also not the mother turning a blind eye, or the victim. The inevitability of subtle re-enactments needs to be acknowledged. What is vital for the therapist is that they maintain a capacity—through reflective practice in its many different aspects—to become aware of these pulls and pushes to action so that they can be thought about and, in time, brought into the therapeutic work for interpretation. If this is not attended to, the re-enactments might become more concrete, and on occasion they can lead to boundary violations, such as sexual contact between therapist and patient.

There is often a sexualized aspect of the work when the therapist and the patient are, in turn, seduced and seduce each other, which might include presenting tantalizing fragments of traumatic memories and an invitation to take up various roles. Exploitation, coercion, guilt, and shame are other common themes played out in the consulting room, leading at times to enactments which need to be understood and thought about without condemnation and hurrying things along. Supervision for therapists is vital to disentangle and understand transference/countertransference phenomena so that the new patterns of more benign ways of relating can emerge in the therapeutic relationship which, with time, can be generalized to the world outside the consulting room.

The request for a gender-specific therapist might also be understood as an example of an invitation for the therapist to take up a particular position. They might feel seduced into agreeing to the request because to refuse might be felt to be cruel or even sadistic. The experience of powerlessness in childhood sexual abuse can continue long into adulthood;[34] can the request for the gender-specific therapist be understood as a first step on a road of empowerment?

Newirth writes:

> the successful treatment of sexually abused patients involves the development of a positive identity as a woman who can experience herself as sexual and desirable without experiencing guilt, shame, or sadomasochistic relatedness.[35]

Some patients might seek condemnation of the abuser, living lives that are a memorial to how damaged they are, stuck with their grievance against the perpetrator, caught up in an endless cycle of repetition compulsion of taking familiar roles in interpersonal relationships, unable to move on. It is an important insight to recognize that becoming better through the process of therapy doesn't mean the past has changed but that it is possible to work through the abuse and move away from it through better integration of traumatic memories in the presence of the mind of another, a mind that is benign and capable of thinking, something that was not available to the patient in the past.

While having such a mind is not explicitly linked to the gender of therapist but more to their capacity to contain unbearable experiences and help the patient to process them, we need to think further about how to understand these requests in a way that facilitates the initial engagement and does not become a barrier to entering treatment.

Discussion

While both the extent and the aftermath of child sexual abuse in boys are becoming more apparent, the overwhelming majority of those who experience it are female which seems to reflect the patriarchal world we still live in, despite all the achievements of the feminist movement. We have chosen in this chapter to focus on three aspects of HCSA: the history of how psychiatry and psychoanalysis have responded to HCSA in their patients; the role of the mother in child sexual abuse; and the request for a gender-specific therapist by a patient with a history of sexual abuse. This has inevitably left many aspects of this topic unexplored and indeed may demonstrate the many unanswered questions we have raised. We hope, however, to have highlighted a number of issues that we believe are central to understanding the response of the individual, the family, the institution, and society to child sexual abuse.

In using the psychoanalytic trauma paradigm, we have shown how the powerful anxieties that are evoked are defended against through defenses of splitting, projection, and projective identification. Trauma disrupts our capacity to symbolize, to use words to think about and to understand what has happened. When words are not available, action is inevitable, and one form of action that commonly holds sway is through the repetition compulsion. Thus, the traumatic experiences are unconsciously and endlessly repeated, with other individuals invited to take up a role in the victim, rescuer, perpetrator, and denying other positions. The dissociative response to trauma, where it is both known and not known, consciously denied and yet endlessly re-lived, perpetuates this endless cycle. We have attempted to describe something of this in the response at a broader historical level, within the family through the role of the mother, and within the therapeutic encounter by specifically looking at a request for a female therapist.

It is our contention that only through a capacity to reflect, to think about, and to understand in the presence of another, can this cycle be disrupted. This needs to therefore be addressed at all levels: within the therapeutic context, within the institutions of psychiatry and psychoanalysis, and within society more broadly. Only then will the powerful splits and polarizations, the dissociative denial, and the repetitions of abuse be fully acknowledged and addressed.

References

1. **The Children's Commissioner** (2015). Protecting children from harm: A critical Assessment of child sexual abuse in the family network in England and priorities for action. London: The Children's Commissioner.
2. **Fergusson DM, Boden JM, Horwood LJ** (2008). Exposure to childhood sexual and physical abuse and adjustment in early adulthood. *Child Abuse & Neglect* **32**:607–19.
3. **Felitti V** (2002). The relation between adverse childhood experiences and adult health: Turning gold into lead. *The Permanente Journal* **6** (1): 44–7.
4. **Kinsey AC, Pomeroy W, Martin C**, and **Gebhard P** (1953). *Sexual Behavior in the Human Female*. Philadelphia, PA: Saunders.
5. **Freud S.** The aetiology of hysteria. In: Strachey J (ed. and trans). *The Standard Edition of the Complete Psychological Works of Sigmund Freud*, Vol. **3**. London: Hogarth, pp. 191–221.
6. **Masson J** (1984). *The Assault on Truth: Freud's Suppression of the Seduction Theory*. New York, NY: Ballantine Books.
7. **Crews F** et al (1995). *The Memory Wars: Freud's Legacy in Dispute*. London: Granta.
8. **Messler Davies J** and **Frawley M** (1994). The impact of trauma on transference and countertransference. In: Messler Davies J (ed.). *Treating the Adult Survivor of Childhood Sexual Abuse: A Psychoanalytic Perspective*. London: Basic Books.
9. **Ferenczi S** (1933). Confusion of tongues between adults and the child. In: *Final Contributions to the Problems and Methods of Psychoanalysis*. London: Hogarth Press, pp. 156–67..

10. **Delap L** (2015). *Child Welfare, Child Protection and Sexual Abuse 1918–1990.* Policy Papers. History and Policy.

11. **Freud, S** (1914). Remembering, repeating and working-through (further recommendations on the technique of psycho-analysis II. In: Strachey J (ed. And trans). *The Standard Edition of the Complete Psychological Works of Sigmund Freud*, Vol. **XII** (1911–1913). London:Hogarth Press, pp. 145–57..

12. **Herman J** (1992). *Traumatic Disorders Part 1 in Trauma and Recovery.* Pandora.

13. *Diagnostic and Statistical Manual of Mental Disorders V.* Washington, DC: American Psychiatric Association Publishing.

14. Kaplan HI, Freedman AM, and Saddock BJ (eds) (1980). *Comprehensive Textbook of Psychiatry.* Baltimore, MD: Williams and Wilkins.

15. **Read J** (1997). Child abuse and psychosis: A literature review and implications for professional practice. *Professional Psychology: Research and Practice* **28**(5): 448–56..

16. **Freud S** (1933). Femininity. In: Strachey J (ed. and trans). *The Standard Edition of the Complete Psychological Works of Sigmund Freud*, Vol. **23**. London: Hogarth, pp. 112–35.

17. **Freud S** (1940). An outline of psychoanalysis. In: Strachey J (ed. and trans). *The Standard Edition of the Complete Psychological Works of Sigmund Freud*, Vol. **23**. London: Hogarth, pp 141–205.

18. **Sanderson C** (2006). *Counselling Adult Survivors of Child Sexual Abuse*, 3rd edn. London: Jessica Kingsley Publishers.

19. **Van der Kolk BA, Perry JC**, and **Herman JL** (1991). Childhood origins of self-destructive behavior. *American Journal of Psychiatry* **148**:1665–71.

20. **Finkelhor D, Hotaling G, Lewis IA**, and **Smith C.** (1990). Sexual abuse in a national survey of adult men and women: prevalence, characteristics, and risk factors. *Child Abuse and Neglect* **14**:19–28.

21. **Sauzier M** (1989). Disclosure of child sexual abuse. For better or for worse. *Psychiatric Clinics of North America* **12**(2):455–69.

22. **Elliott AN** and **Carnes CN** (2001). Reactions of nonoffending parents to the sexual abuse of their child: a review of the literature. *Child Maltreatment* **6**(4):314–31.

23. **Bolen RM** and **Lamb JL** (2004). Ambivalence of nonoffending guardians after child sexual abuse disclosure. *Journal of Interpersonal Violence* **19**(2):185–211.

24. **Alaggia R** and **Turton JV** (2005). Against the odds: the impact of woman abuse on maternal response to disclosure of child sexual abuse. Journal of Child Sex Abuse **14**(4):95–113.

25. **Pintello D** and **Zuravin S** (2001). Intrafamilial child sexual abuse: predictors of postdisclosure maternal belief and protective action. *Child Maltreatment* **6**(4):344–52.

26. **Leifer M, Shapiro JP**, and **Kassem L** (1993). The impact of maternal history and behavior upon foster placement and adjustment in sexually abused girls. *Child Abuse and Neglect* **17**(6):755–66.

27. **Leifer M, Kilbane T**, and **Grossman G** (2001). A three-generational study comparing the families of supportive and unsupportive mothers of sexually abused children. *Child Maltreatment* **6**(4):353–64.

28. **Lewin L** and **Bergin C** (2001). Attachment behaviors, depression, and anxiety in nonoffending mothers of child sexual abuse victims. *Child Maltreatment* **6**(4):365–75.

29. **Herman JL** (1981). *Father–Daughter Incest.* Cambridge, MA: Harvard University Press.

30. **Tormes Y** (1968). *Child Victims of Incest.* Denver, CO: American Humane Association.

31. **Zanarini MC, Williams AA, Lewis RE, Reich B, Soledad VC, Marino MF, Levin A, Yong L**, and **Frankenburg F** (1997). Reported pathological childhood experiences associated with the development of borderline personality disorder. *American Journal of Psychiatry* **154**:1101–06.

32. **Zanarini MC** and **Wedig MM** (2014). Childhood adversity and the development of borderline personality disorder. In: Sharp C and Tackett L (eds) (2014). *Handbook of Borderline Personality Disorder in Children and Adolescents*. Berlin: Springer, pp. 265–76.

33. **Cutajar MC, Mullen PE, Ogloff JR, Thomas SD, Wells, DL**, and **Spataro J** (2010). Psychopathology in a large cohort of sexually abused children followed up to 43 years. *Child Abuse and Neglect* November; **34**(11):813–22.

34. **Baynard VL, Williams LM**, and **Siegel JA** (2004). Childhood sexual abuse: A gender perspective on context of and consequences. *Child Maltreatment* **9**:223–38.

35. **Newirth J** (1992). 'Psychotherapy with sexually abused patient: The use of countertransference'. Paper presented at the 100th Annual Meeting of the American Psychological Association, Washington DC.

36. **Barrie JM** (1904). *Peter Pan*. Toronto: Broadview Press, pp. 179–272.

37. **Freyd JJ** (1996). *Betrayal Trauma: The Logic of Forgetting Childhood Sexual Abuse*. Cambridge, MA: Harvard University Press.

Chapter 12

Old Age, Women, and Dynamic Psychotherapy

Sandra Evans and Jane Garner

I do not wish them (women) to have power over men; but over themselves.

Mary Wollstonecroft
A Vindication of the Rights of Women, 1792

Myths and Stories

Old age, gender, and psychotherapy are all surrounded by sets of false beliefs. This mitigates against understanding. Gender, age, ethnicity, and class are major dimensions of social inequality in human societies as well as important dimensions of social and individual experience. Though their roots lie in biology, gender and age are both understood within a social context. Carney and Gray[1] conclude that feminist scholarship can be used to unmask the elderly mystique, making the personal political. Women in later life may be seen as compounded of the negative myths which surround the feminine and old age. Superstitiously, women may presage ill fortune. First footing at New Year must be a man; for a woman to be the first to enter the house would bring bad luck for the 12 months to come. Miners and fishermen sense impending disaster if they see an old woman on the way to work. Throughout the world there are beliefs in the demonic power of women to transform men and destroy their potency—the 'femme fatale'. In Homer's Odyssey, Circe, the goddess and enchantress of the island of Aeanea, changed men into swine. The female demon varies in detail around the world but however portrayed, they are particular instances of almost universal misogyny.

In Europe and North America pseudoscientific theory and religious fervour translated this hatred into persecutory and murderous deeds against women who were designated witches.[2] Even in the sophisticated twenty-first century where these ideas are eschewed as primitive notions, the image of the *vagina dentata*, ready to mutilate and castrate remains familiar. Women may have laughed at this over the years but they still carry with them this image of a side of themselves which is dark but which also may be powerful. In classical mythology the three Fates were conceived of as old women at a spinning wheel determining men's life spans and destinies. Clotho draws out the thread of life, Lachesis measures it out, and Atropos cuts it off. There was something terrible and inevitable about them such that they could be considered to be above Zeus in status. This duality of women, the weaker sex but with a dark and powerful side, is evident in religions, pseudoscience, art and literature.[3]

Stories may be entertaining, they also inform our world view and personal relationships. Rossiter[4] discusses the nature of the systematic under-recognition of women's work in science which she calls the 'Matthew–Matilda effect'. Parker and Pollack[5] investigated the same phenomenon in art history. This is not simply to accuse chroniclers of bias and prejudice but rather of being bounded by the ideology of the social definitions of masculinity and femininity. In art, the reverential term 'old master' has no female equivalent. 'Old mistress' has a completely different connotation.[6]

There now exists some attempt to redress this imbalance, at least within academic life, with the introduction of the Athena Swan awards for promoting gender equality;[7] however, the portraits of our male ancestors which adorn the walls of universities outnumber portraits of women by almost ten to one. To experience this as a professional woman without some rancour is nigh on impossible. The most toxic aspect of this kind of writing-out of history is the potential for removing young women's aspirations even before they have started out on their careers. The Athena Swan awards attempt to ensure gender equality is afforded more than 'lip service'. Without an Athena Swan accreditation, universities are unable to apply for certain types of research funding, the very life-blood of their existence.

Simone de Beauvoir[8] makes a distinction between female and woman. For her, the male/female distinction is a bald biological fact with no existential significance. However, the category 'woman' is a philosophical question with underpinnings that exist prior to social and political positioning, with meaning ascribed to facts, part 'facts' about the man/woman distinction: to quote her 'one is not born a woman: one becomes one'.

The man/woman distinction is an asymmetric social situation. Hierarchically, she is described in relation to him. It is not only in academic writing where this is noted. Jane Fonda said 'a man has every season, while a woman has only the right to spring'.[9] This echoes the old saying 'a man is as old as he feels and a woman as old as she looks'.

These cultural notions are intertwined with personal meaning. Individuals and their narratives are located culturally, socially, historically, and situationally.[10] This chimes with one psychodynamic perspective, group analysis, which seeks to understand individuals in the context of our social environments and epochs as well as our early nurturing.[11] That men and women are different is not in dispute; the problem arises when differences are given unequal value—'the weaker sex'—or when opinion of differences leads to restrictive identities when women identify solely with their position in society. Difference between men and women can lead to plurality rather than specificity and lead also to object relationships of mutual value.

On a more positive note, the Royal Shakespeare Company performed a women-only trilogy of Shakespeare's works, including *Julius Caesar*, in London in 2016. The part of the thoughtful elder Brutus[12] was played by Dame Harriet Walter, a woman in her sixties able to don the mantel of the respected sage.

For the first time in centuries, the established order of gender binary is being challenged. It is also moving rapidly from a political to a personal issue with individuals announcing that they are not willing to be labelled as either gender. Liberating for some, confusing for others, the anxious suggest that we are moving towards Sodom and Gomorrah, while others are quoting Plato and suggesting it is the natural decline of a democratic world.

Old age also attracts fables which emerge from and influence deeply ingrained fears and attitudes. Old age rarely attracts positive epithets, usually it is denigratory or patronizing—'grumpy old …', 'boring old …', 'sweet old …'. We praise old people not for ageing well but for seeming younger than their years. This negative perception is reflected in the way older people view themselves. Ageing is a wound to one's narcissism and self-esteem.[3,13] This ageism permeates social, economic, and political life. Demographic change in Europe is seen as a challenge for many policy areas, a burden on the (younger) taxpayer. The problems that the National Health Service (NHS) is said to endure are ascribed to the increasing numbers of old people getting frail and ill. There is a failure to explore the potential benefits of old age but there is also perhaps a lazy and ill-considered knee-jerk response to crises. It is easier to blame the elderly.[14]

By contrast, ageing can and should be associated with increased diversity, creativity, continuing psychological development, and sexuality,[15] but these attributes are rarely recognized among unsubtle derogatory attitudes and age-based stereotyping which affects persons' notions of identity. For Carney and Gray,[1] this stereotyping may take four forms—invisible; needy and helpless (and therefore costly); rich and lazy (and therefore greedy); the wise old man (rarely woman). Hopes that the 'baby boomers' may be able to change this substantially have been dashed recently. Pensioner poverty affects women to a greater extent than it does men. The introduction of a change to pension age, although ultimately aiming for equity between the sexes, has been introduced by the UK government in a chaotic and unfair manner for those born in the 1950s.

Cognitive decline, even dementia, is assumed in old age. Although increasing in incidence with age, dementia does not affect 75 per cent of over 80-year-olds. Our brains decrease in weight and volume by 2 per cent per decade but normal ageing is not a straightforward decline in cognitive function. Lifelong verbal and numeric ability is usually preserved. In late life, well-practised skills show little decline; vocabulary and semantic tasks also tend to be stable. There tends to be lifelong stability with no decline of autobiographical memory even in very old age, including theory-of-mind tasks and implicit memory. Older adults use cognitive resources flexibly, involving novel neural regions.[16]

Psychological Changes

Life-event changes tend to occur at the same time and often with unrelenting frequency. With retirement comes a fixed income, a loss of some social contacts, and a need to shift focus and find a different direction. Working women will undoubtedly experience these losses but will they be any better equipped to reshape their lives after retirement than men? They too may be heavily identified with their professional role sufficiently to question their own usefulness after retirement.[17]

Losing friends and contemporaries at the same time as losing one's parents is another aspect of the challenges of ageing. 'Sniper's alley' was the term used to describe one place in the Bosnian War[18] but could equally be given to the years between 50 and

65, the image of people being picked off one by one. Questioning whether one will be next is as much a spur to reconcile oneself to mortality as it is to remaining active and healthy.

Myths also surround psychotherapy. There is currently a decline in the use of psychotherapy, despite evidence for comparable efficacy with pharmacotherapy[19,20] and an enhanced effect of combining the two. When longer-term follow-up is included, effect sizes are larger suggesting that psychodynamic therapy sets in motion psychological processes that lead to ongoing change even after the end of therapy.[21] Prosser and colleagues write of a deep ideological belief that psychotherapy is a psychosocial treatment whereas pharmacotherapy is a biological treatment, therefore pharmacotherapy is a more scientific and valid way to treat a patient.[22] Modern neuroscience demonstrates that this distinction is a myth. Paradoxically both are biological, as evidenced by brain scanning and neurotransmitter changes and both are psychosocial treatments considering attitudes of prescriber and patient and the placebo/nocebo effect. Drug companies advertise and promote their products whereas no group or organization represents psychotherapy in the same way.[22] Freud was a neurologist. When he launched his metapsychology it was with the idea that neurology and psychology would in time be reunited. Although the evidence is clearly available for this reunion[23] and boundaries have become more blurred,[24,25] clinicians tend to maintain their tribal allegiances.

Other dismissive myths about psychotherapy are that it is a vehicle for absurd mumbo-jumbo or relies on magic: sleight of hand/thought. Neither is true. Psychoanalytic psychotherapy provides a framework in which to understand human situations and a way in which people may take more power/control over their lives. It is based on a theory of development, development which continues throughout the life cycle, each developmental phase being dependent on what has gone before. The child is not only father to the man but also grandfather to the old man. Each phase is a preparation for the next. How one reacts to looking more like one's mother (or grandmother) with age depends on early relationships and identifications. In the final stage, towards the end of life in what TS Eliot identifies as 'last the rending pain of reenactment', the old person will naturally reminisce, taking pleasure from some aspects while also feeling regret at not making enough of life, roads not taken or the wrong one travelled. There is no going back, no rewind button; life is irreversible but there can be reconciliation and forgiveness of the self. Self-forgiveness must begin with a degree of understanding. If that understanding is not possible as a solitary task, or undertaken with a close other, then psychotherapy is likely to help. The aim of psychotherapy is to achieve some understanding. Although each person is unique, frequent themes in therapy with older people may be loss, retirement, and increasing dependence. Some may view death as a persecutory or depressive anxiety,[26] but many come to terms with their own mortality in middle life[27] and accept its inevitability with equanimity. Anticipation of the death of an important other may generate more anxiety because it heralds a renewed state of being alone or may rekindle fears of abandonment. Using psychotherapy to consider transitions or to deal with personal problems was not something sought by older persons two or more decades ago; however, the present day cohort of UK-born elders is a generation used to psychoanalytic language. They have a degree of intrinsic psychological mindedness and demand more of their lives at 65 or 75. Our newfound longevity has pushed forward the anticipated frailty and narrowed lives, and 70 can be seen as a time for new beginnings.

Clinical Illustration

Sheila seeks out psychodynamic psychotherapy at the age of 65. Through her general practitioner (GP), she is referred to an IAPT counsellor (Improving access to psychological therapies, a primary care-based stepped service for NHS psychotherapy), but after six sessions she is referred to a private therapist. Her recent widowhood and new diagnosis of osteoporosis are her motivations for looking to the future which she sees as a 'new phase in life for which she would like to feel prepared'. She feels that her son and daughter are frustrated with her timidity and would like to be a different sort of older woman.

Sheila attends weekly therapy where she brings her sense of loss and grief but also a feeling of incompetence and a lack of worldliness. As the therapy progresses, instead of doing what she had anticipated in her contact with her therapist, she brings her childish self, full of worry and fears about a world which she does not feel she understands well. She revisits her growing up in a post-war Britain of austerity and the conservative societal backlash against competent women. It appears that the vituperative response to women in men's jobs was to challenge their femininity, which had had a corrosive effect on Sheila's confidence and her sense of mastery, which had unfortunately persisted into her adult life.

Sheila eventually understands that her holding on to the incompetence and unworldliness was a false self which she retained in order to be acceptable to the men in her life; her father, her brothers, and her husband.[17] She had avoided competing with any man, no matter how much better she was at the things that she thought mattered. She had even allowed her husband to have a better relationship with their children. Now that he was dead, she found herself to be a resentful and dysfunctional person who did not really know what she wanted or how to get it.

The realization of the impact of years of oppressive masculine conservative culture while she was growing up and how they had molded her response to her life made her angry and upset with herself, but it also enabled her to try something different. She began to live in the moment rather than anticipate further decrepitude. Her therapy ended when she had successfully renegotiated her relationship with her son and daughter and her grandchildren. It was almost as though she had emerged as a near fully formed adult who had had her finishing education/ developmental work in her early 70s rather than in her early 20s. She no longer needed to 'prepare herself for old age'; she just needed to allow herself to complete her growing into an adult, emotionally as well as physically and psychologically.

Modern Ageing

Subjective body image and unrealistic expectations for physical perfection are consuming preoccupations for some women whatever the age.[28] In old age with echoes of adolescence Pines (1993) writes that 'the body resumes its important role in a women's life'.[29] Good health can no longer be taken for granted, 'physical ageing thus under-mines omnipotence'. Pleasurable investment in body image in younger life may turn into hypochondriacal concern in later life. The current generation of older women have undoubtedly benefitted from advances in medicine including the use of anti-biotics, psychotropics, antihypertensives, joint replacements, cataract surgery, diag-nostics, and even cosmetic surgery.

It is rare now to see cases of complicated psychosis as a consequence of hypothyroidism—so-called myxoedema madness.[30] Some of the medical profession are moving towards a less dismissive attitude towards old age; illness and pain are treatable not inevitable. Terms such as 'involutional' and 'climacteric' are no longer in use. Pessimism about depression in old age had been generated by further myths and misconceptions but this is countered by an increase in awareness of its treatability by primary care practitioners. It is also unusual nowadays to see older people presenting to secondary care psychiatry with fulminating depressive psychosis and the need for ECT (Electroconvulsive Therapy) is far less than it was 10 to 15 years ago. The authors put this down, in part at least, to earlier effective treatment of depression in primary care. When severe depression does present, however, it is not true that the illness is symptomatically different, more common, more chronic, more difficult to treat, and more often caused by purely psychological factors than depression in younger per-sons.[31] It can and should be treated with medication and with therapy.

Jung[32] was the first of a number of analysts who observed men moving towards fem-ininity and women towards masculinity. This is seen in some somatic characteristics—greater adiposity in men, increased hirsutism in women—but also psychological phenomena with men becoming more 'effeminate' and women more incisive and de-termined. Stereotypes of masculinity and femininity change with advancing years. The loss of generalizations such as 'men are strong and women are beautiful' may be felt as a personal blow to some people.[3] The experience of different cohorts changes as social and economic aspects of the world change. The post-War 'baby boomers' have a very different life experience from their parents and grandparents. It is also possible that some of this new generation of women were protected from the restrictive stereo-typing by the emergence of feminist ideologies in the 1970 and 1980s. Murphy's (sem-inal paper[33] was inspired by Brown and Harris's work[34] on women in the 1960s and 1970s. Many of the social attitudes, the heterocentric assumptions, the class politics, and the economic drivers no longer pertain, at least in relation to the predominantly Anglo-Saxon city dwellers of the new century. The elderly woman with mental health problems today is older, less paranoid, and less prosaically depressed that the woman of 30 years ago. The factors which precipitate mental illness are more democratically distributed between men and women nowadays, such as job stresses, financial worries, and loss of gainful and meaningful employment. Women are almost as likely as men to be suffering from alcohol-related problems; it is not so strange now for women to purchase alcohol for themselves. Addiction to prescription and non-prescribed drugs affects both sexes.[36] It will also be interesting to observe whether the changing techno-logically enabled connectivity of the twenty-first century will impact on older people's sense of social isolation because of positive benefits of new technologies and social network platforms.

Recently, the purchase of cosmetic surgery seems to be increasing for those not accepting the physical changes age brings who wish to look younger than their years. We have a more hedonistic and individualistic society but at the same time a growing capacity to communicate with others, indicated by the growth of communication through social media. There is an increase in divorce, now more socially acceptable, and therefore an increase in single households. More people, both men and women, live alone. Paradoxically, there is a wish to combine greater independence with greater intimacy. The rates for sexually transmitted diseases are increasing in the over 55s. The Internet is an increasing resource for developing relationships; perhaps it is easier to be more assertive online, but it can also dehumanize and commoditize relationships. The willingness to consider divorce or separation in an intolerably broken relationship has also obviated another phenomenon seen in geriatric psychiatry some 15 to 20 years ago. The presentation of warring partners either as an acute emergency or, more commonly, the escape from relationship toxicity into mental illness, has diminished.[37,38]

The economics of national and family life have recently changed. Older people may stop work to provide unpaid care for grandchildren (and for spouses, and with the increase in life expectancy, also for much older parents). Following a decline in intergenerational living in the twentieth century, now for some there is co-residence with unmarried or divorced children, unable to afford their own home, continuing to live with their parents or move back to the parental home. This arrangement may be a practical and financial solution to difficult times but may not be ideal psychosocially for either generation.

Most commonly middle-aged offspring find themselves in a position where they are caring for elderly parents while still bringing up school-age children. It tends to be the women upon whom this task falls, and in Asian and Eastern European families in the United Kingdom, this may also involve looking after the spouse's parent too.

There are also interesting cultural differences in what constitutes old age. In east London where there are a multitude of cultures and over 47 different languages spoken, women as young as 50 are presenting to memory clinics complaining of forgetfulness and expecting a diagnosis of dementia. Women from specific Bangladeshi and eastern Turkish communities are particularly prominent in this cohort, which has been studied and reported.[39] Inevitably, the majority of these women are actually depressed or deeply unhappy. The striking aspect is the fatalistic view they hold of their world. They generally do not speak the host language, English, are often illiterate, and watch cable TV in their own language. They have little access to the host culture and are separated from their own, most particularly from other women of their age or older with whom they would have had daily contact at home.

Intimacy and Sexuality

Intimacy includes the intrapsychic/internal notion of innermost, to do with self-knowledge, and the interpersonal idea of closest, the product of an interaction. The capacity to relate intimately to another, even into late old age, depends on the matrix mother–infant relationship. Intimacy may or may not include sexuality. Likewise, sexuality may or may not include intimacy.[35] Sexuality is culturally reserved for the young. There is widespread distaste/denial of sexuality in old age. This may be incorporated into the view old people have of their own feelings, fantasies, desires, and themselves. So an asexual old age becomes a self-fulfilling prophecy. This attitude pertains more to older women; the lusty old man can be thought of as a charmer with an eye for the ladies. A number of studies conclude that older people are more sexually active either than previously or was previously known. If thoughts of an asexual old age were to be replaced by new myths of the 'sexy oldie' or 'cougars on the prowl', this would be equally untrue and problematic. Older couples are rarely referred for sexual or relationship therapy. For those who can access help the results are encouraging.[37,38]

Attachment styles described by Bowlby[40] persist into old age and are taken into relationships and marriages. Erikson[41], King,[42] and others have delineated developmental tasks and difficulties to be negotiated for a more successful old age. This includes reworking the marital relationship after children have left home. The childless may experience more complex difficulties. The literature about sexuality in old age is mainly statistics about frequency and quantity. Missing is a sense that an aged person's sexual relationships are in the service of a relationship in which tenderness and affection are significant.[43] There is a need for intimate connectedness, whatever the age or sexual orientation. A continuing sex life may be healing to the painful narcissistic wounds of old age for both men and women.

Intimacy may include genital sexuality but beyond penetration it is also about other physical and emotional closeness, conversation, tenderness, empathy, understanding, sharing, and in old age a knowledge of a decades-long relationship including good times and bad times. There is little correlation between quantity and quality in a sexual relationship. Changes in physiology do not render a meaningful sexual relationship impossible. In addition to an individual perspective, couples co-construct attitudes and behaviour in their relationship. The benefits of a stable and intimate relationship may accumulate over the years, with the couple able to treat and acknowledge each other in ways that are not available to the single person starting anew.

Couples with a relationship based on traditional roles may find difficulty if there needs to be more flexibility about tasks because of the physical exigencies of old age. The woman, who from physical or mental frailty can no longer go to the shops, stand at the cooker, carry a tray, or handle the laundry, may feel redundant and resent her partner taking over. Even if old couples no longer attempt genital sexual contact, they have partnership-long sexual knowledge of each other and still have a sublimated sexual relationship based on day-to-day sharing of intimate behaviours. They trust each other.[35] The capacity for trusting others starts at the beginning of life.

Old age is a time of loss. The death of a spouse as the lost object (the important other who impacts strongly on the emotional life of a person) has been seen as the most stressful of life events.[34] The outcome of the bereavement is dependent on many things, but primarily the quality of the relationship with the deceased and whether the deceased can eventually transform into a nurturing internal object.[35] Women tend to marry men who are slightly older than them and have a greater life expectancy. It is still more acceptable for women to live together. Older widows with a previously totally heterosexual life may seek support, companionship, and also a sexual life from other women in similar situations.

Clinical Illustration

Sylvia, a retired State Registered Nurse (SRN) and ward sister in her late 70s, lives with Geoffrey, a university lecturer who is now approaching his 80th birthday. They have been together for 30 years. He left his marriage for her; Sylvia was married to her career.

Over the most recent 12 months, Geoffrey has become short-tempered, frail, and suspicious of Sylvia's continued independence. He has become intensely concerned that she is having an affair with a younger, more virile man. He imagines it is the butcher. Their relationship has always been exclusive. They had no children from their union and their few friends are also getting old. Their social lives are contracting and the intimacy, which they used to enjoy, seems to be in the distant past, leaving Sylvia feeling lonely, isolated, and worried that this is her fault. She feels that she is acting increasingly as Geoffrey's carer but he resents any notion that her ageing is not so dramatic nor difficult as his. This inequality is driving a wedge between them.

Things reach an intolerable pitch when Geoffrey tries to stop Sylvia leaving their flat and in doing so, breaks her arm. They call an ambulance and both are admitted to hospital. The police become involved because of the violence of the assault. In hospital, Geoffrey is seen by the liaison psychiatrist and she is able to make a provisional diagnosis. Geoffrey has probably developed a late-onset paranoid illness with some cognitive impairment. It is likely to be a Lewy body dementia as it is running a fluctuating course and is associated with occasional visual hallucinations and episodes of emotional instability. He can now receive useful drug treatment and the couple can obtain practical help and emotional support. Sylvia is assessed by the psychiatric triage nurse prior to receiving surgery for her arm. She admits she was contemplating a homicide/ suicide and is referred to the old-age psychiatry team where she is treated for depression.

Discussion

This case is illustrative of a common occurrence of women in the caring role, well into late life. Men can find themselves in similar roles too but because women still tend to live longer, it is more often the woman who may be back in a role that she relinquished some three or more decades earlier. What may also happen relatively frequently, particularly in partnerships where one has dementia and the other not, is that the healthier partner finds themselves in a caring role, perhaps one that they had not anticipated and one which can change profoundly the dynamic of the relationship.

In this case, one could ponder on why Sylvia did not seek help for her husband sooner, or why she blamed herself for what was going on in their relationship. One might also consider the potentially catastrophic consequences had the situation not come to the attention of the law and the health system. The psychiatrists will have recognized that Sylvia was suffering from a depressive illness and her treatment is likely to be successful. If however, she were to receive medication only, then the authors might argue that we will not have done enough to support her fully. One can only conjecture at what aspects of Sylvia's early life caused her to choose nursing as a career to the exclusion of all other personal rewards until she met Geoffrey. What aspect of her identity was caught up with caring for him and feeling guilty when things between them were not going well? Why did Sylvia think that the only way out might be to kill him (probably with a drug overdose) and then kill herself? We know that people in the helping professions are often seeking some assistance for a damaged or hurt part of themselves.[17] An important aspect of developing resilience as a doctor or nurse is to dispel the myth that we are somehow superhuman, able to look after everyone else's pain and yet ignore our own. We must also let go of the fantasy that we are the only ones who can help in a given situation; other people's care and attention may not be as good as ours but perhaps it is 'good enough'. A chance for Sylvia to talk to someone professional in a non-judgmental setting might help her make sense of what happened by examining the past. She may come to understand herself better and to be less harsh on herself. This is likely to enhance her recovery, particularly when depression carries much guilt as part of the symptomatology. Feeling guilty is often part of the symptoms but understanding *why* this person feels guilty and helping them to move on makes the task of psychiatry even more interesting.

Conclusion

Psychiatry is a part of medicine, and within psychiatry, psychotherapy enhances our understanding of ourselves and our patients through personal observation, reflection on therapeutic reactions, and the study of mother–infant and other relationships. The arts can and should be used further to understand ourselves and our patients as well as the effects of ageing and disease. Certain types of psychotherapeutic discourse, ones which have their roots in the understanding of ourselves as adults, as coming from what we experienced as children and infants and others, ones which see how our thinking processes, both conscious and unconscious, are affected by the socio-political and cultural climate of our environment, all lend themselves to the understanding of illness and ageing. The authors of this chapter have endeavoured to demonstrate how this understanding both enriches and enhances our work as clinicians, and helps us to come to terms with the fragility of our own as well as our patients' lives.

Psychiatry is a satisfying career for all genders. It is one in which women do well both in terms of numbers but also in developing their careers and getting promoted to senior positions. Old age psychiatry and psychotherapy are important specialties. There is so much yet to discover and so much we can do to help people.

References

1. **Carney GM** and **Gray M** (2015). Unmasking the 'elderly' mystique. Why it is time to make the personal political in ageing research. *Journal of Ageing Studies* **35**:123–34.
2. **Bierdermann H** (1992). *Dictionary of Symbolism: Cultural Icons and the Meanings Behind Them.* New York, NY: Facts on File Inc.
3. **Baldwin R** and **Garner J** (2016). Anxiety and depression in women in old age. In: D Castle and K Abel (eds). *Comprehensive Women's Mental Health.* Cambridge: Cambridge University Press, pp. 247–67.

4. **Rossiter MW** (1993). The Matthew–Matilda effect in science. *Social Studies of Science* **23**:325–41.

5. **Parker R** and **Pollack G** (1981). *Old Mistresses: Women, Art and Ideology* London: Routledge and Keegan Paul.

6. **Gabhart A** and **Broun E** (1972). *Walters Art Gallery Bulletin* **24**:7.

7. ECU (2005) <http://www.ecu.ac.uk/equality-charters/charter-marks-explained/>.

8. **de Beauvoir, S** (1989). *The Second Sex* (HM Pashley trans and ed.) (1989) Vintage.

9. **Jane Fonda** (1989), *Daily Mail*, 13 September. London: Daily Mail Associated Newspapers.

10. **Spreckels J** (2002). What discourse analysis reveals about elderly women, sex and the struggle with societal norms. *Narrative Inquiry* **12**(1):145–53.

11. **Foulkes SH** (1964). *Therapeutic Group Analysis*. London: Allen & Unwin.

12. **Walter H** (2012). *Brutus and Other Heroines: Playing Shakespeare's Roles for Women*. London: Nick Hern Books.

13. **Hess N** (1987). King Lear and some anxieties of old age. *Psychology & Psychotherapy* **60**(Sept):209–15.

14. **Oliver D** (2015). Minding our language around care for older people and why it matters. *BMJ Blog* 7 May 2015. <http://blogs.bmj.com/bmj/2015/05/07/david-oliver-minding-our-language-around-care-for-older-people/>.

15. **Garner J** (2009). Considerably better than the alternative: Positive aspects of getting older. *Quality in Ageing* **10**(1):5–8.

16. **Shafto M**, **Tyler L**, **Dixon MJ**, **Taylor**, **Rowe J** (2014) The Cambridge Centre for ageing and neuroscience study protocol: A cross-sectional lifespan multidisciplinary examination of healthy cognitive ageing. *BMC Neurology* **14**(1):204.

17. **Winnicott DW** (1960). Egodistortion in terms of true and false self. In: Winnicott DW (ed). *The Maturational Processes and the Facilitating Environment*. London: Hogarth, pp 140–152.

18. **Burns JF** (1992). 'Racing through snipers' alley on ride to Sarajevo'. *New York Times*, 26 September, 1992.

19. **Schedler J** (2010). The efficacy of psychodynamic psychotherapy. *American Journal of Psychiatry* **65**: 98–109.

20. **Huhn M**, **Tardy M**, **Spineli LM**, **Kisling N**, **Forstl H**, **Pitschel-Walz G**, **Leucht C**, **Samara M**, **Dold M**, **Davis JM**, **Leucht S** (2014). Efficacy of pharmacotherapy and psychotherapy for adult psychiatric disorders: A systematic overview of meta-analyses. *JAMA Psychiatry* **71**:706–15.

21. **Taylor D**, **Carlyle J**, **McPherson S**, **Rost F**, **Thomas R**, and **Fonagy P** (2012). Tavistock Adult Depression Study (TADS): A randomised controlled trial of psychoanalytic psychotherapy for treatment-resistant/treatment-refractory forms of depression. *British Medical Council Psychiatry* **12**:60 24–5.

22. **Prosser A**, **Helfer B**, and **Leucht S** (2016). Biological v psychosocial treatments: a myth about pharmacotherapy v psychotherapy. *British Journal of Psychiatry* **208**: 309–11.

23. **Schore AN** (1997). A century after Freud's project: is a rapprochement between psychoanalysis and neurobiology at hand? *Journal of the American Psychoanalytic Association* **45**: 807–40.

24. **Fitzgerald M** (2015). The neurology–psychiatry divide: A thought experiment. *British Journal of Psychiatry Bulletin* **39**(3) 134–5.

25. **Reilly TJ** (2015). The neurology–psychiatry divide: A thought experiment. *British Journal of Psychiatry Bulletin* **39**(3) 105–7.

26. **Segal H** (1958). Fear of death: Notes on the analysis of an old man. *International Journal of Psychoanalysis* **39**:173–81.

27. **Knight BG** (1986). *Psychotherapy with Older Adults* London: Sage.

28. **Garner J** and **Bacelle L** (2004). Sexuality. In: Evans S and Garner J (eds). *Talking Over the Years: A Handbook of Psychodynamic Psychotherapy with Older Adults.* Hove: Brunner-Routledge, pp. 247–63.

29. **Pines D** (1993). *A Woman's Unconscious Use of Her Body; A Psychoanalytical Perspective.* London: Virago.

30. **Asher R** (1972). Myxoedema madness. In: Asher R (ed.). *Talking Sense.* Edinburgh: Churchill Livingstone.

31. **Blazer D** (1997). Depression in the elderly: Myths and misconceptions. *Geriatric Psychiatry* **20**(1):111–19.

32. **Jung CG** (1931). The Stages of Life *CW8*, London: Routledge & Kegan Paul, pp. 387–403.

33. **Murphy E** (1982). The social origins of depression in old age. *British Journal of Psychiatry* **141**:135–42.

34. **Brown G** and **Harris TO** (1972). *The Social Origins Of Depression. A Study of Psychiatric Disorder in Women.* London: Routledge.

35. **Garner J** and **Bacelle L** (2016). Intimacy and sexuality in old age. In: Fenieux CG and Rojas R (eds). *Sexo y psicoanálisis. Una mirada a la Intimidad Adulta.* Santiago, Chile: La Pólvora Editorial Imprint, pp. 247–63.

36. **Carlisle Maxwell J** (2009). Epidemiology and Demography of Non-Prescription Drug Use. In: Chrome I, Tzy-wu L, Rao RT, and Chrome P (eds). *Substance Misuse and Older People.* Wiley.

37. **Evans S** (2004a). Sex and death: the ramifications of illness and aging in older couple relationships. *Journal of Sexual and Relationship Therapy* **19**(3): 319–35.

38. **Evans S** (2004b). Elderly couples and their families. In: Evans S and Garner J (eds). *Talking Over the Years: A Handbook of Dynamic Psychotherapy with Older Adults.* Hove: Brunner-Routledge, pp. 231–46.

39. **White L** and **Evans S** (2015). Demographics and intervention possibilities in a female Turkish-speaking sample. Paper presented at the *17th IPA International Congress* Berlin, 13–16 October.

40. **Bowlby J** (1969). Attachment. In: Bowlby J (ed). *Attachment and Loss*, Vol **1**. London: Hogarth Press.

41. **Erikson E** (1959). *Identity and the Life Cycle.* New York, NY: International Universities Press.

42. **King P** (1980). The life cycle as indicated in the psychoanalysis of the middle aged and elderly. *International Journal of Psychoanalysis* **61**:153–60.

43. **Berezin MA** (1976). Normal psychology of the ageing process revisited. Sex and old age: A further review of the literature. *Journal of Geriatric Psychiatry* **9**: 189–209.

Chapter 13

A Woman who Made a Difference: An Interview with Nori Graham

Amanda Thompsell

Introduction

Anyone involved in dementia care will have heard of Nori Graham. Over a long career in psychiatry beginning in the 1970s, she combined the demands of National Health Service (NHS) clinical practice with her work for the Alzheimer's Disease Society (now the Alzheimer's Society), becoming chairman of the Alzheimer's UK, and subsequently chairman of Alzheimer's Disease International. Despite reaching NHS retirement age more years ago than she might care to admit, she has never retired and continues to operate an extensive portfolio of jobs concerning older people's issues and in the field of dementia care.

I was lucky enough to work as a junior trainee for Nori when she was still practising as a consultant at the Royal Free Hospital. Interviewing her for the purposes of this book, I found her energy and passion for her field to be undiminished. This interview provides insights from the frontline of old age psychiatry over the last half-century; it takes in developments within the NHS, the charitable sector, and the private sector.

Nori was brought up in Manchester. Although her household was one steeped in science (her parents, Jewish refugees from Russia, were theoretical chemists, and her aunt was a doctor), at school (Manchester High School for Girls) her strengths seemed to be more in the arts than the science subjects. Nevertheless, she was determined to read medicine and was accepted by Somerville College at Oxford. Her clinical training was undertaken at University College Hospital, London. Nori's early career was in general practice but before long she made the move into psychiatry. She trained at Goodmayes Hospital followed by Friern Hospital, and then as senior registrar at the Royal Free Hospital. She became a consultant in old age psychiatry in 1981, at first part-time and then full-time at the Royal Free Hospital, and continued in that role until 2000. During this time, she pioneered an innovative model of care which was a truly multidisciplinary service, attracting interest from all over the world, and inspiring a large number of people working with her to follow in her footsteps.

From 1984 to 1994 she was chairman of the Alzheimer's Society, UK, and subsequently was chairman of Alzheimer's Disease International (1996–2002).

She was an active member of the executive of the old age section of the World Psychiatric Association and contributed to a number of international guidelines.

After reaching NHS retirement age and finishing her term as chairman of Alzheimer's Disease International, she worked as medical advisor to Nightingale House, a 200-bedded care home in Clapham, for 9 years. She also kept busy performing testamentary capacity assessments and was made an honorary fellow of the Association for Contentious Trust and Probate Specialists, to which for many years she gave annual seminars. For two years she was co-chair of the working party on older people's issues for the Centre for Social Justice. Subsequently, she became a member of the partnership Board of the Age Action Alliance and until recently chaired the working group on Public Health and Active Lifestyles. In 2013 she was appointed Medical Director of Red and Yellow Care, a specialist private sector healthcare company focusing on the assessment, diagnosis and post-diagnostic care of people with dementia and other mental health problems. She recently stepped down from this role.

At present she continues working for the Alzheimer's Society as a Dementia Friend Champion providing training sessions for Dementia Friends. Since 2013 she has served as a non-executive director of Care UK. She has just completed four years as a co-opted member of the Executive of the Royal College of Psychiatrists Faculty of Old Age Psychiatry. She remains an Honorary Vice-President both of the Alzheimer's Society and of Alzheimer's Disease International.

Amongst her publications, the one she co-authored with James Warner and is now most proud of is *Understanding Alzheimer's Disease and Other Dementias*.[1]

Nori's outstanding contribution to old age psychiatric care has been widely recognized and marked by an Honorary Doctorate (D. Univ. Public Services, Open University 1996), the inaugural lifetime achievement award from the Old Age Faculty of the Royal College of Psychiatrists (2004), an Honorary Fellowship of the Royal College of Psychiatrists (2005), and the International Psychogeriatric Association award for distinguished service (2013)

Interview

Nori's Career and the Development of NHS Old Age Psychiatry

Who Were the key Influential Figures in Your Career?

I have met so many inspirational figures but I would like to mention two members of my family and several colleagues.

Within my family, my father was very influential. He was always certain that medicine was a good career for a woman as it would allow her to stand on her own two feet. He was also very clear that I should go to Oxford, and his belief in, and expectations for me, certainly provided the necessary motivation. Later on, ever since I first met him at medical school in London, my husband, Philip Graham has been consistently supportive of the roles and responsibilities that I have taken on. I don't think I would have been able to juggle my various commitments without his complete support and encouragement.

I have been privileged to be trained by and to work with many great doctors. The late John Horder, later President of the Royal College of General Practitioners, was originally my trainer in general practice but he later became a colleague and close friend. He modelled a psychological approach to medical history taking. I learned from him the powerful benefits that come from really knowing your patients; he practised person-centred care before that was a buzzword.

Tom Arie was the consultant who taught me psychiatry at Goodmayes. Particularly empathetic and warm, he took me on domiciliary visits and showed me the value of home visits in providing a fuller picture of the environment in which the patient lived. He stressed especially the importance of listening to the relatives and enlisting their support in care. I was very impressed by how he went out of his way to reward his staff with praise, seeking out staff to tell them how well they had done their job (Figure 13.1).

Like many women, I benefitted hugely from the ability to do my training on a part-time basis while my children were small. For this opportunity I owe a debt of thanks to Gerald Russell, a psychiatrist who was willing to look at different ways of training and who put great effort in the development of a part-time training scheme. I shall always be indebted to Anthony Mann for his research experience, his ability to listen and offer wise advice, and his encouragement at all times. He introduced me to Barry Gurland in the United States, and as a result together we built up a series of useful transatlantic exchange visits and seminars over several years.

When I became a consultant, one of my closest colleagues was Archie Young, Professor of Geriatric Medicine at The Royal Free Hospital. He and the late Jerry

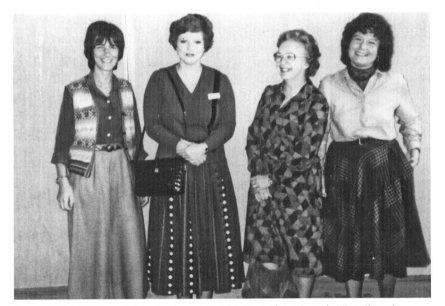

Figure 13.1 1975 Tom Arie's Goodmayes' 'girls': Nori, Elaine Murphy, Zoe Slatterly, Elizabeth Taws

Morris, Professor in Public Health, remain lasting influences on my life and on my attitudes to the influence of lifestyle factors on both physical and mental health.

For reasons I give later I would like to mention George Cyriax (who sadly died in July 2016), a close friend in the business world who introduced me to an entirely different perspective in the running of an organization.

Tell me Something About how you Have Seen Old Age Psychiatry Develop as a Specialty

The history and early development of old age psychiatry are well described in the Guthrie Trust witness seminar 'Development of Old Age Psychiatry from the 1960s until 1989.[2] In the early 1970s, larger numbers of very able, pioneering psychiatrists including Tom Arie and Brice Pitt established services and inspired trainees like me to go into the specialty. A peer support group was set up and eventually mutated into first the Section and then the Faculty of Old Age Psychiatry.

When I first started in the field my colleagues said to me: 'There is nothing you can do for elderly people, you won't get many requests so you do not need any beds'. I may have started with virtually no resources but I developed a vision and I knew what I wanted to do. By example, I was able to demonstrate how valuable a service for the elderly mentally ill could be. As I showed the need so the service grew. *The Rising Tide*, a 1982 Health Advisory Service publication,[3] laid out guidelines for psychiatric services for the elderly. I took that as my road map and a guide to requests for additions to my service. I worked on having a close and supportive relationship with the managers of the hospital and the psychiatric department as well as with colleagues in social services, primary care, and the local voluntary sector.

What Were the Factors in the Growth of the Specialty?

As I mentioned, the original catalyst was the pressure on medical and general psychiatric beds, meaning something had to be done. However, getting something *good* to be done required psychiatrists with an interest and commitment to old age as a specialty who through the force of their personalities could persuade others of the need. Researchers like Martin Roth, Felix Post, Klaus Bergmann, and Raymond Levy provided findings that demonstrated the need for and the value of the service.

What Factors Were There Holding Back the Specialty and How Did You Deal With Them?

Inevitably, doctors in other disciplines were worried about losing their own resources, including medical staff, to old age psychiatry, but persistence and a slow, gentle approach managed to convince them we were not a threat. After I was appointed to be the Old Age Consultant in Psychiatry to the Hampstead District I made it my business to meet general practitioners (GPs) and listen to what they wanted and to explain what we could and could not offer. GPs are crucial and we hospital-based doctors need to align ourselves to primary care and acknowledge that the increasing contribution of primary care to our field is likely to increase.

There are Currently Recruitment Issues not Just for Psychiatry as a Whole But Specifically for Old Age Psychiatry at All Trainee Levels. How Do You Think These Can Be Overcome? What Helped in the Past?

I agree there is a recruitment problem. I see this being partly down to bad press and partly to the intolerable degree to which bureaucracy has increased. Despite the problems in recruitment, it is important to maintain standards and only appoint people who meet the criteria. The fact is that old age psychiatry has so much to recommend it: there is an increasing number of elderly people in the population and our specialty is one of the few remaining generalist specialties. To practice it you really do have to see the whole person. Compared to general psychiatry, for example, there is much less emphasis on personality issues and drugs and alcohol disorders. I have always found that attractive and I believe others do too. I firmly believe that recruitment can increase with inspiring, enthusiastic teachers and enjoyable training opportunities. It would be useful if juniors routinely experienced more old age psychiatry during their rotation. In the end, if the specialty is exciting, lively people will want to work in it.

Career and Thoughts on What Makes for Career Success

What Piece of Advice Would You Give to Someone Considering Starting in Old Age Psychiatry?

First, be ready to work in a team. One person cannot do everything and this is an area where a mix of skills and disciplines is needed.

Second, try early on to take any opportunities offered to you to do some research, especially if this is in the community. With encouragement from Gerald Russell, I spent two years on a research project led by Enid Levin at the Institute of Social Work which involved assessing 150 families and interviewing patients' relatives at length about the problems associated with dementia.[4] When I became a consultant and worked in care homes, Anthony Mann invited me to join him in some research in the Camden homes and the issues that I encountered there were the subject of my first paper.[3] As a result I ended up with some first-hand knowledge in these areas and this turned out to be very useful to me in my career.

How Did You Drive Your Career Forward?

I don't think there is one general plan that works for everybody, but for me some of the important factors were that I was generally clear about what I wanted and how to achieve it. Listen to others and be on the lookout for new ideas. I have been a shameless networker, using both formal and informal links.

Once you are in a leadership position, think about your team. I have always tried to make sure that my team are kept informed of changes and consulted them before any changes were made so they felt engaged with the plans. I also believe in going out of my way to recognize and praise good practice when I see it.

Having a varied portfolio is a key factor in keeping stimulated. Taking part in research, playing a role in the voluntary sector, teaching all disciplines, presenting at conferences, a little private work all help to produce new and exciting ideas and bring one in touch with many different people. Then one thing leads to another!

Finally, as you come towards the end of your tenure in any particular job, secure your legacy by good succession planning. Nobody goes on forever.

How Have You Found the Opportunities for Women Doctors at Different Times?

I have never found being a woman a disadvantage in itself. Like many women, there have been stages in my career when I really needed to be able to work part-time. Initially, there was not the opportunity to train part-time—you either did voluntary work or were a clinical assistant—but in the late 1970s part-time specialist training began and this allowed me, at some cost to my sleep, to combine training/working and motherhood.

How Did You Deal with Juggling Your Career and Raising Children?

I was lucky. In addition to a supportive husband I always had a lot of help. I made a point of having someone to clean the house and somebody different to look after the children. I was incredibly lucky in the people I found to look after the children; they were always mature mothers usually with grown up children.

Once I had children I became, to some extent, a different person. My priorities changed. I realized that I wanted them to succeed more than I wanted to be successful myself and, for a while at least, I became less ambitious. However, this did not remain the case forever. I remember one day when I was sitting in a staff room I asked about the membership exam and a colleague said 'Don't bother with the exam. You don't really need it'. That so incensed me that I went home and started studying. I found it quite a challenge but Philip was very supportive and good at entertaining the children and taking then away from time to time for a few days which all helped.

What are the Key Lessons that You Have Learnt Through Your Career?

Don't overextend yourself financially (if you can possibly help it) so that you have to stay in a job you do not like or work at private practice if you don't really want to.

Don't expect to change the world all at once. Allow time for change. It is better to start something small and develop it slowly.

Don't take on too much administration

Look outwards. Listen to everyone. Visit all the GPs in your patch. Have a good relationship with the managers. Develop good relationships with social services/voluntary organizations/other disciplines/colleagues.

There is great reward in helping younger people flourish and develop in their career path. Your trainees today are your friends and colleagues tomorrow.

Look after yourself as well as other people. That means keeping fit, finding time to lead a full social life, and taking enjoyable holidays.

What was One of the Hardest Choices You Had to Make?

Deciding whether to stand as chair of the Alzheimer's Society.

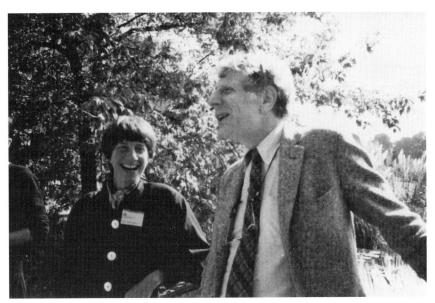

Figure 13.2 AGM of the Alzheimer's Society, Bath 1998. Jonathan Miller (President) and Nori (Chairman).

I was encouraged to become a member of the Alzheimer's Society by an old friend, Jonathan Miller, who was President (Figure 13.2). At his suggestion, Christine Kirk, the retiring Chairman, asked me if I would consider standing. I was frankly astonished but my loyal and longstanding secretary, Marilyn Greenfield, a great supporter of the voluntary sector, urged me to take this suggestion seriously saying it was a 'good thing' to get involved in the voluntary sector. How wise those words were!

Nori's Work with the Alzheimer's Society and Alzheimer's Disease International

How did the Vision of the Alzheimer's Society Come About?

The Alzheimer's Society (originally the Alzheimer's Disease Society) was started in 1979 by two women whose husbands both had dementia at a relatively young age. They contacted each other through a newspaper and got together with a couple of doctors and formed a group. Gradually the group enlarged and a charity was started and branches began to spring up around the country. The way the carers came together in each branch varied. A great spur to the developing momentum and profile was when Jonathan Miller became President and Gordon Wilcock the Chairman. At the same time in Canada and the United States, there was the beginning of a sense that carers needed support and to be able to talk about dementia and national charities developed there too.

What Were the Key Factors in Growing the Society into a Bigger Movement?

When I took over as Chairman the organization was in poor shape and my immediate tasks were to find out what the problems were, find a permanent treasurer because there wasn't one, appoint a new Executive Director, and sort out the structure and finance of the organization. Before my arrival, the Society had been supported by a grant from the Department of Health and Social Security (DHSS). However, the output from the Society had begun to be very unsatisfactory and the immediate threat was that the grant would be removed. I persuaded an old friend George Cyriax, economist and successful business man, to be the Treasurer. His appointment proved to be key to the success of the organization. He taught me the basic principles of business. Most importantly, he taught me that raising money was not, in fact, the first priority. The first priority was to have a clear idea what the money was needed for. Raising money then became a whole lot easier.

We appointed a brilliant new Executive Director, Noreen Miller (now Siba), who came with very valuable experience after 11 years as Executive Director of Contact a Family.

We totally restructured the Society. I had a full-time NHS Consultant job so for me this new full-time voluntary job was one I did in the evenings, nights, and weekends. What is more it was a vertical learning curve for me because running a business (not for profit), chairing meetings, sacking and appointing staff was entirely virgin territory.

The first major task was to clarify the aims of the organization. The aims we agreed to focus on, which to a great extent remain the same to this day, were:

 ◆ the provision of information (helpline, fact sheets, regular newsletters, training materials)

 ◆ making the Society a membership organization and facilitating members to meet each other in support groups

 ◆ raising public awareness

 ◆ encouraging research, and

 ◆ fund-raising.

Without achieving clarity in our aims and objectives and stronger financial discipline, I think the Society might well have gone under as our grant was under severe threat.

After three years Noreen left to start a family and we were able to attract Harry Cayton to become our Chief Executive. He came from many successful years as Director of the National Deaf Children's Society. Together we developed a strategy for fund-raising including appointing a legacy officer. I am proud to say that the Society has never looked back. From about £300,000 in the bank in 1987 its income today is over £90 million.

How did you Promote the Alzheimer's Society?

We promoted the Society in a really professional way with dissemination of information through conferences, media coverage, factsheets, newsletters, and training materials. Availability of good professional material is a proven route to greater awareness and recognition by families, professionals, and governments. The Society was greatly helped in the early years by Jonathan Miller who had a real genius for communication and took an active part in many of the programmes seen on television. Another way we promoted the Society was through involving family members, many of whom showed great courage in telling their stories in public. Their courage helped to raise awareness and gave comfort and support to others. Nowadays, people with dementia play an active part themselves in promoting the Society.

I personally actively discussed and tried to increase awareness of the Alzheimer's Society at every opportunity. In the early years I used to raise the subject of the Alzheimer's Society at every executive meeting of the Old Age Faculty. People got very tired of me but eventually the tide turned and colleagues would come and reassuringly tell me about their involvement with their local organizations.

How did Alzheimer's Disease International (ADI) Start and What did You Do There?

Alzheimer's Disease International started in 1984 with five jurisdictions—England and Scotland, Canada, the United States, Australia, and France. My involvement with this organization grew gradually. I became increasingly involved in the international setting, and Brian Moss from Australia and the outgoing chairman suggested that I put my name up to become chairman as I was about to complete seven years as Chairman in the United Kingdom. I realized that it would be a daunting task as fund-raising for an international charity I knew to be a huge challenge. However, I felt I had learned so much about how to set up and run a charity that it would be good to try to share this with other interested countries. So I agreed and got elected in 1996.

The Head Office of ADI was in Chicago and I realized that if I were to become Chair, the day-to-day administration would need to move to London to ensure effective coordination. I achieved this with the help of the Alzheimer Society London branch offering us a room.

As chairman of the international organization, I took the same approach as I had at national level. I listened to people and clarified the aims and objectives and got the right staff with the right skills. Our aims were to support national Alzheimer associations and increase global awareness about dementia. It required some slimming down of the organization with the abolition of some sub-committees. We ran a tight ship of three staff, with an excellent Chief Executive, Elizabeth Rimmer, a former lawyer. I had an executive committee with representatives from all over the world, with particularly strong support from Henry Brodaty.

During the 6 years that I was chairman membership grew from 25 to 66 national members. There are now 83 members. We secured an official relationship with the World Health Organization and developed financial and academic viability. An annual conference is held once a year in a different part of the world and members meet and share ideas, skills, and materials, and obtain update information (Figure 13.3). We initiated Alzheimer University courses to help new national Alzheimer associations learn how to set up and run their organization.

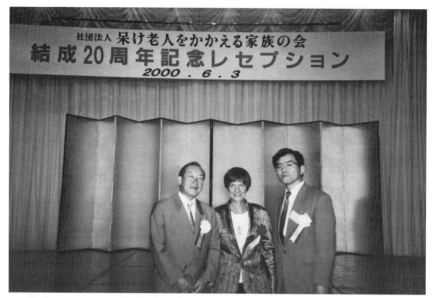

Figure 13.3 Kyoto 2000, 20th Anniversary of Alzheimer Association Japan (AAJ). Mr Kunio Takami (President AAJ), Nori (Chairman ADI), Dr Yoshio Miyake (Vice president AAJ).

I feel that one of my greatest achievements was to encourage the development of the 10/66 research network led and masterminded by Martin Prince. This work has been focused on low- and middle-income countries and has, over its 18-year existence, produced prevalence and incidence figures and data on caring arrangements which our members have been able to use to lobby their governments. ADI is extremely proud of its part in the support of this work which is referenced worldwide.

How did You Encourage People to Follow Your Lead?

Being enthusiastic and excited about what I was doing. Having a positive attitude to problems and involving young people as much as possible. I am a strong believer in the importance of rewarding good work.

What are the Top Skills That You Feel Influence Change?

Being clear about your aims and objectives and having a coherent plan. You need to know, and have all those engaged in a venture know, why you are there, what are you doing, and why you are doing it.

Inspire. People need encouragement and regular individual support and to be reminded of the importance of what they are doing and recognized for their efforts and successes.

Have a good team of skilled individuals around you to support you, and make sure the right people are doing the right job.

Run an efficient office.

What Were the Hardest Challenges that You Had to Overcome in Your Work for Alzheimer's?

One of the hardest challenges was around fundraising. You had to make sure you did things to get money, but it costs money to raise the money so there is something of the chicken and the egg about this. During my time as chair of Alzheimer's Society in England, we did not accept money from drug companies and were very successful in finding alternative sources of money. However, when it came to Alzheimer's Disease International, that was a quite different story. Individuals and companies generally want to give money to their own country, not to other countries, so I had to swallow my feelings and make friends with the drug companies.

Another challenge was selecting the right staff. Selecting the right staff and being prepared to confront staff who, even after discussion and further training, turn out not to be right for their jobs in a way that is fair and just are key leadership skills.

Looking Over Your Career, Have You Any Reflections About the Roles of Voluntary Organizations in Healthcare Generally?

It is important that voluntary organizations are recognized as being key to supporting health and social care services. They are an essential independent voice. It is easier for them to be innovative and take risks.

Large voluntary organizations are now much more centralized than they used to be. That has meant both gains and losses. It is important to liaise with politicians and obtain recognition and respect as an organization, but the bigger you get the greater the risk of losing contact with what's happening on the ground and it can be more difficult to get the support of volunteers.

Issues tend to arise when the role of the voluntary organization becomes blurred, such as when they are contracted by local authorities who retain considerable control over their activities. There is also an issue in our society about the nature of volunteering. This should be seen as an activity that all citizens undertake as part of their lives.

Thoughts on Care Home Provision for the Elderly Mentally Ill.

What are Your Views on Care Homes That Provide Care for Older People with Mental Health Problems? How They Have Changed?

Currently, my work as a non-executive director of Care UK frequently takes me into care homes and I have been giving this matter a great deal of thought. In the past, the NHS controlled all long-stay wards in mental hospitals and that was where people with mental health problems were expected to be. Whilst there were many disadvantages in this approach, it was a protected environment and patients were supported by a psychiatrist and multidisciplinary staff team. When these institutions closed, the money went to placing the patients into residential and nursing homes run by local authorities. With much encouragement from central government local authorities handed this responsibility over to the private sector.

Most residents in care homes now have significant mental health issues. In particular, a large proportion of residents have dementia, but despite the obvious need there is usually little regular input from specialists in mental health.

Have You Any Reflections on the Key Ingredients Needed to get the Optimal Care for Those With Mental Health Issues in Care Homes?

To make a difference you need to have trained care home staff with training provided on an ongoing basis and this should not be just a tick-box exercise. You also need to have a manager who understands mental health issues, leads from the front, and has access to a back-up system from local services.

The other essential ingredient to achieve optimal care is to have a regulatory system fit for purpose. We need external regulation but it needs to operate with more carrot and less stick.

Final Thoughts: Life Beyond Retirement

Why Have You Carried on Working in Retirement?

I have been lucky to have had such tremendous training and immensely varied experience. I still have an enormous interest in improving life for those older people suffering from mental illness. I have also found myself taking an interest in older people's issues more generally. I still want to change the world! I remain in good health and can't see that reaching any particular number of candles on my cake provides an excuse for not continuing to contribute where I can. I am a great believer in the importance of being physically and mentally active as you get older, if personal circumstances allow it. I have loved everything that I have done and I have often found that one thing leads to another if you are open to new challenges. I also have to say that people have been particularly kind to me and continue to ask me to become involved in new work. In the last three years, new opportunities have come up for me in both the voluntary sector and in the private sector. I am so lucky and so privileged.

What Three Things are you Most Proud of?

Leaving aside my family, in my working life:

1. I am thrilled to be able to watch the people who worked with me when they were young develop and continue the work we started together while themselves moving onwards and upwards.

2. I am proud of the community-orientated multidisciplinary service for older people with mental health problems which I started in north Camden in London. Whilst this service has adapted to changing times, it continues very successfully to this day.

3. The Alzheimer's Society has never looked back since I was able to steer it out of troubled waters with the support of a team that was unique in its combination of business, personal, and professional skills. It is difficult to believe this now but when I started in the field, most people hadn't heard of the Society. I think I may have contributed just a little to this growing awareness of a disease which all need to know about and, if that is indeed the case then I feel very proud.

References

1. **Graham N** and **Warner J** (2014). *Understanding Alzheimer's Disease and Other Dementias*. London: Family Doctor Books.
2. **Hilton C, Arie T**, and **Nicholson M** (2010). A witness seminar: the development of old age psychiatry in Britain 1960–1989 Themes, lessons are highlighted. *International Journal of Geriatric Psychiatry* **25**:596–603.
3. **Health Advisory Service** (1982). *The Rising Tide*. London: NHS Advisory Service.
4. **Levin E, Sinclair I**, and **Gorbach P** (1989). *Families, Services and Confusion in Old Age*. Aldershot: Avebury.

Eluned Woodford-Williams
12 September 1913 to 25 November 1984

Itunuayo V. Ayeni

Life

Dr Eluned Woodford-Williams was born in Cardiff in 1913, the eldest of four daughters. Her early life was spent in Liverpool; she attended Liverpool College initially before her family moved to Wales when she transferred to Cardiff High School. It was during this time that she decided to pursue a medical career.

In 1933 she matriculated at the Welsh National School of Medicine and obtained a Bachelors degree, BSc. She moved to London, attending University College London, where she completed her clinical medical training. After graduating she worked as a medical officer at Alder Hey Children's Hospital in Liverpool. In 1938 she obtained a Diploma in Child Health. She then moved to Redhill and worked at the local hospital before obtaining Membership of the Royal College of Physicians, Diploma of the Royal College of Obstetricians and Gynaecologists, and MD (Doctor of Medicine, a postgraduate medical degree).

In the 1950s she became senior registrar and first assistant to Oscar Olbrich. This move became pivotal to her career and was fundamental in establishing geriatric medicine and old age psychiatry in the United Kingdom.

Career

Dr Woodford-Williams pioneered a holistic approach to caring for older people (Figure P5.1). She worked at the interface of geriatric medicine and old age psychiatry. She understood the overlap between mental and physical health and the fact that social stressors may masquerade as physical illness. She believed that older people required the same standard of medicine as younger patients, that the specialty of geriatrics is about understanding the social aspect of the patient's life, and the need to work with voluntary organizations and health authorities.

Dr Woodford-Williams demonstrated that the specialty was about the health of ageing and the aged and the special application of general clinical medicine. She implemented age-based admittance of all patients over 65 years, irrespective of needs, for comprehensive geriatric assessment, and taught that the reintegration of mental health social workers into healthcare was crucial for elderly patients.

In 1958 she was pivotal in successfully organizing the European Clinical Section of the International Association of Gerontology, following the sudden death of the previous secretary, Oscar Olbrich. She was appointed to the directorship of the National Health Service Health Advisory Service in 1973 and collaborated with Barbara Castle (Minister for Social Services) in developing policies aimed at improving care for older people. Later she had an active role in Faculty of Old Age Psychiatry, Royal College of Psychiatrists, and the education of 'psychogeriatricians'. She was awarded Commander of the British Empire (CBE) in 1979 and became a Fellow of the Royal College of Psychiatry in 1983 for services to Old Age Psychiatry.

Principles and Favourite Quotations

'Diagnosis in the aged is diagnosis in the young plus something else.'

'No standard method of treatment is applicable to the aged.'

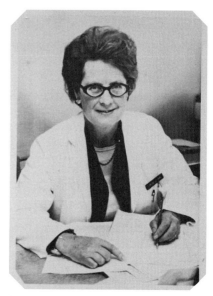

Figure P5.1: Image of Dr Eluned Woodford-Williams— Pioneer of the holistic approach to the care of older people.
© Royal College of Psychiatrists

'Furthermore, in the aged, environmental factors, especially the social, frequently precipitate the breakdown in health.'

'By careful balancing of clinical medicine with concern of social background it is possible to deal with the needs of the aged sick.'

'Greater accuracy in prescribing is also needed because the margin of safety is reduced by the diminished response to stress.'

Major Papers and Publications

Woodford-Williams E (1958). Beds for the aged. *British Medical Journal*. **2**(5098):741.

Woodford-Williams E (1960). The clinical medicine of old age. *Proceedings of the Nutrition Society* **19**(2), 120–25. DOI:10.1079/PNS19600033.

Woodford-Williams E and Exton-Smith AN (1962). Aspects of geriatric psychiatry, haematology, nutrition and cancer in old age. 3rd Meeting of the European Clinical Section of the International Association of Gerontology, The Hague, September 1961: Part II. Basel: Karger.

Woodford-Williams E, Alvarez AS, Webster D, Landless B, and Dixon MP (1964). Serum protein patterns in 'normal' and pathological ageing. *Gerontology* **10**:86–99. DOI:10.1159/000211396.

Woodford-Williams E and Alvarez AS (1965). Four years' experience of a day hospital in geriatric practice. *Gerontologia Clinica* **7**(2–3):96–106.

Woodford-Williams E, McKeon JA, Trotter IS, Watson D, and Bushby C (1962). The day hospital in the community care of the elderly. *Gerontologia Clinica* **4**:241–56. DOI:10.1159/000244750.

Woodford-Williams E (1966). Respiratory tract disease: Diagnosis and management of pneumonia in the aged. *British Medical Journal* **1**(5485):467–70.

Woodford-Williams E and Coakley D (1979). Effects of burglary and vandalism on the health of old people. *The Lancet* 314(8151)1066–7.

Bibliography

Hilton C (2005) The clinical psychiatry of late life in Britain from 1950 to 1970: An overview. *International Journal of Geriatric Psychiatry* **20**(5):423–8.

Hilton C (2008) The provision of mental health services in England for people over 65 years of age. *History of Psychiatry* **19**(3):297–320.

Irvine RE (1985). Eluned Woodford-Williams. *British Medical Journal* **VIII**:550.

Royal College of Physicians (2016). Eluned Woodford-Williams. <http://munksroll.rcplondon.ac.uk/Biography/Details/4876>.

Philp I (2015). The contribution of geriatric medicine to integrated care for older people. *Age and Ageing* **44**:11–15.

Woodford-Williams E and Exton-Smith AN (1962). Aspects of geriatric psychiatry, haematology, nutrition and cancer in old age. 3rd Meeting of the European Clinical Section of the International Association of Gerontology, The Hague, September 1961: Part II. Basel: Karger.

Woodford-Williams E (1960). The clinical medicine of old age. *Proceedings of the Nutrition Society* **19**(2):120–5. DOI:10.1079/PNS19600033.

Chapter 14

A Woman the Government Feared: Barbara Robb (1912–76)

Claire Hilton

Introduction

'Mrs Robb has always been a terrible danger to [the government] ... I knew we had to de-fuse this bomb,' wrote Richard Crossman,[1] a fine compliment from the Secretary of State for Social Services (1968–70) to a woman who emerged from the shadows to fight for improvements in the care of older people. Barbara Robb published *Sans Everything: A Case to Answer* in 1967.[2] The slim volume comprised two parts. The first contained short accounts by staff and patients' relatives about degrading and undignified care which they witnessed in psychiatric and geriatric hospitals. Part two provided suggestions from experts about how to make improvements. The Ministry of Health and the hospital management hierarchy gave *Sans Everything* a hostile response, but many psychiatrists, nurses, voluntary organizations, and the media welcomed it. Subsequently, formal committees of inquiry investigated the *Sans Everything* allegations.

Sans Everything achieved 'bestseller' status in the first week of publication. Soon after, Mabel Franks, previously unknown to Barbara, wrote to her. Franks compared Barbara to Francis Chichester, recently returned from his solo circumnavigation of the globe:

> I consider your achievement far more commendable than that of Chichester. Granted he is a very brave man and we all admire his courage, but your courage is of a noble kind for it will benefit humanity in the future ... you had the guts and moral fibre to pursue this matter and bring it right into the open.[3]

Who was Barbara Robb? Why did she take on the cause of older people on long-stay wards? What gave her the 'uncrushable belief in the need to expose what was going on'?[4] How did she build the fearsome reputation Crossman described? Finally, why has she been forgotten?

The theme of women runs through this story. Elderly women occupied a dispropor-tionate number of beds (over age 75 years: 4 per cent of female population, 25 per cent of female psychiatric hospital beds).[5] Many other women were involved, including as nurses, campaigners, and journalists, all championing, or reporting on, the work of caring, a role traditionally ascribed to them.

Barbara: Nettles and Dock Leaves

Barbara Robb (née Anne) was born in Yorkshire in 1912, into an upper-class recusant Roman Catholic family. Barbara was fond of her grandfather, Ernest Charlton Anne (Figure 14.1), and, alongside her deep faith, carried his words with her throughout life: once, as a child, stung by nettles, he told her that 'everything in life is like the nettles; there are always dock leaves if only you look hard enough'.[6]

The family included some forthright women role models. Elizabeth Anne, a Benedictine nun, died in a French Prison in 1791 'for the faith'.[7] Great-grandmother Barbara Charlton, a life-long commentator on people and their behaviours, wrote her memoirs.[8] Grandmother Edith Anne, an opera singer early in life, later wrote and published novels.[9] Aunt Ernestine Anne played in the first Yorkshire women's cricket team, tried to live as a nun, and wrote a history of the family home, Burghwallis Hall, near Doncaster.[10] Another aunt, Emily Wood, was a magistrate and, during the Second World War, a commandant in the Voluntary Aid Detachment nursing service.[11]

Barbara wanted to be a ballet dancer and performed with the Vic–Wells company, the predecessor of the Royal Ballet.[12] An ankle injury meant a career change, so she went to the Chelsea College of Art to study theatre design. There she met Brian Robb (1913–79). They married in 1937. During the Second World War (Figure 14.2), Barbara had

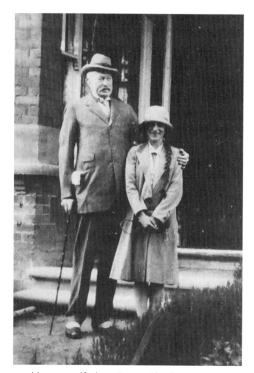

Figure 14.1 Barbara and her grandfather, Ernest Charlton Anne, c. 1922.
Reproduced with permission from Elizabeth Ellison-Anne.

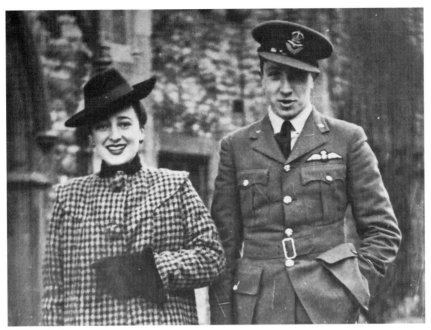

Figure 14.2 Barbara and her brother, Pilot Officer Robert Anne.
He was killed in action, June 1941. Reproduced with permission from Elizabeth Ellison-Anne.

various jobs including helping socially deprived teenage boys. This sparked an interest in Jungian psychotherapy. She taught herself the techniques, and according to Victor White, psychotherapist and Dominican monk, undertook a 'remarkable self-analysis'. White corresponded with Carl Jung for over a decade, and through that link, Barbara visited Jung in Switzerland in 1951. Jung and White commented on her appearance and personality. Jung said, she was 'an eyeful and beyond' and an intuitive introvert who 'decidedly leaves you guessing'. White called her 'quite a corker' and sought Jung's advice on how to 'deal with' her.[13] Their sentiments echoed her effect on other men. Kenneth Robinson (Minister of Health, 1964–68) and Crossman both described her as 'strange'.[14] A former *Sunday Times* journalist said in 2015 that politicians 'really didn't know the beast they were battling with. They totally underestimated her.'[15]

Barbara and Brian lived in a tiny cottage in Hampstead, each floor 'cabin-cruiser' size.[16] They had no children. Barbara worked as a psychotherapist and Brian as an artist, illustrator, and cartoonist. Their marriage was 'near perfect'.[17] Their home, in 1965, became Barbara's campaign headquarters.

Discovering the Long-Stay Wards

From the 1890s, the government ignored warnings about the increase in older people in the asylums and overcrowding on the long-stay wards. From the 1940s, social science and medical evidence indicated that accurate psychiatric diagnosis and clinical and social interventions, in hospitals and in the community, could improve the mental well-being of older people and reduce the need for institutional care. Hospitals and local authorities seldom adopted these recommendations which contradicted widespread stereotypical assumptions of decline in old age rather than recovery. Little interest from the medical profession, lack of public demand, government fear of the perceived insurmountable 'burden' of more older people living longer, and lack of allocated financial resources to activate plans, contributed to the deteriorating situation in the psychiatric hospitals.

Amy Gibbs (1891–1967), a psychotherapy patient of Barbara's, was admitted to Friern Hospital in north London in October 1963. She expected a short admission for 'anxiety' to sort out medication which was making her muzzy-headed. In December 1964, a mutual acquaintance informed Barbara that Amy was still in hospital and wanted to see her. Convinced that Amy was not a 'mental patient', Barbara thought it would 'not be improper' to visit.[18]

This was Barbara's first visit to a psychiatric hospital. Built in 1851, Friern was huge and forbidding. It had 2,250 beds. An unwelcoming, dimly lit corridor over one-third of a mile long linked most of the wards. The lights could go off unexpectedly[19] as the electricity supply needed upgrading.[20] Barbara was stunned when she saw Amy. Since they last met, 14 months earlier, Amy had changed from being plump, upright, and active to being thin, stooped, frail, and inactive. She wore hospital clothes and her hair was cut in the same 'pudding-bowl' style as the other patients. She had neither dentures nor spectacles. Most patients lacked these necessities, hearing aids, and other personal possessions, depriving them of independence and dignity. Most were 'sat as if sunk in torpor'.[21] None had bedside lockers. Visitors were rare. Staff were unfriendly and unhelpful.[22] The experience contradicted Barbara's expectations and government rhetoric that the National Health Service (NHS) was 'the best health service in the world'.[23]

Amy worried about complaining as she feared punishment for doing so.[24] Staff lacked understanding of patients' emotional needs. They teased patients unkindly, chastized or slapped them for being incontinent,[25] and patients were generally in bed by 7 p.m. Barbara visited one evening and found five still up: 'one of the five sat on a commode; another minus most of her clothes, was receiving treatment nearby. No attempt was made to use screens'.[26] Barbara was appalled by the undignified care she witnessed, and began to write what she called her 'Diary of a Nobody' as 'I felt that I would never have another really easy moment unless I did everything I could to try to right this situation'.[27]

1965: The Campaign Begins

Barbara took Brian and some friends to visit Amy. One friend, Lord Strabolgi, was a hereditary Labour peer. Strabolgi sent a copy of the Diary to Kenneth Robinson in early April 1965, who promised to investigate.[28] In May, Strabolgi arranged for Barbara to meet Geoffrey Tooth, head of mental health at the Ministry of Health. She expected to hear the result of the investigation but instead found that nothing had been done. Barbara also learnt from Tooth the term 'stripping', referring to removing all personal possessions, including spectacles and dentures.

Barbara and Strabolgi did little more until Amy was discharged to a residential home which Barbara had found for her. Then, no longer fearing that Amy might be punished for their interference in her care, Strabolgi addressed the House of Lords. He described stripping, lack of activities, staff discouraging visitors, 'appalling' food, serving the last meal of the day as early as 3.30 p.m., and

> an atmosphere of humiliation and neglect. The patients are ... 'pulped.' They lose all sense of self-respect. Worse than this, many are cowed and frightened. All just vegetate and seem lost to the world. And they are lost to the world. There is nothing more relentless than the State machine when it gets the helpless into its maw.[29]

The press seized the story and Strabolgi received numerous letters of concern describing similar conditions elsewhere. Robinson reprimanded Strabolgi for causing 'unfavourable publicity'. Barbara wrote to Robinson that the way to avoid such publicity was 'to firmly remove the faults that occasioned' it.[30]

Creating AEGIS

It was clear that the problems were not confined to Friern. Barbara formed a small pressure group, AEGIS (Aid for the Elderly in Government Institutions). In Greek mythology, aegis was a symbol of protection carried by Athena and Zeus. It was not a name for an organization likely to admit defeat. AEGIS's advisors included: psychiatrists Russell Barton, Tony Whitehead, and David Enoch; Professor of Social Administration, Brian Abel-Smith, at the London School of Economics; social rights campaigner Audrey Harvey; CH Rolph, journalist with the *New Statesman*; and Phyllis Rowe, vice president of the Royal College of Nursing. AEGIS also worked closely with Mary Applebey (National Association for Mental Health, NAMH, later Mind), and Helen Hodgson, founder of the Patients Association. Barbara told her campaign plans to a doctor, probably Brian's brother Douglas: he 'turned pale green and said "For God's sake, don't do it!"' and described how hospital staff collude with each other and tell lies.[31]

AEGIS wrote to *The Times*. Signatories to the letter included three peers.[32] The letter described AEGIS's findings of undignified care of older people in long-stay wards and sought further information. It also mentioned a lack of confidence in the Ministry's ability to investigate or improve the situation. Soon after this, the Ministry wrote to Regional Hospital Boards (RHBs) about allowing patients to retain their aids and personal possessions.[33] Around the same time, the RHB in charge of Friern investigated and found numerous problems on the wards but took no action to remedy them.[34] The RHB chairman refused to tell AEGIS the outcome of the investigation. He wrote to Barbara: 'I have your letter of 18th December and have no comment to make.'[35] Barbara described his response as 'short and sour'.[36] It was pivotal to her campaign: she decided then to publish the Diary.[37]

Writing and Publishing *Sans Everything*

After *The Times* letter, patients, their relatives, and hospital staff wrote to AEGIS in 'an avalanche of anguish'. Barbara answered every letter personally.[38] Some of these letters, alongside the Diary, created 'the case' for *Sans Everything*. The book also gave 'some answers' to the problem at hand. Tony Whitehead provided the medical answer: effective comprehensive psychogeriatric services, as at Severalls Hospital, Colchester. An architect described a scheme to build housing for rent on spare hospital land, a financial answer. Abel-Smith stated the need for better funding and gave an administrative solution: improved complaints procedures, and a hospitals' inspectorate and independent ombudsman to help monitor and maintain standards.

While Barbara created the book, the Ministry of Health demonstrated lack of awareness of how to undertake inquiries into complaints. During 19 years of the NHS, it instigated a mere 6 statutory inquiries, none directly concerning patient care.[39] For *Sans Everything*, it prejudged the allegations, and planned non-statutory inquiries, considering the allegations as probably unsound rather than serious.[40] The RHBs would appoint the committees: Barbara doubted they could be truly independent. As non-statutory inquiries, the Council on Tribunals, the advisory public body set up to ensure that inquiries were open, fair, and impartial, would not provide oversight. Abel-Smith likened the Ministry's plan to appointing the Coal Board to investigate the Aberfan Disaster, the colliery tip collapse which killed 116 children and 28 adults in 1966, for which the Board was found negligent.[41]

In June 1967, the national press paved the way for publication of *Sans Everything*. *The Sunday Times* featured a three-quarter-page spread about it which generated correspondence.[42] The *Nursing Mirror* reported on its survey indicating that nurses feared reprisals if they voiced concerns.[43] A television programme about *Sans Everything* on the day of publication gave Kenneth Robinson the last word: 'I am absolutely sure, that the care of our old people in our geriatric and psychiatric hospitals is as good as anything in the world.'[44] In another BBC broadcast, the interviewer asked Robinson about ill-treatment: 'Are you satisfied that it has been reduced, now, almost to non-existence?' Robinson replied: 'That is my belief and I hope that any enquiries we can make will bear that out.'[45] His stance was unlikely to encourage unbiased investigations. The press criticized Robinson's lack of knowledge and concern about poor care, and his attitude to the allegations.[46] Dennis Hobden MP (Labour) wrote to Barbara: 'I long ago gave up [on] Kenneth Robinson. There has been nothing but evasion and covering up by Hospital Management Committees from top to bottom.'[47]

A Witness, Her Allegations, and an Inquiry

Space in this chapter only permits analysis of one *Sans Everything* report and the subsequent RHB inquiry into its allegations. Joyce Daniel's report offers a good illustration of what happened. In 1964–65, Daniel ('Adeline Craythorne': Barbara gave her authors pseudonyms, to protect them from victimization), a widow in her 50s, worked as an auxiliary nurse on a long-stay female geriatric ward at St Lawrence's Hospital at Bodmin. Her allegations included: staff swearing at patients, hitting them, and handling them roughly; communal bathrooms where 44 patients were bathed in a single morning; patients 'locked in the lavatory to keep them out the way'; and staff making crude remarks about patients in their earshot. When she complained about staff behaviour towards patients, she was taken off duties with patients and transferred to cleaning copper pipes in the bathroom. Her colleagues said that her comments created an unpleasant work atmosphere and that nurses should be loyal and act as a unified body.[48] Daniel resigned.

George Polson, a senior barrister, chaired the committee of inquiry. He asked leading questions: 'You have never seen anything like that at all, have you?'[49] He did not probe criticisms which existing staff made, such as when a nurse admitted that he witnessed unkind behaviour but 'rightly or wrongly, it is as well to let certain things that I do not like pass'.[50] The committee chillingly highlighted disregard of patients' lives when it asked the nursing superintendent, but did not challenge, what would happen on a locked, unstaffed ward at night in an emergency: 'Assistance has been summoned in the case of one upstairs ward and a night nurse down in the ward below with a patient banging on the floor. Apart from that we are dependent upon a patient in the ward being able to use the telephone.'[51]

Before questioning Daniel, one lawyer declared his bias: 'quite frankly I anticipate that some of the allegations in the book may very well not be quite so impressive after cross examination'.[52] He attacked minor errors in Daniel's report, such as the number of patients on the ward: Daniel said there were about 70,[53] the ward report books said about 60, and the lawyer commented: 'Well, it is a little artistic licence. She is a poet, after all'.[54] Daniel's concern, that the ward was severely overcrowded, was considered trivial compared to the inaccuracies. Another lawyer, representing hospital management, described her as 'sentimental and sloppy and perhaps soft, this has had an influence on her which it … has not had on other people'.[55] Personally discrediting Daniel automatically condemned her evidence. At the end of the first day Daniel wrote to Barbara: 'I cannot convey the air of hostility'.[56]

Daniel alleged that patients drank from the lavatory pans but senior staff explained: 'there are always in every psychiatric hospital patients who drink from toilet pans'.[57] Staff attributed patients' fears and flinching to them not understanding why certain things were done to them[58] rather than because of inadequate explanations, slapdash, uncaring, or harsh nursing practices. Staff did not modify practices according to patients' needs. The committee rejected Daniel's concern about lack of 'scented soap' for bathing patients. That seemed a minor complaint until explored in the context that staff washed patients with the Lifebuoy soap used to scrub the floors.[59] It reinforced the evidence that patients were not treated as human beings.

Even on the worst wards some staff were caring and criticized harsh nursing practices. Other staff, aware of the deficits, feared speaking out. Senior staff justified demeaning and disrespectful practices, which reinforced their continuation. They ignored their detrimental effects on patients, visitors, and staff. The committee exonerated a ward sister who swore at and hit patients when stressed: it did 'not think she would ever deliberately ill-treat' any patient,[60] a subjective verdict which implied that disrespectful behaviour towards patients was acceptable if unintentional or if it occurred when work was stressful. The committee overlooked published principles of good psychiatric practice used elsewhere in the NHS,[61,62] and its obsequiousness to the hierarchical system of hospital management precluded candid scrutiny.

In the final published report,[63] five paragraphs of the 'summary of findings' praised staff for high standards of work. The other four attacked Daniel personally, accusing her of misinterpreting, misunderstanding, and distorting her observations, that her judgements were 'manifestly unsound' and her 'sentimental approach' conflicted with the 'objective attitudes' of other staff. Daniel's treatment alone justified Barbara's concern about anonymity for her witnesses. The report concluded: 'we have no hesitation to say that in our unanimous opinion there is no substance whatever in the allegations of cruelty by staff',[64] and 'the standard of psychiatric and psychogeriatric services provided in the hospital might well be emulated by the rest of the country'.[65] These conclusions, based on the evidence, are mindboggling. Lack of knowledge of good practice, leading questions, deferring to seniority, condoning low standards for older people, and uncritical endorsement of 'the best health service in the world' contributed.

Max Beloff, Professor of Government and Public Administration at Oxford, commented in 1967: 'with our close-knit political-administrative network ... most inquiries are so manned that they turn out to be nothing but the system looking at itself, and finding more to admire than to blame'.[66] Crossman described the Sans Everything inquiry committees as 'fairly well rigged'.[67]

The White Paper

The Ministry of Health compiled a single White Paper[68] comprising reports from all seven inquiries conducted by the RHBs. Only one committee of inquiry considered a Sans Everything author-witness as reliable, upholding his complaints: the Ministry relegated that committee's brief report to the last two pages of the White Paper, a location likely to be overlooked by readers. The other reports discredited the Sans Everything witnesses and cleared the hospital staff of wrongdoing. Most identified some problems but these were based on inspections of the hospitals rather than on the Sans Everything allegations. The White Paper made 48 recommendations for improvements.

Kenneth Robinson announced in the House of Commons that the inquiries proved that most of the allegations in Sans Everything were 'totally unfounded or grossly exaggerated', that the committees reported 'very favourably on the standard of care provided', and 'the White Paper should discourage anyone from making ... ill-founded and irresponsible allegations in future'. Some MPs criticized Sans Everything for causing distress and wasting public money with 'wild and irresponsible allegations'.[69] A Ministry of Health press release concurred with Robinson's statement,[70] leading to national newspapers exonerating the hospitals. However, when the full White Paper became available later the same day, journalists made abrupt U-turns in their judgements, with fresh reports vindicating Sans Everything. Rolph wrote about the journalists deceived by the Ministry: 'I don't remember hearing pressmen so angry'.[71]

Crossman wrote in his diary: 'Robinson mis-handled her [Barbara] and instead of treating Sans Everything sensibly Kenneth set up committees of investigation into her charges and then published a White Paper as a non-controversial document to answer her, which it didn't'.[72] Robinson expected that the Sans Everything White Paper would 'demolish Mrs Robb'.[73] Barbara had astonishing strength of character. Despite the humiliation of public discrediting, she persisted with the campaign, helped by her faith, Brian, friends, and the AEGIS advisors.

Other Allegations and Their Outcomes

Responses to *Sans Everything* revealed malpractice in other hospitals, including 'smouldering discontent' at Whittingham Hospital in Lancashire.[74] Barbara, anonymously, received pages torn from a ward report book at South Ockendon Hospital in Essex describing injuries probably inflicted on a patient by staff.[75] This highlighted Barbara's reputation for dealing with complaints, emphasizing the need for an official, independent ombudsman to do the same. AEGIS thus triggered the inquires at Whittingham and South Ockendon. Other disturbing reports emerged, including deaths of patients, leading to convictions for manslaughter of three staff at Farleigh Hospital near Bristol. A nauseating *World in Action* television documentary about Powick Hospital, *Ward F13*, exposed undignified batch-living of 78 elderly women, and valiant over-worked nurses.[76]

David Roxan's article on *Sans Everything* in the *News of the World*[77] triggered letters of concern about other hospitals, including Ely Hospital in Cardiff. Roxan forwarded them to the Ministry.[78] For Ely, Robinson set up an inquiry chaired by Geoffrey Howe, an outstanding lawyer. He represented Coal Board managers at the Aberfan Inquiry and was deeply affected by the experience. Howe conducted the Ely Inquiry in line with Council on Tribunals guidance. He weighed all the evidence meticulously, including the reliability of the whistle-blower, nursing auxiliary Michael Pantelides. Allegations were comparable with those in *Sans Everything*, but the Ely committee upheld the allegations, including appalling abuse of patients, victimization of staff who complained, and inadequate management at all levels. Howe wanted the full report published. Crossman, fearful of Howe's legal skills and Barbara's media relationships, agreed. He announced the findings and plans to establish an inspectorate, the Hospital Advisory Service, on 27 March 1969.[79]

Crossman genuinely wanted to improve the long-stay mental illness and 'mental handicap' hospitals and transferred some funds to them. He accepted that criticism could help developments. When an undercover journalist working at Friern published his report, Crossman wrote: 'naturally the hospital staff are furious with the *Daily Mail* for smuggling a reporter into Friern … But I fear this is the kind of trick which must be used in order to shake the public out of its apathy.'[80]

The Impact

A year after publication of the Ely Report, Labour lost the General Election to the Conservatives, but the momentum of Crossman's programme continued. The Department of Health and Social Security (DHSS) established both an NHS ombudsman and the Davies Committee into hospital complaints procedures.[81] Alongside clinicians, the DHSS created blueprints for developing services for mental handicap and for older and younger adults with psychiatric illness.[82] All these outcomes were attributed to the Ely Inquiry, forgetting that Barbara's work initiated it, and that, helped by her Fleet Street allies, she put pressure on the DHSS to act. The Council on Tribunals, which upheld Barbara's complaints about the *Sans Everything* inquiries, also contributed to new NHS policies based on their analysis of those inquiries.[83]

AEGIS helped to end the culture of secrecy in psychiatric hospitals. It helped to develop guidance to manage violence in them. It inspired the NAMH and other voluntary organizations to adopt more forceful campaigning roles. *Sans Everything* influenced nurses to be less submissive and more assertive.[84] It affected the lives of doctors, such as Tom Arie, whom it encouraged to apply for a consultant psychiatrist post working with older people in a psychiatric hospital in 1968.[85] Barbara inspired Enoch to set up a study group comprising geriatricians and psychiatrists whose deliberations, published in 1971,[86] inspired more geriatrician–psychiatrist collaboration. Members of Enoch's group were among the earliest activists in the Group (now Faculty) for the Psychiatry of Old Age at the Royal College of Psychiatrists.

AEGIS only existed because of Barbara, but she did not function in isolation. She drew repeatedly on the expertise of the AEGIS advisors. In the complex field of health service policy development, AEGIS could not produce changes single-handedly. However, it influenced DHSS policy, by identifying issues, suggesting answers, and using the media to increase awareness and stir up public and professional support. AEGIS operated relentlessly from 1965 until 1974, and then more modestly until Barbara's death two years later. Barbara never tried to create a large organization. AEGIS remained small, elite, and independent. Independence gave Barbara freedom to be more publicly outspoken than was possible for academics, doctors, lawyers, and politicians who might jeopardize their careers by doing so. In 1974, when Mrs Castle, Labour Secretary of State for Social Services, invited Barbara to join the Central Health Services Council, an advisory body to the DHSS, Barbara and her AEGIS advisors agreed that 'AEGIS functions best as a totally independent body, and has the best hope of being of service to the Secretaries of State and to the public by continuing in that capacity'.[87] AEGIS's style also fitted Barbara's personality: 'I'm better suited to Walls of Jericho than to Trojan Horse tactics.'[88]

Reflections

It is notable that the *Sans Everything* and Ely whistle-blowers were mainly NHS staff without professional training, middle-aged, in post for a short time, and with a variety of previous life experiences. At Whittingham and Farleigh, student nurses played important roles in raising concerns. In 2017, these professionally inexperienced clinical team members are the least likely to be asked for their opinions on standards of care, but the NHS needs to value their insights and fresh approach to solving problems.

Several factors contributed to Barbara being forgotten. These include: official discrediting of *Sans Everything*; overshadowing by the Ely Inquiry; Barbara's distaste for self-grandstanding; her untimely death followed by Brian's health deteriorating and his death three years later; and being eclipsed by people more formally prominent and ambitious within government and political circles. Her reputation as 'a thorn in the flesh of certain hospital authorities in whose flesh a thorn was long overdue'[89] was hardly conducive to those in power wanting to remember her. If Barbara had destroyed her archive, as she initially planned, we would know significantly less about her today.[90]

Barbara inspired many people during her lifetime, including doctors, nurses, journalists, academics, politicians, and the author-witnesses. Barbara's energy and commitment to improve conditions for older people in psychiatric hospitals matched the dedication of Elizabeth Fry (1780–1845), the prison reformer, and Florence Nightingale (1820–1910), who professionalized nursing. All three were appalled by the inhumanity they witnessed in institutions and set their minds to eliminating it. All were upper class, of independent means, with strong religious inspiration, and spent years trying to make improvements. Barbara, like her predecessors, broke the chain of the establishment condoning inhumane practices. None of them provided all the answers but they made crucial contributions, relieving much suffering. Scandals recur, in prisons,[91] hospitals,[92] and in the care of older people.[93] We do not live in a utopia. Societies include vulnerable individuals and others who can exploit or abuse them. Inhumanities persist and need fresh campaigns and inspiration, and Barbara's story may inspire future generations. Fifty years since *Sans Everything* was published, it is rightful to recognize Barbara's place in history. As Abel-Smith said: 'For one woman ... to suddenly do so much in such a short period—and tragically, to die so soon—is a remarkable story.'[94]

Acknowledgements

I am grateful to the Wellcome Trust for a Leave Award for Clinicians and Scientists in Medical Humanities (108519/Z/15/Z) which allowed me to undertake this study.

References

1. **Crossman R** (1977). *The Diaries of a Cabinet Minister. Vol 3. Secretary of State for Social Services 1968–1970*. London: Hamilton and Cape, p. 727.

2. **Robb B** (1967). *Sans Everything: A Case to Answer*. London: Nelson.

3. Mabel Franks to Robb, July 1967, AEGIS/2/10 (AEGIS archive at London School of Economics).

4. **Anne Robinson**, interviewed by author, November 2015.

5. **Brooke E** (1967). *A Census of Patients in Psychiatric Beds 1963*. London: Her Majesty's Stationery Office, p. 24.

6. **Allen A** (1967). 'One woman who refused to pass by ..'. *Sunday Mirror*, 9 July.

7. Plaque at Burghwallis Hall.

8. **Charlton L** (ed.) (1949). *The Recollections of a Northumbrian Lady 1815–1866. The Memoirs of Barbara Charlton of Hesleyside, Northumberland*. London: Jonathan Cape.

9. e.g. **Allan EF** (1897). *A Woman of Moods*. London: Burns and Oates.

10. **Anne E** (*c*. 1970). *Burghwallis and the Anne Family*.

11. **Lundy D.** 'Emily Wood', <http://www.thepeerage.com/p30395.htm#i303949>.

12. **Anon** (1976). 'The patients' campaigner'. *Hampstead and Highgate Express*, 25 June.

13. **Lammers A** and **Cunningham A** (eds) (2007). *The Jung–White Letters*. London: Routledge, pp. 168–70.

14. Kenneth Robinson, interviewed by Margot Jeffreys. In: *Oral History of Geriatrics as a Medical Specialty*. British Library Sound Archives. This is a single unpublished cassette recording held in the collection.

15. **Anne Robinson**, interviewed by author, November 2015.

16. **Anne Robinson**, interviewed by author, November 2015.

17. **Harvey A** (1976). 'Mrs Barbara Robb'. *The Times*, 28 June, p. 17.

18. **Robb B** (undated). 'Record of a campaign'. 1:4, AEGIS/1/1.

19. **Robb B** (1967). *Sans Everything: A Case to Answer*. London: Nelson, p. 78.

20. North West Metropolitan Regional Hospital Board (NWMRHB), meeting, 13 November 1967, 11 (LMA).

21. **Robb B** (1967). *Sans Everything: A Case to Answer*. London: Nelson, p. 72.

22. **Robb B** (1967). *Sans Everything: A Case to Answer*. London: Nelson, pp. 70, 88.

23. 'Mental health service'. *Hansard* HC Deb 19 March 1965 vol 708 cc1645–719:1656.

24. **Robb B** (1967). *Sans Everything: A Case to Answer*. London: Nelson, pp. 73–4.

25. **Robb B** (1967). *Sans Everything: A Case to Answer*. London: Nelson, p. 88.

26. **Robb B** (1967). *Sans Everything: A Case to Answer*. London: Nelson, p. 74.

27. **Allen A** (1967). 'One woman who refused to pass by …'. *Sunday Mirror*, 9 July.

28. Strabolgi to Robinson (draft letter), July 1965, AEGIS/7/8.

29. 'Community care'. *Hansard* HL Deb 07 July 1965 vol 267 cc1332–410:1398.

30. Robinson–Robb correspondence, 5–9 August 1965, AEGIS/1/1.

31. Robb to Russell Barton, 21 July 1966, AEGIS/1/20.

32. **Strabolgi, Beaumont, Heytesbury, Abel-Smith B, Ardizzone E, Harvey A, Hewetson J, Robb B, Sargent W,** and **Woolgar D** (1965). 'Old people in mental hospitals'. *The Times*, 10 November.

33. Ministry of Health to Regional Hospital Boards, 17 December 1965, in NWMRHB, minutes, 14 February 1966 (LMA).

34. NWMRHB (1966). Report of the committee of inquiry on Friern Hospital, 7 January 1966, Mental Health Committee, minutes and papers. London: LMA; NWMRHB (1968). Report of an independent committee of enquiry into allegations concerning Friern Hospital in a book entitled *Sans Everything*. London: LMA, p. 32.

35. Maurice Hackett to Robb B. 29 December 1966, AEGIS/A/1/A.

36. Robb, 'Record of a campaign' 2:71, AEGIS/1/2.

37. Robb, 'Chronology' 29 December 1965, AEGIS/2/14.

38. Robb, 'Record of a campaign' 8:5, AEGIS/1/8.

39. Ministry of Health, Section 70 inquiries, MH 159/213. The National Archives (TNA), Kew.

40. Mr Hales to 'Secretary', 4 July 1967, MH 150/350. TNA.

41. *24 Hours*. BBC1, 28 July 1967, transcript, AEGIS/1/6.

42. **Young H** (1967). 'The old in hospital'. *Sunday Times*, 4 June.

43. **Anon** (1967). 'First response to last week's editorial'. *Nursing Mirror*, 23 June, pp. 287–8.

44. *24 Hours*. BBC1, 30 June 1967, AEGIS/1/6.

45. *24 Hours*. BBC1, 28 July 1967.

46. **Allen A** (1967). 'One woman who refused to pass by …'. *Sunday Mirror*, 9 July.

47. Dennis Hobden to Robb, 25 April 1967, AEGIS/2/3.

48. **Daniel J** (Pseudonym: Adeline Craythorne) (1967). In: Robb B (ed.) *Sans Everything: A Case to Answer*. London: Nelson, pp. 37–43.

49. St Lawrence's, 26 September 1967, 65–6, MH 159/226. TNA.

50. St Lawrence's, 26 September 1967, 52–3, MH 159/226. TNA.

51. St Lawrence's, 15 September 1967, 44, MH 159/226. TNA.

52. St Lawrence's, 30 October 1967, 54, MH 159/228. TNA.

53. **Robb B** (1967). *Sans Everything: A Case to Answer.* London: Nelson, p. 39.

54. St Lawrence's, 19 November 1967, 8–9, MH 159/229. TNA.

55. St Lawrence's, 22 November 1967, 92, MH 159/229. TNA.

56. Daniel to Robb, 'Wednesday'. AEGIS/2/10.

57. St Lawrence's, 25 September 1967, 83, MH 159/226. TNA.

58. St Lawrence's, 31 October 1967, 12, MH 159/227. TNA.

59. St Lawrence's, 19 November 1967, 20, MH 159/229. TNA.

60. South Western Regional Hospital Board. 'Report of the committee of inquiry concerning St Lawrence's Hospital Bodmin' 9, MH 159/227. TNA.

61. **World Health Organization** (1959). *Mental Health Problems of Aging and the Aged.* Geneva: World Health Organization, p. 10.

62. **Post F** (1965). *The Clinical Psychiatry of Late Life.* London: Pergamon Press.

63. **Ministry of Health** (1968). *Findings and Recommendations Following Enquiries into Allegations Concerning the Care of Elderly Patients in Certain Hospitals* Cmnd. 3687. London: Her Majesty's Stationery Office.

64. **Ministry of Health** (1968). *Findings and Recommendations Following Enquiries into Allegations Concerning the Care of Elderly Patients in Certain Hospitals* Cmnd. 3687. London: Her Majesty's Stationery Office, p. 78

65. **Ministry of Health** (1968). *Findings and Recommendations Following Enquiries into Allegations Concerning the Care of Elderly Patients in Certain Hospitals* Cmnd. 3687. London: Her Majesty's Stationery Office, p. 81

66. **Beloff M** (1969). 'Defining the limits of official responsibility'. *The Times,* 11 September.

67. Richard Crossman, manuscript of diary, 12 November 1969, JH/69/39 (University of Warwick Modern Records Centre, UWMRC).

68. **Ministry of Health** (1968). *Findings and Recommendations Following Enquiries into Allegations Concerning the Care of Elderly Patients in Certain Hospitals* Cmnd. 3687. London: Her Majesty's Stationery Office.

69. 'Sans Everything (Reports of Inquiries)'. *Hansard* HC Deb 09 July 1968 vol 768 cc213–16.

70. Ministry of Health, press service, 9 July 1968, AEGIS/B/3.

71. **Rolph C** (1968). 'Whiter-than-white paper'. *New Statesman,* 19 July.

72. **Crossman R** (1977). *The Diaries of a Cabinet Minister. Vol 3. Secretary of State for Social Services 1968–1970.* London: Hamilton and Cape, p. 727.

73. Crossman, 16 July 1968, 151/68/SW (UWMRC).

74. **Department of Health and Social Security** (1972). *Report of the Committee of Inquiry into Whittingham Hospital.* Cmnd. 486. London: Her Majesty's Stationery Office.

75. Robb, 'Record'. 9: introduction, AEGIS1/9/1.

76. *Ward F13,* World in Action. Granada Television, 21 May 1968.

77. **Roxan D** (1967). ' "Old folk beaten in hospital" allegation'. *News of the World,* 25 June.

78. Ministry of Health press office, 27 July 1967, MH 150/350. (TNA).

79. 'Ely Hospital, Cardiff: Inquiry Findings'. *Hansard* HL Deb 27 March 1969 vol 300 cc1384–93.

80. **Crossman R** (1971). 'London diary'. *New Statesman*, 22 October.

81. **Department of Health and Social Security** (1973). *Report of the Committee on Hospital Complaint Procedures*. London: Her Majesty's Stationery Office.

82. **Department of Health and Social Security** (1971). *Better Services for the Mentally Handicapped*. London: Her Majesty's Stationery Office; Department of Health and Social Security (1971). *Hospital Services for the Mentally Ill* HM(71)97. London: Her Majesty's Stationery Office. Department of Health and Social Security (1972). *Services for Mental Illness Related to Old Age* HM(72)71. London: Her Majesty's Stationery Office.

83. Alistair Macdonald to Robb, 13 January 1969, AEGIS/2/9.

84. **Anon** (1968). 'Tug of war at nurses' Commons protest'. *Daily Telegraph*, 14 December.

85. Tom Arie, email to author, April 2009.

86. **Enoch MD** and **Howells J** (1971). *The Organisation of Psychogeriatrics*. Ipswich: Society of Clinical Psychiatrists.

87. Robb to Department of Health and Social Security, 30 April 1974, AEGIS/1/10/D.

88. **Anon** (1976). 'The patients' campaigner'. *Hampstead and Highgate Express*, 25 June.

89. **Rolph C** (1987). *Further Particulars*. Oxford: Oxford University Press, p. 180.

90. Robb to FJ Charlton, 19 August 1970, AEGIS/1/10/B.

91. 'Teenage prison abuse exposed'. *Panorama*. BBC1, 11 January 2016.

92. **Mid Staffordshire NHS Foundation Trust** (2013). *Mid Staffordshire NHS Foundation Trust Public Inquiry* HC.947. The Stationery Office.

93. 'Behind closed doors: Elderly care exposed'. *Panorama*. BBC1, 30 April 2014.

94. **Brian Abel-Smith**, interviewed by Hugh Freeman (1990). *BJPsych Bulletin* **14**:257–61. DOI: 10.1192/pb.14.5.257.

Chapter 15

Change and Continuity in Psychiatry: One Woman's Reflections

Claire Murdoch

Change and Continuity

Change and continuity have marked my three decades of working in psychiatry. So much has changed since I entered mental health nurse training at Friern Barnet Hospital in 1983. An eminent consultant psychiatrist told me during my first week that I would hear a lot of stuff and nonsense about the hospital closing, but not to worry, it never would. Seven or eight years later I was privileged to be one of those asked to speak at the closing ceremony. Issues of rights and responsibilities, freedom, care, or custody, funding, stigma, innovation, and great passion have all been constants throughout a time of incredible change.

Today we are still grappling with how best to co-ordinate care in community settings for those with the most complex disorders; how to maximize independence without losing people to loneliness and a life of poor quality. People with a serious mental illness are dying scandalously earlier than they should from physical ill health. As social care services struggle to fund all but their statutory responsibilities, issues of housing occupation and social support for those living in the community require urgent attention. On the other hand, the user voice and innovation has never been more powerful. Innovations such as Recovery Colleges, collectives, peer support workers, and alternative models of crisis care and prevention proliferate. The *Five Year Forward View for Mental Health*[1] is setting an exciting and important development agenda, and awareness of mental health has never been greater. There is a sense of being on the precipice of a new era in psychiatry and while the pressures are great, there is much cause for optimism. This is because across the country, collaborations of clinicians, patients, carers, and commissioners are determined to drive progress forward. Even as we look to the future, we can draw lessons from the past and the institutions we were proud to close.

Asylum Days

The early 1980s were an incredible point in history during which to train in psychiatry, in a big Victorian asylum. It was a potent mixture of institutions, tradition, hierarchy, and routine alongside a growing expectation that Friern Barnet Hospital would close, routines were to be abandoned for individualized care, wards would be unlocked, bath books and weight books discarded, and uniforms set aside. It was a strange contradiction to feel that as a student nurse, you were low down the hierarchy with seemingly little power, and yet you were an agent of change. It was true of the other professions as well. We were there to learn and challenge. It was like existing in a parallel universe, one which didn't yet exist.

The strange thing about the institutional aspects of life at Friern is that there was so much opportunity to press for change and to question the status quo. It was a place of great love and expertise and I witnessed the best and worst aspects of care there. The space and beautiful grounds were a valuable part of the asylum which we miss today. My own tactic for walking a tightrope between past conventions and the promise of the future was to ensure that my uniform, time-keeping, and adherence to the sensible rules was impeccable. I also worked hard at my studies and strove to be an excellent nurse. I believed that doing all of these things gave me licence to challenge or change and, in turn, demand change.

> There was a sense of order which reminded me of the hymn 'All Things Bright and Beautiful' by Cecil Frances Alexander in 1845.

The rich man in his castle,
The poor man by his gate,
God made them high and lowly
And ordered their estate.

Much of the initial appearance of life within Friern was of this Victorian order and hierarchy, but things were definitely changing and the scope to create something new and better was manifest. Powerful and increasingly well-organized patient lobbies were developing both inside and outside the 'system'. Amongst the professions there was a sense of learning all we could from a dying system of care which had offered a great deal but which was now clearly of a bygone age, even as we studied it.

Being a woman in psychiatry at that time is hard to disentangle from being a nurse. The men in my nurse training group wore white coats and were called 'Mr'. The women wore little J-cloth dresses and funny paper hats (when we did our general training at the Royal Free) and I was definitely 'Nurse Murdoch'. The first time I wore a uniform I felt like a doll. Fashion at that time entailed lots of long, black, flowing dresses, so our uniforms felt skimpy and exposing.

I remember Margaret Thatcher visiting Friern Hospital during my first few weeks there. The miner's strike and the Griffiths Report[2] on introducing general management into the NHS and austerity both led to loud demonstrations greeting the Prime Minister as her car rolled into the hospital. I protested too. The limousine sped through the main gate in an instant and the chanting crowd were left dissatisfied that their protest had not amounted to much. Shortly after her arrival, I was on the famous long hospital corridor, having just left the school of nursing, and there, in the distance, coming towards us was Margaret Thatcher with the hospital unit general manager and two aides. Slowly but steadily they approached us; only the sound of muffled conversation and clacking of heels broke the silence inside the hospital. Outside, angry protesters could still be heard. Finally, the small group of dignitaries drew level and Margaret Thatcher stopped and said hello. From nowhere I heard myself ask her loudly 'have you come here for something to help you sleep at night?' She was rushed away by the hospital unit general manager and I was summoned to a meeting the next day. The lecturer, who had been dispatched by the unit manager, said that he had been sent to extract an apology from me. I refused to give one; he left and we carried on as before. I took this as a signal that the hospital might seem disciplinarian and rule-bound but that there was scope for staff to challenge things and to be outspoken too. The next day's newspaper reported the visit and the protest and referred to a young patient in the corridor who had challenged the Prime Minister. I would love a copy of that clipping, but alas it's long gone.

Training

As student nurses much of our syllabus[3] was very traditional and included diagnosis, treatments, medication and side effects, the use of Electroconvulsive Therapy (ECT), basic observations, giving injections, a significant amount of physical healthcare, hydration, nutrition, anatomy, aseptic technique, how to give a bed bath, last offices, how to construct hospital bed corners, and so on. Every three months we underwent assessments and exams. However, the training also addressed communication and basic counselling skills, family therapy, choice, individualized care, social systems, and, of course, the Mental Health Act 1983. The nursing process was introduced. The setting of goals and outcomes were seen as a new thing to help personalize care. However, resistance by longer-serving staff members was tangible. The process was seen as a bureaucratic paper exercise by many staff, yet another challenge to order and systems that had managed patient care for 100 years. It took two or three years to make it standard practice and student nurses, trainee doctors, social workers, and therapists were all part of implementing change.

Changing Principles of Care

A myriad issues were fought over on the battleground of progress. Milk and sugar was added to tea pots on some wards without offering patients any choice; bed times, bath times, and therapy times were all strictly regimented. We challenged restrictive regimes such as these all the time.

They no longer exist to quite the same extent but many of the underlying issues of choice, routine, care, freedom, and responsibility are very much alive today. We still debate what is the role of social care, how we ensure meaningful contributing lives, how we stop people being lonely and unsupported or relapsing too seriously. Whose responsibility are these? When does freedom become neglect?

One of the key lessons we were taught as student nurses was not to read patient notes too early on. See the person, talk to them, listen to them, and only then read their notes. They are people first; not just a diagnosis.

This was never a more important principle than when caring for long-stay patients. We undertook two rehabilitation placements of three months each during our three-year, three-month RMN (Registered Mental Nurse) training. People on these wards had often been admitted decades previously with a diagnosis of 'moral deficiency'; perhaps they had become pregnant while an unmarried teenager or had stolen something, for example.

Harry's Life

I still vividly remember a man I will call Harry. Admitted 70 years earlier, often cata-
tonic for weeks or months at a time, he was mute, gentle, and totally endearing. In the
three months I worked on his ward I found that we made a connection by sitting at the
piano together. I would play a note and he would respond and on a good day it would
be the other way around. He was painfully slow and it could take an hour and a half
to coax him from his chair to the piano and to sit together for 45 minutes or so. It felt
like a connection. I felt as though it mattered but I didn't understand why. Towards
the end of the three months Harry was admitted to the Royal Free with an obstructed
bowel, and one morning at 3 a.m. I took a call from the hospital reporting that he had
passed peacefully away minutes earlier. I was alone on the ward (25 rehab patients
were asleep) and pulled out Harry's files for the first time. There were vast volumes of
papers, a life-time in manila folders. I then discovered that he had been committed
to hospital at the age of 14 (dying at the age of 86) for stealing sheet music. Over the
decades he had been given insulin coma therapy, cold bath treatments, and ECT. His
family did not visit him. His catatonia meant that he had spells without moving volun-
tarily, was able to hold strange postures for days on end if permitted (waxy flexibility).
He had also experienced weeks of mania during which he had no sleep, food, or drink.
I have often wondered whether our connection over the piano was linked to a long
distant love of music. At three in the morning I sat and wept for Harry, his life, his loss,
all because he stole a few sheets of music.

Opportunities for an RMN

When I qualified as an RMN I left Friern to work in the modern, permissive environment of the Royal Free Hospital (RFH) in the adult acute wards. There were 40 beds on
the second floor of the tower and no garden. The staff group (all disciplines) was largely
youthful and progressive and patient care was of a high standard. During my training
I had worked at the RFH in the acute wards, in out-patient services for children, and
on the eating disorder unit and older adult services. I had also worked on a medical
and surgical ward. The majority of the training had been hospital-based but I had also
had placements in a day hospital, with a health visitor, in general practice, and with
Community Psychiatric Nurses (CPNs). These community services were very much in
the minority, but were expanding as plans for hospital closures advanced. There was
a movement towards more multidisciplinary working and the dispersal of power. The
hierarchy was shifting.

After only 11 months as a staff nurse at the RFH I was offered a job as a ward sister
back at Friern Hospital. I couldn't resist as it felt like a golden opportunity to put into
practice so many of the things I had wanted to do as student nurse. This early promotion reflected, amongst other things, that being a woman was no impediment to my
career. What was valued at that time (1988/89) was a drive to challenge and change
things. Thus, I became a sister of a 26-bedded acute ward. This ward was in Halliwick,
a modern 1960s building, in the grounds of Friern. It was a unit with a reputation for
progressive treatments in the 1960s, including the use of lysergic acid diethylamide
(LSD) therapy. At the time I became sister of Oak Ward, the Halliwick day hospital was

developing progressive treatments for people with personality disorder and it really did feel like a major change was coming.

My main memories of my time on Oak Ward are characterized by how hard it was to make even small changes and how important identity was for both the team we created and our patients, especially when, after a year or so, we had to move into the main hospital. I had support from hospital management and other young doctors and clinical colleagues to make changes, but resistance was huge. For example, we wanted to create one nursing team with a single culture. Three separate teams operated on early, late, and night shifts, our shift structure at the time. Each team had a different way of doing things. The night staff never came on to days. This and other changes introduced were intensely resisted. Some staff left to work on other wards as they couldn't stand the interruption to their own routines. On the other hand, many staff came to work on the ward because they wanted to provide care in a different way. It was an exciting time because finally several of us had our own ward to manage and we were determined to do things differently, very much encouraged by the consultants too. I became aware that much of the rest of the hospital were challenging what we were doing. One day I was told by a colleague that I had become known as 'that girl' throughout the hospital. Quite soon this became shortened to 'TG'. I had arrived! By this time, I was a 28-year-old woman and the none too subtle put-down, calling me a girl, was not lost on me. As more new and willing staff joined the team, it was really exciting to realize that we had the power and the determination to make changes. The daily patients' meeting was an important part of what these changes should be and the whole multi-disciplinary team (MDT) was behind them.

What's in a Name?

The hospital closure programme began in earnest and the plan was to retrench staff to work in the main hospital and close down all other buildings on the land, then to empty the hospital from the furthest wings, slowly consolidating patients and staff into the centre. Oak Ward was moved to Ward Six in the main hospital. Both staff and patients feared that the moving to the old hospital would lead to the return of old routines and institutionalized treatments. As a symbol of our new emerging ways, patients and staff determined to continue to call the ward Oak Ward, rather than Ward Six.

We were aware that Chekhov had written a short story, *Ward No. 6*, in 1892[4] that explored the philosophical conflict between Ivan Gromov, a patient, and Audrey Ragin, the director of the asylum. Our push for our own identity and freedoms was not a new one. Opposition to our name for the ward by the rest of the hospital came hard and fast. The whole team would repeatedly make signs for the ward (patients, nurses, the occupational therapists, even doctors) which were, repeatedly, torn down, sometimes several times a day. We used copious supplies of paint and paper, courtesy of a ward-based occupational therapy fund. Switchboard staff refused to acknowledge us if we phoned up as Oak Ward: 'No ward of that name here'. The pharmacy box left the ward daily to be restocked with 'Oak Ward' clearly labelled on it and was returned with a big 6 where the name had been.

I appealed to the Unit General Manager to take action. He responded: 'But what if there's a fire? The brigade won't know where to find you. People could die.' So

I proposed that we called ourselves Ward Six Oaks, placing us firmly between Wards 5 and 7 on the map if disaster struck. We reached an impasse. We would not stop calling ourselves Six Oaks Ward, making the signs, telling patients and relatives, the world! Still the hospital would keep on ripping up the signs, ignoring us, and continuing to call the ward by number. I wrote to management a final time, setting out the case to keep our name (with the 6 in it) and how important the name was to patients and staff. I made it clear that we would not stop using our new name. A letter finally came back after three or four months of battling, giving us permission to call the ward Six Oaks Ward. We were jubilant; I cried again. Of course, in the scheme of things, this was minor, but what it symbolized mattered deeply to us. Today this continues to remind me of the vital principle of individuality as we push for greater standardization of clinical outcomes.

The naming of the ward is just one of so many examples of a clash between the receding Victorian world and a new and emerging world where everyone, staff and patients, have licence to demand change. I felt that we were increasingly powerful and that we should share that power with patients. I didn't understand the full extent of the power shift that was required or that would come over the next three decades or so. This shift is still occurring today, with more to come. The shift in power base afforded me incredible professional opportunities, despite being a nurse, working class, and a woman. I have never felt constrained by the psychiatric community.

The Rabbit Lesson

Before leaving my days as a ward sister at Friern, I need to tell the story of the rabbits. One day Reg, the gardener, said 'would you like a couple of rabbits for the patients?' We had a huge enclosed garden bordered by two other wards. I had no intention of asking permission to adopt these rabbits because I was sure we'd have been denied it. However, soon the 3 rabbits, which were a huge success with the patients and staff alike, became 20 rabbits and then 60 and then.... Holes and subsistence appeared in the garden; everyone wondered where the rabbits had come from and we needed to find a solution quickly. One of the team found 'the Rabbit lady', and she came every couple of months or so to take the rabbits we all rounded up by chasing them and capturing them with hospital sheets. She released them into the wild. I should not have accepted the rabbits without some forethought, and it took me years before I confessed to the authorities that I was the one that took them on. It was perhaps one of many examples of naivety and inexperience on my part. I will be forever grateful for a prevailing regime that valued innovation, challenge, and new ideas, that it forgave mistakes, thus creating the conditions for thinking, experimentation, and risk. All are conditions for progress.

Preparing for Community Living and Care

The period of closure saw a great deal of thought given to the long-term patients. Every single one that I was aware of was rehomed in supported living arrangements or nursing homes. This included a couple of people from Six Oaks Ward, which was mainly an acute, short-stay ward. This rehousing heralded another period of awakening for us as we began to understand privations we had allowed patients to experience. Was it because I was a woman that I was so touched by the fact that people who'd been in hospital for decades were choosing curtains, buying duvets and duvet covers to replace hospital blankets, choosing colour schemes for their rooms—private rooms not dormitories—tea pots, cups and saucers, and other domesticating touches?. I was greatly moved by this awakening in both patients and staff.

I was honoured to have been asked to speak at the closing ceremony of the hospital. Hundreds of people attended, including bishops and other dignitaries. It was a momentous event; somewhere I still have the speech I gave. I know I spoke about standing on the brink of a new era in mental health care, understanding that we still had much to do in terms of new approaches to community-based care. As we closed the era of the institution, I acknowledged that the hospital had seen much love, kindness, and innovation, but it had also experienced deep sorrow. I paid homage to the thousands of people who had been cared for in Friern Barnet Hospital and expressed my hope that their legacy would guide us all into a better future.

By the time the hospital closed in the early 1990s, I was a matron at the Royal Free Hospital, having transferred Ward Six Oaks there as part of the closure programme. While the policy of rehoming the long-stay patients was largely successful, in my opinion insufficient thought had been given to the support patients now in the community would need to achieve maximum independence. The next generation of community services and policies were born. The Care Programme Approach (1990) (CPA)[5] was introduced, an attempt to coordinate care for people with more complex needs. I remember the policy being greatly resisted by many clinical colleagues at the time. It was seen as being bureaucratic top-down intrusion. However, in truth, we had not thought sufficiently about care coordination, occupation, and complexity following the closure of the hospitals. The quality of people's lives, not the very long-stay patients who were well catered for but rather those with relapsing conditions, or newly identified as having serious mental illness, were too little considered. I saw excellent examples of individual care but we did not have a well-developed system of community assessment, treatment, and support.

Discovering Community Care

I used to attend community mental health team (CMHT) meetings where very unwell and vulnerable people were discussed, and if the team had made attempts to engage which had been refused it was quite common to discharge the person back to their GP until (or unless) they wanted to engage. Freedom had gone too far.

There was no sense of assertive outreach, intervention, or of assessing risks against the benefits. There were, however, examples of innovation and flexibility such as work with schools, new mothers, counselling services, and primary care support. There was little proscription, regulation, inspection or policy, other than CPA and a push towards integration with social care. Strangely, in the 1990s, my guess is that there was more support for primary care and wider social institutions in understanding and managing mental health conditions, but services for the seriously mentally ill were underdeveloped.

I remember pressing all consultants and team leaders at some point in the mid-1990s, by which time I was lead nurse and service manager at Camden and Islington NHS Community Trust. I urged them to implement the Care Programme Approach, by now well established. We had also seen the tragic death of Jonathan Zito in 1992 and the Clunis Report that followed in 1994.[6] The failings in coordinating the care of someone clearly unwell, vulnerable, and at high risk brought into sharp relief the imperative to have systems in place to improve and coordinate care. I remember receiving a particularly hostile barrage from one consultant whom I knew well who was incensed that I, as a nurse and a manager, was being seen fit to direct care. This was an unusual attack. With hindsight, we were having to learn a very different approach to psychiatry and the issues of the rights, responsibilities, and freedoms were still very much as alive as they had been in past institutions. Do I think I had a harder time because I was a woman and not a doctor in this instance? Yes. Do I also think we have let the bureaucracy of the CPA process get out of hand? Definitely.

Mental Health Service Innovations

Throughout the 1990s and early 2000, I remained in Camden and Islington, my job changing, promotions coming but I always retained my nurse leadership role. During that decade there was plenty of scope for me to innovate and I worked with some dynamic and committed professionals and patient groups. Race, gender, and old age featured heavily in the policies and practices of mental health at that time.

Three examples of forward-looking practice in our area during that period were:

♦ The BME (black and minority ethnic) third sector attending all S136 detentions (psychiatric assessments of people causing a disturbance in a public place and thought by police to be mentally ill) of African Caribbean people in Accident and Emergency departments in order to seek alternative solutions to detention.

♦ The establishment of the Drayton Park Crisis House for women; a single side of A4 paper written by me and a determined female Trust Chair saw us win £1.5 million to set up a unique service creating a unit which is still successful today and run by a phenomenal nurse who trained with me back in Friern. It is a service that thinks about the needs of women, their children, abuse the women may have experienced in the past, their illnesses and current social situations, and has created a nurturing environment and a different therapeutic approach.

♦ An inspirational (and scary) psychiatrist called Nori Graham and I set up a group called Spotlight which was a learning journal group around the needs of older people with mental illness, good practice, and innovation in old age psychiatry. It was multidisciplinary, met one lunchtime a month, and continued for many years, providing a real platform to shine a light on the needs of an all-too-often-forgotten group in society, older people with mental illness. Throughout my career I have found old age psychiatrists to be some of the warmest, most creative colleagues to have worked with, many of them have been impressive women—and men, of course.

MH Services and Me: If the Shoe Fits, Wear It

The 1990s were a busy time for me personally. I got a first-class honours degree in social policy after studying for four years part-time while working full-time. I got married, had two babies (now 19 and 22) and had 3 months' maternity leave from work with each. I remember with my first child in particular (1994); I was reluctant to tell anyone at work that I was expecting a baby until I was five-and-a-half months' pregnant and nature was taking matters into her own hands. I was concerned that people would think that I was not serious about my career. Was this because, as a woman, I seem to have perpetual imposter syndrome? Was it because I wanted to keep up with the men and not be thought frail? The truth is I don't know why I was so worried. When I did disclose my news everyone, including the then Chief Executive, was amazing.

It has felt good to have worked in mental health all of these years and looking back, several factors lead me to where I am, but none have been more influential than my upbringing.

Number five of six children, I grew up in a loving but incredibly poor household. We had no electricity upstairs, an outside loo, no bath (other than the tin one that hung on the wall of the outside toilet), no central heating, and one cold tap in the kitchen. I lived as if in a Monty Python sketch. Coming home from school one day at the age of 16 to find my mum crying and my dad pacing the floor brought me the news that the environmental health officer had appeared, uninvited, and declared our rented house unfit for human habitation. We were rehoused in a council house with central heating, hot water, electricity in every room, and a bath. This was sheer bliss!

Deep social responsibility, justice, kindness, and a pride in the NHS, which both my parents believed in and supported staunchly, were other factors in my upbringing. These may help explain how I fell into mental health nursing and came to relish the fight for progress and equality, a fight alongside the like-minded, often in hostile and challenging circumstances, who largely held the same values.

After A Levels, I spent the years until I was 23 acting, dancing, travelling, chambermaiding, waitressing—anything but settle down in a proper job. I didn't know what I wanted to do other than 'help people'. Eventually an advert in a women's magazine captured my imagination. It had pictures of four people and asked which one had mental illness and asked whether you had the right skills and values to help them by becoming a mental health nurse. It appealed to my innate belief that anyone could have a breakdown and that we needed to challenge the stigma attached to this condition. A random advertisement stimulated an interest that turned into the next 30 years of my life.

Twenty-First Century

As I come towards the end of this chapter I am aware that I still have the years between 2000 and 2017 to cover. I give this less time as it still feels very present and alive, not yet history, not yet synthesized in my thinking. I have just completed a thrilling decade as Chief Executive of Central and North West London NHS Foundation Trust and, prior to that, from about 2000 on I was the Director of Nursing and Operations in the same Trust. People continue to develop community models of service which seek to push the boundaries of coordination of care, professional and individual freedoms, and life before and beyond services. I am humbled by the work of staff colleagues and those we care for daily.

It is an incredible privilege to be working nationally on the mental health agenda and also to be leading an integrated NHS Trust. Still a registered mental health nurse, I want to inspire people to come and work in the NHS and mental health and community services. We have a long way still to go. However, across the country there are colleagues, partners, service users, and citizens who are passionate and hungry for yet more change. There is 'no health without mental health,'[7] and the time for innovation, new models of care, a growing evidence base, and a determination to implement it is here.

Throughout my career there have been times when well-meaning people have asked me why I didn't become a doctor. The simple truth is that it never occurred to me, respectful as I am of my medical colleagues. I am proud to be a nurse and the last three decades have afforded me incredible opportunities to spend time with impressive people, patients, policy-makers, and professionals. I have never felt restricted because I wasn't a psychiatrist. The silver buckle my parents gave me when I qualified is one of my most treasured possessions.

The thing that still really rankles is those people who tell me 'you could be the chief executive of an acute Trust'. Although I am full of admiration for the work my colleagues do and I enjoy working with them, I reject what the statement belies. The Victorian hierarchies are long gone but we still have a way to go before full equality in healthcare and wider society is achieved for mental health. The statement 'you're good enough to work in acute hospitals' implies that work there is more important and deserving of the best talent. However, notwithstanding our long-term battle with the stigma of mental illness, it has been tremendously rewarding being a small part of an incredible common cause and getting this far. I am looking forward to the next thirty years.

References

1. **NHS England** (2016). *Five Year Forward View for Mental Health.* London: NHS England.
2. **Griffiths, Sir Roy** (1983). *NHS Management Inquiry Report.* London: Department of Health.
3. **English National Board for Nursing, Midwifery and Health Visiting** (1983). Royal College of Nursing Archives, held by the Nursing and Midwifery Council
4. Wilks R (ed. and trans) (2002). *Ward No 6.* London: Penguin.
5. **Department of Health** (1990). *Care Programme Approach.* London: Department of Health.
6. **Clunis Inquiry Team** (1994). *The Report of the Inquiry into the Care and Treatment of Christopher Clunis*: Norwich: Her Majesty's Stationery Office.
7. **Department of Health** (2011). *No Health Without Mental Health: A Cross-Government Mental Health Outcomes Strategy for People of All Ages.* London: Department of Health.

The Disappeared

Third form, I remember you, Lorraine,
in your Wonderbra and gaping shirt,
larking around, strewing Opal Fruits
and Spangles, jokes and paper planes.

Later we all stopped seeing the funny side,
but you went further, transforming
from real to virtual, pursuing lightness.
We hadn't a name for it, back then, Lorraine,

so far out in the seventies, and only after the mocks
we noticed you'd gone. They say you went up Bodmin,
to the bin. They say you were fatted and slowed
on Largactil and ECT, and married a longstay

with silvery scars on neck and wrist. That's all
the proof we have of you, sweet-scattering Lorraine,
the only girl in physics, with your baggy cardigans,
your tiny diagrams of neat opposing forces, your talk

of instability and subatomic spin. How dense
we were, back then: with what momentous speed
you must have been propelled in search
of smaller, weightless, elementary.

Emily Wills

Lisbeth Hockey and Annie Altschul

Nikita Hyare

Introduction

When looking at the impact of women on mental health practice, it is imperative that we draw attention to the people who have the most contact with patients: nurses. Two very important women in nursing, particularly mental health nursing, are Lisbeth Hockey and Annie Altschul. Both had profound influences on the roles of nurses. They were particularly interested in improving research opportunities for nurses, developing the teaching nurses received, and encouraging them to improve their practice in imaginative ways such as community care and valuing the therapeutic relationship.

The Life of Lisbeth Hockey (1918–2004)

Lisbeth Hockey (Figure P6.1), like Altschul, originated from Austria and migrated to England in the 1930s where she flourished in the field of nursing.[1,2,3] She was known throughout her childhood as being very inquisitive and a problem solver. It was this curious mind and her parents' push that

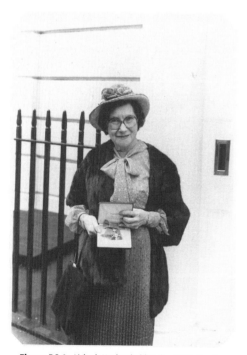

Figure P6.1: Lisbeth Hockey holding her OBE after the ceremony at Buckingham Palace, 4 December 1979.
© Royal College of Nursing

drew her to subjects such as philosophy, and ultimately a career in medicine.[3] Lisbeth started to train as a doctor in Austria. However, once the Nazi regime began she was encouraged by her parents to emigrate as they did not support Hitler.[3,5]

Lisbeth arrived in England, unable to speak English and in need of a job. She worked as a governess for a year and became fluent in the language. Lisbeth wanted to continue the training she began in Austria but realized this would not be possible. Like many other women aspiring to medical careers at that time, and finding their paths blocked, she turned to a career in nursing.[4,5]

When Lisbeth started training as a nurse she was shocked at the education nurses were receiving. She felt hospitals were too rigid in their practice, and nurses were expected to be submissive beings, not questioning or improving the treatment around them. She used her passion for people to push herself through the remainder of her training.[5] Despite the strong belief that nurses should not educate themselves, Lisbeth rebelled. She received several qualifications throughout her entire career, something which is mirrored in the nurses of today.[5] Although she suffered from a stroke when she was elderly, she maintained her strength and cared for herself throughout most of her recovery.[4]

The Life of Annie Altschul (1919–2001)

Annie Altschul (Figure P6.2) was born to a Jewish family in 1919 in Vienna. Her childhood was pleasant, and she was surrounded by a vibrant environment.[6] As a teenager, she was exposed to the concept of 'psychoanalysis' when she worked as a counsellor in a camp for children. Furthermore, Annie learnt more about the group who followed the teachings of Alfred Adler. His school of thought had more of a social emphasis, which chimed with Annie. This experience influenced the choices she made in her later career.[7]

Annie studied maths in Vienna and moved to England just before the Second World War where she worked as a nanny. She had intended to return to Vienna but started her nursing studies and fell in love with psychiatric nursing to which she eventually devoted her career.[2]

Favourite Quotations

'Basic to care is empathy; a nurse extends this empathy not only to her patients and their families but also to her medical, paramedical and domestic colleagues. Without empathy the nurse's contribution

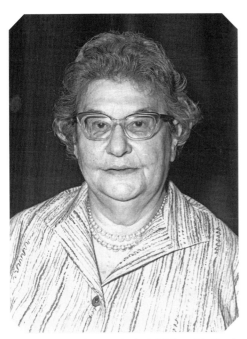

Figure P6.2: Professor Annie Altschul, Fellow of the Royal
College of Nursing, London.
© Royal College of Nursing

developing future community nurses, and became
the 'Director of Nursing research in the University
of Edinburgh' in 1971.[4] Her impact on nursing research led to her receiving an Order of the British
Empire,[4,5] and a 'Fellowship at the Royal College
of Nursing in 1980.'[5] She subsequently became an
'Honorary Fellow of the Royal College of General
Practitioners,' due to her role in enhancing nursing
in general practice.[4,5] Lisbeth received two international degrees from universities in Canada and
Sweden.[4,5] Although she received many accolades,
Lisbeth never distanced herself far from the crux of
research, reaffirming the important contribution she
has made to nursing.[5]

The Career of Annie Altschul

Annie initially trained at Ealing Hospital where
she was disappointed by the attention placed on
minor details that rarely affected patient care.[6]
She then continued her psychiatric nurse training
at the Maudsley Hospital and eventually was employed there as a psychiatric nurse and tutor. During
this time, Annie met many famous psychiatrists
including Maxwell Jones who specialized in treating
shellshock using 'talking therapy' as his treatment
of choice. Jones' approach throughout his career
focused on the social rehabilitation of patients, and
this influenced Annie greatly.[6,7,11]

Annie then undertook further training enabling her
to tutor at the Maudsley.[6,11] In addition to this, she
obtained a psychology degree (1951), demonstrating
her work ethic and determination.[2,6,11] In 1958 she
obtained a scholarship to observe how nurses were
trained in psychiatry in America. Here she learnt the importance of forming a connection with psychiatric patients. Through careful communication she discovered
nurses could adapt the strength of this connection at
different points of the patient's journey, thus improving
their outcome. Back in England she tried to implement
this but felt the education system was not receptive to
her ideas. Annie vocalized this and was corroborated
by a report in 1968, which influenced nursing education for many years.[6] She was appointed 'Professor of
Nursing' at the University of Edinburgh in 1976[2,6] and
published many books and papers throughout her life-
time. Her most famous is *Psychiatric Nursing* (1957)
which became one of the most important resources
for nursing students.[2,6,11] Subsequently she received
many accolades for her work, including becoming a
'Fellow of the Royal College of Nursing'.[6]

to care in the changing setting would not deserve
mention.' Lisbeth Hockey[9]

'It is impossible to prevent relationships occurring,
either by disapproving or by worrying about non-
specific dangers or by injunctions to treat everyone
alike. The existence of relationships needs to be acknowledged. If nurses became conscious of their
feelings towards patients and had the opportunity
to discuss this without feelings of guilt, understanding and control of relationships and conversion
into therapeutic relationships might occur.' Annie
Altschul[10]

The Career of Lisbeth Hockey

The most important influence Lisbeth had on
nursing and medicine was her passion for research.
While she was a student she carefully tried to discover the origin of bedsores. She was discouraged
by her seniors, who informed her it was not her
role to ask questions. This further motivated her to
delve into nursing research, looking for solutions
to problems.[5] Once qualified, Lisbeth worked hard
to gain further skills in the field of nursing. This included training in managing febrile patients and
those in the community.[5] She was responsible for

*Principles of Lisbeth Hockey
and Annie Altschul*

One of Lisbeth's key principles was the importance
of nursing in the district setting, emphasized by

Continued on next page

the fact she was President of the 'International Conferences for Community Health Nursing Research.'[8] To this day, a majority of psychiatric patients are treated in their own homes. Lisbeth also highlighted the importance of adaptation in nursing. She spoke about patients increasing demand due to improving technology, the diversity that now existed, and the fact that higher education in nursing increased the responsibility placed on nurses.[9]

Annie Altschul also had an important role in developing community health services. Early in her career she developed firm beliefs that good social constructs led to good health and happiness. She was certain that society should support those less fortunate and passionately supported the National Health Service.[6] In addition, she carried out many studies. Her most famous study was entitled 'Relationships Between Patients and Nurses in Psychiatric Wards.'. This research concluded that many patients benefitted from good relationships. However, many nurses believed that these attachments may affect their ability to work. Annie disagreed and published evidence which supported this.[10]

Annie also suffered from severe depression and was treated as an in-patient. She spoke about this experience in 'Wounded Healers',[2,7] and organized protected time for nurses to consider how they felt about cases and their own personal well-being.[7] Her opinion that clinicians should reflect on work-based experiences allowed healthcare practitioners to refine their own clinical practice[11] and is similar to the work of the Balints.

References

1. Dopson L (2004). *Lisbeth Hockey. Independent*, 24 June 2004. <http://www.independent.co.uk/news/obituaries/lisbeth-hockey-730639.html>. [cited 13 September 2016].
2. Barker P (2002). Obituary: Annie Altschul. *Guardian*, 8 January 2002 <https://www.theguardian.com/society/2002/jan/08/mentalhealth>.
3. Mason K (2005). Dr Lisbeth Hockey, 1918-2004. <https://www.yumpu.com/en/document/view/40373697/lisbeth-hockey-full-biography-school-of-nursing-midwifery-and->.
4. *The Scotsman*. Lisbeth Hockey. 2004. <http://www.scotsman.com/news/obituaries/lisbeth-hockey-1-536639>.
5. McIntosh J (2004). Dr Lisbeth Hockey. *Primary Health Care Research and Development* **5**(4):367–8. <https://doi.org/10.1191/1463423604pc226xx>.
6. Nolan P (1999). Annie Altschul's legacy to 20th century British mental health nursing. *Journal of Psychiatric and Mental Health Nursing* **6**(4):267–272. <http://onlinelibrary.wiley.com/doi/10.1046/j.1365-2850.1999.00209.x/epdf>.
7. Winship G, Bray J, Repper J, and Hinshelwood R (2009). Collective biography and the legacy of Hildegard Peplau, Annie Altschul and Eileen Skellern; the origins of mental health nursing and its relevance to the current crisis in psychiatry. *Journal of Research in Nursing* **14**(6):505–17. DOI: 10.1177/1744987109347039.
8. Tschudin V (2002). Interview with Lisbeth Hockey. *Nursing Ethics* **9**(2):122–5. <http://journals.sagepub.com/doi/pdf/10.1191/0969733002ne492xx>.
9. Hockey L (1977). The nurse's contribution to care in a changing setting. *Journal of Advanced Nursing* **2**(2):147–56. DOI:10.1111/j.1365-2648.1977.tb00187.x.
10. Altschul A (1971). Relationships between patients and nurses in psychiatric wards. *International Journal of Nursing Studies* **8**(3):179–87. <http://dx.doi.org/10.1016/0020-7489(71)90026-5>.
11. *The Scotsman* (2002). Professor Annie Altschul. <http://www.scotsman.com/news/obituaries/professor-annie-altschul-1-591892>.

Chapter 16

Reducing the Risk of Dementia

Joanne Rodda

Introduction

It is estimated that there are around 35 million people in the world with dementia and that this figure will double every 20 years until at least 2050. Dementia affects more than 1 person in 9 of those over the age of 65 and 1 in 3 of those over the age of 80. At any given age, women are a little more likely than men to develop Alzheimer's disease, although not other types of dementia. Despite this, there are many more women than men living with dementia because life expectancy is higher in women. This, combined with the higher likelihood of women becoming carers for people with dementia, means that they are disproportionately affected.[1]

Recent reports based on data from large studies of different populations have suggested that a third or more of cases of dementia in the United Kingdom, Europe, and the United States of America can be attributed to risk factors that may be modifiable, a finding which has huge implications in terms of the possibility of reducing the prevalence of dementia in the future.

What is Dementia?

Rather than being a disease in its own right dementia is a syndrome that can be caused by many different diseases. A syndrome is a group of symptoms that consistently occur together. These symptoms may be present in a variety of different patterns, but central to the syndrome of dementia is a deterioration in a person's cognition and ability to perform normal day-to-day activities. Cognition is the term given to the mental processes that allow us to make sense of and interact with the world and this includes perception, attention, memory, language, judgement, problem-solving, and many other skills.

The most common types of dementia are Alzheimer's disease, vascular dementia, dementia with Lewy bodies, and frontotemporal dementia, and there are many other rarer forms.

Alzheimer's disease is the most common type of dementia. The key pathological findings in the brain are of amyloid (insoluble protein deposits outside the brain cells) and neurofibrillary tangles (abnormal protein tangles inside brain cells). No-one knows exactly why these changes happen. The first symptoms of Alzheimer's disease are typically short-term memory problems which later progress to affect other cognitive domains and day-to-day abilities.[2]

Vascular dementia is often said to be the second most common cause of dementia, although it often occurs together with Alzheimer's disease. Vascular dementia is caused by cerebrovascular disease (i.e. disease of the blood vessels of the brain), which covers a wide variety of different problems. Vascular dementia may occur due to a single stroke, although more usually it is caused by multiple strokes and damage to smaller blood vessels in the brain.[3]

Dementia with Lewy bodies (DLB) is related to Parkinson's disease, and the microscopic changes (Lewy bodies) seen in the brain tissue are the same in both conditions. People with DLB experience symptoms that may include the movement symptoms of Parkinson's disease (e.g. tremor, stiffness, slowing down of general movement), visual hallucinations, and marked fluctuations in levels of attention and awareness. Dementia due to Parkinson's disease has the same symptoms as DLB, but the timing is different; in Parkinson's disease the movement symptoms are present well before any cognitive symptoms. Parkinson's disease and DLB are related and exist on a spectrum of disease rather than being two completely different conditions.[4]

Frontotemporal dementia (FTD) is less common than the other main types of dementia and tends to affect a younger age group (generally 50–65 years). There is atrophy (shrinkage due to cell death) of the frontal and/or temporal lobes of the brain which results in a range of different clinical syndromes which particularly affect behaviour and language.[5]

When the brains of people with dementia are examined after death, it is common to find pathological brain changes caused by two or more of Alzheimer's disease, cerebrovascular disease, and dementia with Lewy bodies/Parkinson's disease. It is estimated that more than half of all people with dementia have two or more identifiable types of brain pathology, and the overlap may be due to shared risk factors and/or synergistic mechanisms in disease pathology.[6]

When Does a Mild Memory Problem Become Dementia?

People don't go to sleep one day and then wake up the next with a neurodegenerative dementia. For example, in Alzheimer's disease, pathological brain changes build up for 10 to 15 years before a person starts to experience early cognitive symptoms, followed later by frank dementia with clear impairments in activities of daily living.

In the early 2000s, the concept of 'mild cognitive impairment' (MCI) became accepted as a term to define cognitive decline (representing a change from previous cognitive ability) without impairment in activities of daily living. Anyone with MCI has an increased risk of developing dementia (estimated at 10–15 per cent per year), and the highest risk is in amnestic MCI (characterized by deficits in short term memory +/- other cognitive domains) and progression to Alzheimer's disease.[7]

Dementia and Genetics

A small proportion of people with dementia have familial conditions which result from the inheritance of a rare genetic mutation from a parent. For most people, genetic factors make up a much smaller part of their overall risk for dementia and relate to genetic variation rather than inherited mutations. Genetic variation is what makes us different from each other, for example in eye and hair colour. The APOE gene is the most important source of genetic variation in terms of determining Alzheimer's disease risk, but other genetic variants have been linked to risk of Alzheimer's disease and other dementias.

Despite these findings, even people with both parents affected by dementia have only a slightly increased risk of dementia themselves compared to the general population. This is because dementia is very common, and genetic variation accounts for only a part of our overall risk of developing the condition. Research suggests that elimination of the APOE risk gene would reduce the number of new cases of dementia or mild cognitive impairment over the next seven years by 7.1 per cent.[8]

Cognitive Reserve

Cognitive reserve is a measure of how much damage a person's brain can tolerate before they develop cognitive impairment (i.e. how much 'spare' cognitive function they have). It is linked to education, as well as to overall brain health and ongoing cognitive activity; it is not fixed and is something that we can add to throughout our lives. Any insult to the brain may reduce our cognitive reserve, including neurodegeneration, head injury, cumulative effects of high alcohol intake, and stroke.

A Note About the Evidence: Epidemiological Studies Versus Clinical Trials

Much of the evidence regarding modifiable risk for dementia comes from epidemiological studies. These are studies of a population which record information over a period of time without any specific intervention. This allows researchers to look at a range of different factors (e.g. age, sex, ethnicity, dietary habits, blood pressure) and outcomes (e.g. heart disease, diabetes, dementia) and see what relationships exist. Statistical methods allow us to tease out the relevant importance of each individual risk factor or cluster of risk factors, but these studies do not allow us to find out for sure that risk factor X causes condition Y, or that treatment of X will prevent Y.

The accepted gold standard of evidence for a medical intervention is a randomized controlled trial (RCT). In such trials, participants are randomly allocated to either a control (placebo) or a treatment group. This type of study allows us to determine whether or not a certain intervention is effective (e.g. treatment of high blood pressure and prevention of stroke), but they are intensive and expensive and generally last for months rather than years. This is relevant in terms of dementia risk factor modification because it may require many years to assess the efficacy of any intervention. A key challenge in converting evidence from epidemiological studies regarding dementia risk into evidence from RCTs is that the period of time needed for a risk or protective factor to take effect may well be far longer than the period over which it is practically possible to conduct a RCT.

What is the Overall Effect of Modifiable Risk Factors on Dementia Risk?

There has been a great deal of focus in recent years on risk factors for dementia that we can do something about. It seems clear that many health and lifestyle factors, particularly in middle life, are crucial. A detailed analysis of data from existing studies looked at the population attributable risk (PAR) for different modifiable factors for Alzheimer's disease (Table 16.1).[9] The population attributable risk is the difference in the rate of Alzheimer's disease in groups exposed versus not exposed to the risk factor. The risk factors that were investigated were diabetes, midlife hypertension, midlife obesity, physical inactivity, depression, smoking, and low educational attainment. Diet was excluded from the analysis because there was too much diversity between the studies to make the analysis meaningful. Some of the risk factors are not independent of each other (e.g. lack of exercise is associated with obesity and hypertension), and therefore the investigators performed complex statistical analyses to account for this. Based on these adjustments, they calculated that overall almost a third of cases of Alzheimer's disease in the United Kingdom may be attributable to potentially modifiable risk factors. Further analyses suggested that a 10 per cent reduction per decade in each of the seven risk factors studied could reduce the worldwide prevalence of Alzheimer's disease in 2050 by 8.3 per cent, equating to 200,000 cases of Alzheimer's disease.

Table 16.1 Risk factors and attributable risk for Alzheimer's dementia

Risk factor	Population attributable risk	Number of attributable cases in the United Kindom in 2010
Diabetes	1.9%	14,000
Midlife hypertension (high blood pressure)	7%	53,000
Midlife obesity	6.6%	50,000
Physical inactivity*	21.8%	166,000
Depression	8.3%	63,000
Smoking	10.6%	80,000
Low educational attainment**	12.2%	93,000
All risk factors combined	52.0%	395,000
All risk factors adjusted combined***	30.0%	228,000

Data for the population attributable risk for different risk factors for Alzheimer's disease in the United Kingdom. *Physical inactivity was defined as not doing 20 minutes of vigorous activity for at least 3 days per week or moderate activity for at least 5 days per week. **Lower secondary education or less. ***Adjusted for risk factors being non-independent.[9]

Reproduced from *Lancet Neurology*, 13(8), Norton S, Matthews FE, Barnes DE, Yaffe K, Brayne C, Potential for primary prevention of Alzheimer's disease: An analysis of population-based data, pp. 788–94, Copyright (2014), with permission from Elsevier

Midlife Hypertension (High Blood Pressure)

Aside from age, hypertension is the most important risk factor for cerebrovascular disease and is associated with an increased risk of dementia of almost any cause. The mechanism is likely to relate to the disruption of the structure and function of blood vessels and the impact of the resulting ischaemic damage on cognitive function. It is possible that there is also an effect relating to enhanced development of Alzheimer's disease pathology itself, but this mechanism remains unclear. Systolic hypertension (^{3}160 mmHg) during midlife appears to be particularly important in terms of dementia risk.[10,11] A 2016 statement by the American Heart Association concluded that there was consistent evidence that midlife hypertension is associated with mid- and late-life cognitive impairment but that there was insufficient evidence from clinical trials on which to base recommendations for treatment for cognitive health. However, treatment of hypertension is appropriate in order to safeguard vascular health, and as a consequence, brain health.[12]

Antioxidants

Vitamin E is an antioxidant found in a wide range of food, including nuts, seeds, sunflower oil, safflower oil, red peppers, asparagus, avocado, mango, and papaya. In the Chicago Health and Aging study of 1041 people aged over 65 and followed for 6 years, high vitamin E intake was associated with reduced risk of Alzheimer's disease over the study period.[13] In the Rotterdam study of 5395 people aged over 55, people with a high intake of dietary vitamin E were 25 per cent less likely to develop dementia than those with the lowest level of intake.[14] Conversely, vitamin E supplements (tablets) have not been shown to reduce Alzheimer's disease risk. This may be because vitamin E is found in several different forms in food, and supplements do not replicate this.

The role of vitamin C in dementia risk is less clear, with some epidemiological studies suggesting that it may be helpful and others suggesting no benefit. Research is ongoing into other antioxidant supplements including coenzyme q10, organic selenium, lipoic acid, and beta carotene, but there is no clear evidence of benefit in terms of reduced dementia risk at present.

Fish Oils and Omega 3 Fatty Acids

Docosahexanoic acid (DHA) and eicosapentanoic acid (EPA) are long chain omega 3 fatty acids found in fish oils. Alpha linoleic acid (ALA) is a short-chain omega 3 fatty acid found in plant oils (e.g. nuts, seeds, green leafy plants), from which the body can synthesize EPA and DHA.

Normal ageing results in the depletion of long-chain omega 3 fatty acids, and reduced levels of DHA have been found in the brains of people with Alzheimer's disease. Epidemiological studies suggest that people who regularly consume fish oils in their diet are less likely to develop Alzheimer's disease in later life. Furthermore, DHA supplementation can reduce markers of inflammation, which is thought to be important in the development of many neurodegenerative conditions. Other molecular mechanisms, and the association of omega 3 fatty acids with a reduced risk of cerebrovascular disease, are also likely to be important. Despite this evidence, no RCTs to date have shown that supplementation of omega 3 fatty acids in cognitively normal individuals or in people with Alzheimer's disease is beneficial in terms of cognition, although there is preliminary evidence of benefit in people with MCI.[15]

Vitamin B12 and Folate

Vitamin B12 is found is fortified foods as well as in meat, fish, and dairy products. Folate is found in dark-green vegetables and in legumes, and in fortified food products. Vitamin B12 and folate are both required for function of the brain and nervous system and for production of red blood cells. Deficiency of one or both can result in specific neurological disorders and anaemia, and can be due to either inadequate dietary intake or to problems in absorption from the gastrointestinal tract (more common in older people). It is common for doctors to routinely measure B12 and folate levels and to correct any identified deficiencies.

Vitamin B12 is involved in the metabolism of homocysteine, and low plasma levels of vitamin B12 are associated with high plasma homocysteine. Folate (vitamin B9) is also known to play an important part in the metabolism of homocysteine although no relationship between folate and homocysteine levels has been identified. Several epidemiological studies have shown an association between both high homocysteine and low vitamin B12 levels in the blood in mid and late life, and an increased risk of cognitive decline and Alzheimer's disease.

RCTs have not demonstrated any effect of vitamin B12 supplementation on cognitive function in people with or without cognitive impairment, or with or without vitamin B12 deficiency and despite normalization of plasma homocysteine levels. Similarly, there is no clear evidence of cognitive benefits with folate supplementation. The VITACOG study, however, reported that supplementation with vitamins B12, B6, and folate over a two-year period in people with mild cognitive impairment was associated with significantly lower rates of brain atrophy than in a placebo group.[16]

General Dietary Patterns

There is no single food or nutritional supplement which on its own has been shown to convincingly reduce our risk of dementia, and the overall content of our diet is likely to be more important. There has been a great deal of attention paid to the 'Mediterranean diet', based on the observation that people living in the Mediterranean region have amongst the highest life expectancies in the world and a low incidence of Alzheimer's disease. There is no definitive rulebook for the Mediterranean diet but it is generally accepted that it includes high levels of fresh fruit and vegetables, wholegrains, beans, nuts, seeds, some fish and poultry, and little red meat, dairy products, or sweet treats. The primary oil used is olive oil. The MIND diet study investigated a variation of this diet and reported an association with a slower decline in cognitive scores, such that strong adherence to the MIND diet was associated with the equivalent of 7.5 years' less cognitive decline when compared to weak adherence.[17] Other observational studies have shown similar positive associations and this type of diet also appears to be protective against other conditions including heart disease and stroke.[18]

The protective effect of the Mediterranean diet is likely to be due to both the presence and absence of many different factors. Monounsaturated fat in olive oil, the intake of polyunsaturated fats (including DHA and EPA) and the mix of micro- and macronutrients in the components of the diet may all play a part. Notable for their absence are simple sugars and trans and saturated fats, all of which are associated with adverse health outcomes.

Obesity

Epidemiological studies have consistently reported an association between midlife obesity and risk of dementia.[9] Obesity also increases the risk of diabetes, heart disease, stroke, some cancers, and many other adverse health outcomes. The relationship between obesity and dementia is not completely understood, and a controversial 2015 paper based on review of general practitioner records for nearly 2 million people reported that midlife obesity was related to a reduced risk of dementia, whilst being a normal weight or underweight increased the risk.[19] The published commentary on this paper was extensive, and criticisms included the exclusion of the majority of patient records due to lack of body mass index (BMI) measurements and the variable and inconsistent recording of dementia diagnoses.

The relationship between obesity and dementia risk may depend on life stage, and in later life high BMI may have no effect or even be protective in terms of dementia risk.[20] It has been suggested that this relationship reflects the decline in weight that may precede the development of Alzheimer's by up to 10 years before the development of cognitive symptoms. The nature of the changing relationship between obesity, dementia, and life stage remain a matter of speculation until further data are available. There can be no doubt, however, that reducing midlife obesity is a key public health priority.

Diabetes

Diabetes is associated with an increased risk of Alzheimer's disease as well as all-cause dementia.[20] It is also associated with an increased risk of cerebrovascular disease which itself causes cognitive impairment and may promote the development of Alzheimer's disease pathology. Long-term high blood glucose levels (hyperglycaemia) may have a direct effect on brain neurones via osmotic insults (related to the flow of water across cell membranes), oxidative damage, and unregulated activation of microglia (the resident immune cells in the brain). It is also possible that insulin resistance reduces the ability of the brain to clear amyloid. People with type 2 diabetes have been shown to have significantly higher rates of brain atrophy than people without diabetes.

The ACCORD-MIND trial found that improvements in HbA1c (a measure of blood glucose control over a period of weeks/months) were associated with less cognitive decline.[21] Other data from treatment trials are less clear. There is no doubt that for overall health, careful monitoring and treatment of diabetes is extremely important. Although it seems intuitive that this treatment would have a knock-on effect in terms of cognitive protection, there are not enough data from clinical trials at present to confirm this.

Depression

Depression both in mid and late life has been repeatedly demonstrated to be associated with an increased risk factor of dementia. It appears likely that depression is itself
a risk factor for dementia but can also be present as a prodrome to or as part of the
symptomatology of dementia. The mechanisms of this complex relationship are unknown, but several theories exist. Cerebrovascular factors play a role in depression,
Alzheimer's disease, and vascular dementia, whilst Alzheimer's disease and depression
also share genetic risk factors. Depression may directly reduce cognitive reserve (and
so increase risk of dementia) due to damage to the brain during depressive episodes
secondary to neuroinflammation and high levels of cortisol (a hormone released in
response to stress). There is evidence of atrophy of the hippocampus and prefrontal
cortex in prolonged depression.[22]

Depression appears to be a risk factor for dementia but the information available
does not tell us whether treatment of depression affects this risk. Initiatives and current guidelines already exist for the identification and treatment of depression, and
access to psychological therapies is becoming more readily available. Other potential
interventions aimed at reducing dementia risk, for example social interaction and exercise, are also known to have a positive effect on depressive symptoms.

Smoking

Heavy smoking in middle life may double the risk of later dementia, but stopping
smoking may reduce the risk to levels comparable to people who have never smoked.[23]
The relationship between smoking and dementia risk probably relates in part to cerebrovascular damage and the overall burden of chronic disease. The finding of an association between smoking and thinning of the cortex (grey matter) of the brain suggests
that there is also an effect on neurodegenerative processes.[24]

Alcohol

There is some evidence from meta-analyses of epidemiological studies that low or moderate intake of alcohol is associated with a reduced risk of cognitive decline and dementia.[11] This evidence is not, however, strong enough to justify advising people who
do not drink to start doing so. High levels of alcohol can directly cause cognitive impairment, and no 'safe' level of drinking has been established. The CAIDE (Cardiovascular
risk factors, Aging and Dementia) midlife healthy diet index includes alcohol intake of
1–24g per week for women, which is equivalent to two glasses of wine per week.[25]

Exercise

Physical inactivity may be the single most important modifiable risk factor for dementia and numerous epidemiological studies have shown that regular exercise in
midlife is associated with reduced risk of dementia.[9]

Many studies have demonstrated a positive effect of exercise on cognitive function
in healthy middle-aged and older adults without cognitive impairment. The most well-
documented effects have been on executive function but there is also some evidence of

improvements in memory.[23] A 2015 Cochrane review concluded, however, that their analyses of data from studies to date had not shown a convincing relationship between exercise and improved cognition and that larger trials were needed.[26] Even if this is the case, benefits of midlife physical activity exercise on cognition may be seen far later in life in the form of protection of the brain from neurodegenerative disorder and cerebrovascular disease. In support of this are findings suggesting that exercise is associated with brain changes detectable in neuroimaging. Several studies have reported increases in grey matter in frontal brain regions and hippocampus, whilst functional MRI studies have shown differences in activation patterns of the cortex in exercise versus non-exercise groups,[27,28] which would be in keeping with enhanced executive functions.

The association between exercise and reduced dementia risk is probably partly due to effects on cardiovascular health, cerebral blood flow, and reduced risk of type 2 diabetes and obesity. It is also likely that there are other mechanisms at play. Brain-derived neurotropic factor (BDNF) is a protein which acts in the brain to support the survival of neurones and to promote the growth of new neurones and their connections. Several studies have reported that BDNF release is increased during exercise, but the long-term effects of exercise on BDNF and other neuroprotective factors are not clear. Whatever the mechanism, there is evidence that exercise has positive effects on brain structure and function and that midlife physical activity is protective against dementia and many other adverse health outcomes in later in life. Midlife physical inactivity, however, is a huge public health concern.

The positive associations between exercise and reduced dementia risk are probably driven by aerobic exercise, although in terms of overall health and successful aging, programmes which include aerobic activity, strength, and balance exercises are linked to the most positive outcomes.

Crystallized Intelligence and Cognitive Training

Crystallized intelligence refers to knowledge and experience gained during our lifetime and is something that we can add to throughout our lives. Years of education, cognitively demanding occupations, and cognitive activity outside work (e.g. reading, writing letters, learning a language) all contribute to our crystallized intelligence. All of these factors have been associated with a reduced risk of dementia, which probably relates to increased cognitive reserve. The greatest amount of evidence exists from studies which have used years spent in education as a proxy measure for crystallized intelligence (probably because it is easy to measure). There is evidence that any cognitive activity in mid and late life reduces dementia risk such as reading, writing letters, studying a language, going to evening classes, playing chess, or any of a wide range of activities during which we use and stretch our cognitive processes. A 2014 consensus of experts concluded that cognitive inactivity was a crucial and modifiable risk factor for dementia.[20]

A range of studies of different cognitive training interventions in healthy adults have reported improvements in cognitive performance, and appear to be most effective in group settings. Whether this benefit translates into a reduced risk of dementia is unknown. Based on the available evidence, the best advice that we can give people at present is to engage in enjoyable and stimulating cognitive activity on a regular basis.

Multimodal Strategies for Preventing Dementia

The health and lifestyle factors that affect dementia risk overlap and interact, and the best evidence for modifying dementia risk may come from interventions that adopt a holistic approach. The FINGER trial is one of few positive RCTs of an intervention which has shown a positive effect on cognition in older people. The intervention was an intensive two-year programme during which cognitively healthy older adults attended group and individual sessions to help them to maintain a healthy diet, participated in a tailored exercise programme with access to organized group activities, and took part in a cognitive training programme. The cognitive training programme also included group and individual sessions, and the group sessions for different parts of the study formed the social component. Participants saw a nurse and physician at several points during the two years and tailored recommendations and treatment were provided based on national guidelines. Compared to the control group who received regular health advice, the intervention group showed significant benefit in overall cognition. Dropout rates were low and adherence to the programme was high.[29] This study points us towards active interventions, and not just the passive provision of lifestyle advice, if we are serious about affecting meaningful changes in future dementia prevalence.

Conclusions

There is a wealth of evidence to support an association between dementia risk and many health and lifestyle factors including exercise, diet, cognitive activity, smoking, diabetes, depression, and social activity. The interactions between these factors and our overall physical health and well-being are complex. It is unrealistic to expect that we can generate evidence from clinical trials to elucidate the complex interplay of these factors clearly, whose protective or deleterious effects may relate to years or even decades of exposure. A key time for action may well be midlife, and the effect of at least some factors on dementia risk may be lessened or absent in later life. There is sufficient evidence at present for public health authorities to focus on enabling people to engage in physical and cognitive activity, stop smoking, maintain healthy eating along the lines of a Mediterranean or similar diet, control blood sugar and blood pressure, and avoid excessive alcohol consumption. None of these messages are new, and if this knowledge is to be converted into behavioural change, active programmes providing opportunities to engage in all facets of healthy activity, rather than passive advice, may be the most successful strategy. Rather than looking at individual problems with individual solutions, we need to view health and health behaviour as a continuum. We may not be able to prevent dementia but we have an opportunity to reduce the risks.

References

1. Rocca WA, Mielke MM, Vemuri P, and Miller VM (2014). Sex and gender differences in the causes of dementia: A narrative review. *Maturitas* October; **79**(2):196–201.
2. Scheltens P, Blennow K, Breteler MM, de Strooper B, Frisoni GB, Salloway S, and Van der Flier WM (2016). Alzheimer's disease. *Lancet* 30 July; **388**(10043):505–17.

3. **O'Brien JT** and **Thomas A** (2015). Vascular dementia. *Lancet* 24 October; **386**(10004):1698–706.

4. **Walker Z, Possin KL, Boeve BF**, and **Aarsland D** (2015). Lewy body dementias. *Lancet* 24 October; **386**(10004):1683–97.

5. **Bang J, Spina S**, and **Miller BL**. Frontotemporal dementia. *Lancet* 24 October; **386**(10004):1672–82.

6. **Schneider JA, Arvanitakis Z, Bang W**, and **Bennett DA** (2007). Mixed brain pathologies account for most dementia cases in community-dwelling older persons. *Neurology* **69**(24):2197–204.

7. **Eshkoor SA, Hamid TA, Mun CY**, and **Ng CK** (2015). Mild cognitive impairment and its management in older people. *Clinical Interventions in Aging* **10**:687–93.

8. **Ritchie K, Carrière I, Ritchie CW, Berr C, Artero S**, and **Ancelin ML** (2010). Designing prevention programmes to reduce incidence of dementia: Prospective cohort study of modifiable risk factors. *British Medical Journal* 5 August; **341**:c3885.

9. **Norton S, Matthews FE, Barnes DE, Yaffe K**, and **Brayne C** (2014). Potential for primary prevention of Alzheimer's disease: An analysis of population-based data. *Lancet Neurology* August; **13**(8):788–94.

10. **Kivipelto M, Ngandu T, Laatikainen T, Winblad B, Soininen H**, and **Tuomilehto J** (2006). Risk score for the prediction of dementia risk in 20 years among middle aged people: A longitudinal, population-based study. *Lancet Neurology* September; **5**(9):735–41.

11. **Xu W, Tan L, Wang HF, Jiang T, Tan MS, Tan L, Gulati M, Kamel H, Knopman DS, Launer LJ, Saczynski JS, Seshadri S, Zeki Al Hazzouri A, American Heart Association Council on Hypertension, Council on Clinical Cardiology, Council on Cardiovascular Disease in the Young; Council on Cardiovascular and Stroke Nursing, Council on Quality of Care and Outcomes Research**; and **Stroke Council** (2015). Meta-analysis of modifiable risk factors for Alzheimer's disease. *Journal of Neurology, Neurosurgery, and Psychiatry* December; **86**(12):1299–306.

12. **Iadecola C, Yaffe K, Biller J, Bratzke LC, Faraci FM, Gorelick PB, Gulati M, Kamel H, Knopman DS, Launer LJ, Saczynski JS, Seshadri S, Zeki Al Hazzouri A, American Heart Association Council on Hypertension**, Council on Clinical Cardiology, Council on Cardiovascular Disease in the Young, Council on Cardiovascular and Stroke Nursing, Council on Quality of Care and Outcomes Research, and Stroke Council (2016). Impact of hypertension on cognitive function: A scientific statement from the American Heart Association. *Hypertension* December; **68**(6):e67–94.

13. **Morris MC, Evans DA, Tangney CC, Bienias JL, Wilson RS, Aggarwal NT**, and **Scherr PA** (2005). Relation of the tocopherol forms to incident Alzheimer disease and to cognitive change. *American Journal of Clinical Nutrition* February; **81**(2):508–14.

14. **Devore EE, Grodstein F, van Rooij FJ, Hofman A, Stampfer MJ, Witteman JC**, and **Breteler MM** (2010). Dietary antioxidants and long-term risk of dementia. *Archives in Neurology* July; **67**(7):819–25.

15. **Thomas J, Thomas CJ, Radcliffe J**, and **Itsiopoulos C** (2015). Omega-3 fatty acids in early prevention of inflammatory neurodegenerative disease: A focus on Alzheimer's disease. *Biomedical Research International* 172801. <http://dx.doi.org/10.1155/2015/172801>.

16. **Health Quality Ontario** (2013). Vitamin B12 and cognitive function: An evidence-based analysis. *Ontario Health Technology Assessment Series* **13**(23):1–45.

17. Morris MC, Tangney CC, Wang Y, Sacks FM, Barnes LL, Bennett DA, and Aggarwal NT (2015). MIND diet slows cognitive decline with aging. *Alzheimers Dementia* September; **11**(9):1015–22.

18. Swaminathan A and Jicha GA (2014). Nutrition and prevention of Alzheimer's dementia. *Frontiers in Aging Neuroscience* **6**:282.

19. Qizilbash N, Gregson J, Johnson ME, Pearce N, Douglas I, Wing K, Evans SJW, and Pocock SJ 2015). BMI and risk of dementia in two million people over two decades: A retrospective cohort study. *Lancet Diabetes Endocrinology* June; **3**(6):431–6.

20. Deckers K, van Boxtel MP, Schiepers OJ, de Vugt M, Muñoz Sánchez JL, Anstey KJ, Brayne C, Dartigues JF, Engedal K, Kivipelto M, Ritchie K, Starr JM, Yaffe K, Irving K, Verhey FR, and Köhler S(2015). Target risk factors for dementia prevention: A systematic review and delphi consensus study on the evidence from observational studies. *International Journal of Geriatric Psychiatry* March; **30**(3):234–46.

21. Cukierman-Yaffe T, Gerstein HC, Williamson JD, Lazar RM, Lovato L, Miller ME, Coker LH, Murray A, Sullivan MD, Marcovina SM, Launer LJ, Action to Control Cardiovascular Risk in Diabetes–Memory in Diabetes (ACCORD-MIND) Investigators (2009). Relationship between baseline glycemic control and cognitive function in individuals with type 2 diabetes and other cardiovascular risk factors: The action to control cardiovascular risk in diabetes-memory in diabetes (ACCORD-MIND) trial. *Diabetes Care* February; **32**(2):221–6.

22. Bennett S and Thomas AJ (2014). Depression and dementia: Cause, consequence or coincidence? *Maturitas* October; **79**(2):184–90.

23. Baumgart M, Snyder HM, Carrillo MC, Fazio S, Kim H, and Johns H (2015). Summary of the evidence on modifiable risk factors for cognitive decline and dementia: A population-based perspective. *Alzheimers Dementia* June; **11**(6):718–26.

24. Cho H, Kim C, Kim HJ, Ye BS, Kim YJ, Jung NY, Son TO, Cho EB, Jang H, Lee J, Kang M, Shin HY, Jeon S, Lee JM, Kim ST, Choi YC, Na DL, and Seo SW (2016). Impact of smoking on neurodegeneration and cerebrovascular disease markers in cognitively normal men. *European Journal of Neurology* January; #**23**(1):110–19.

25. Eskelinen MH, Ngandu T, Tuomilehto J, Soininen H, and Kivipelto M (2011). Midlife healthy-diet index and late-life dementia and Alzheimer's disease. *Dementia and Geriatric Cognitive Disorders Extra* January; **1**(1):103–12.

26. Young J, Angevaren M, Rusted J, and Tabet N (2015). Aerobic exercise to improve cognitive function in older people without known cognitive impairment. *Cochrane Database of Systematic Reviews* April **22**(4):CD005381.

27. Hötting K and Röder B (2013). Beneficial effects of physical exercise on neuroplasticity and cognition. *Neuroscience and Biobehavioural Reviews* November; **37**(9 Pt B):2243–57.

28. Huang P, Fang R, Li BY, and Chen SD (2016). Exercise-Related changes of networks in aging and mild cognitive impairment brain. *Frontiers in Aging Neuroscience* **8**:47.

29.. Ngandu T, Lehtisalo J, Solomon A, Levälahti E, Ahtiluoto S, Antikainen R, Bäckman L, Hänninen T, Jula A, Laatikainen T, Lindström J, Mangialasche F, Paajanen T, Pajala S, Peltonen M, Rauramaa R, Stigsdotter-Neely A, Strandberg T, Tuomilehto J, Soininen H, and Kivipelto M(2015). A 2 year multidomain intervention of diet, exercise, cognitive training, and vascular risk monitoring versus control to prevent cognitive decline in at-risk elderly people (FINGER): A randomised controlled trial. *Lancet* 6 June; **385**(9984):2255–63.

Whose Life is it Anyway? Life and Death in the Court of Protection

Clementine Maddock

How do you make decisions for another person, especially when that decision may result in a person's death? There is no easy answer, and every situation is specific to the individual. As medicine has evolved, patients who would hitherto have been untreatable can now be kept alive through medical technologies such as artificial ventilation and clinically assisted nutrition and hydration. Every patient attending hospital should be given life-sustaining treatment but when the prognosis becomes clear and the patient is diagnosed as being in, for example, a persistent vegetative state, is it in the best interests of that person to continue to receive treatment? At what point, if ever, is it acceptable to stop such treatment once it is started? These are dilemmas that clinicians, families, and ultimately the courts have to resolve.

An unconscious patient is clearly unable to express any preference for whether or not they consent to continuing treatment. However, what about situations where a conscious patient is refusing potentially life-saving interventions? If the person has capacity to refuse treatment, then they may do so, even if others may consider it an unwise decision.[1] The only exception is provided by section 58 of the Mental Health Act 1983 (MHA) if treatment is necessary for mental disorder. If there is doubt as to whether a person has capacity to make a decision to refuse potentially life-saving treatment, the case may ultimately be referred to the Court of Protection (CoP), which will determine if the person has capacity, and if not, consider what is in the patient's best interests.

These cases bring into sharp focus the conflict between the sanctity of a human life versus personal autonomy and self-determination. This chapter will explore the development of case law with respect to life and death decision-making where a person is judged as being unable to make a decision or where decision-making capacity is in doubt.

The Bland Case and Stopping Life-Sustaining Treatment

The Bland[2] case raised, for the first time, the question: in which circumstances, if any, can a doctor lawfully discontinue life-sustaining treatment, including nutrition and hydration, without which the patient will die? Anthony Bland was a 17-year-old Liverpool Football Club fan who went to support his team at the Hillsborough stadium on 15 April 1989. He suffered devastating injuries in the disaster that unfolded that day. Although Mr Bland's brainstem was functioning, meaning that reflexive functions of the body such as breathing, heartbeat, and digestion continued, he was unable to see, hear, feel, or communicate in any way, and there did not appear to be any element of consciousness. He was diagnosed as being in a persistent vegetative state. After three years in this condition, Mr Bland's family, treating clinicians, and independent experts all agreed that there was no hope of recovery and sought a declaration from the court that it would be lawful to withhold artificial nutrition and hydration and other life-sustaining measures.

Lord Goff of Chievely, considered the principles of sanctity of life versus the right to self determination as follows:[3]

> the fundamental principle is the principle of the sanctity of human life —a principle long recognised not only in our own society but also in most, if not all, civilised societies throughout the modern world ... But this principle, fundamental though it is, is not absolute ...We are concerned with circumstances in which it may be lawful to withhold from a patient medical treatment or care by means of which his life may be prolonged. But here too there is no absolute rule that the patient's life must be prolonged by such treatment or care, if available, regardless of the circumstances.
>
> First, it is established that the principle of self-determination requires that respect must be given to the wishes of the patient, so that if an adult patient of sound mind refuses, however unreasonably, to consent to treatment or care by which his life would or might be prolonged, the doctors responsible for his care must give effect to his wishes, even though they do not consider it to be in his best interests to do so ... To this extent, the principle of the sanctity of human life must yield to the principle of self-determination, and, for present purposes perhaps more important, the doctor's duty to act in the best interests of his patient must likewise be qualified.
>
> Ibid at 863 and 864

Lord Goff confirmed the position that a doctor treating a patient who is unable to make a decision may do so in the patient's best interests, and established the question to be answered in Mr Bland's case as[4]

> not whether it is in the best interests of the patient that he should die. The question is whether it is in the best interests of the patient that his life should be prolonged by the continuance of this form of medical care.
>
> Ibid at 868

The House of Lords decided that the object of medical treatment and care was to benefit the patient, that doctors have no duty to provide futile medical treatment,[5] and that it was not in Mr Bland's best interests to continue with clinically assisted nutrition and hydration. The judgment was handed down on 4 February 1993 and Mr Bland died on 3 March 1993, having been in a coma for nearly four years. However, the decision raised legal, ethical, and moral dimensions about the value to be placed on a human life, and the distinction between allowing a person to die versus prolonging a life.

Right to Life Versus Self-Determination: Anorexia Nervosa

Psychiatrists are entering a brave new world. While patients with anorexia nervosa may be forcibly fed as treatment for their mental disorder under the MHA, the question has become whether we should be treating such patients when they are clearly objecting to treatment, and continual interventions are futile?

E's case[6] required the courts to decide, for the first time, whether life-sustaining treatment was in the best interests of E, a lady with severe anorexia nervosa who, while lacking capacity, was aware of her situation and was refusing force-feeding, even with the knowledge that this would lead to her death. Anorexia nervosa is characterized by a morbid fear of weight gain, behaviour aimed at weight loss, and a grossly disordered body image in that the sufferer, while being noticeably underweight to others, sees themselves as fat. Force-feeding can be extremely unpleasant and uncomfortable for the patient, especially one who is objecting, and may involve insertion of a nasogastric feeding tube through the nose and into the stomach, or a PEG (percutaneous endoscopic gastrostomy) tube which requires an incision into the stomach, with associated risks of infection.

E was seriously sexually abused between the ages of 4 and 11 years. Her parents were not aware of this until many years later. At the age of 11 she began to control her eating. By the age of 13, she was binge-eating with self-induced vomiting and was drinking alcohol. E was admitted to a specialist unit for 9 months at age 15 to treat her weight loss, following which she returned to school, completed A levels, and entered medical school. She was a high achiever until she began drinking heavily and was involved in an unhappy relationship. She didn't complete her training and between the ages of 26 and 30 she spent half her time in specialist eating disorder or alcohol treatment units. In 2012, when the case was heard, E was aged 32 and had been living in her own flat for the previous 2 years, with emergency admissions for medical and psychiatric care, under the MHA, on 10 occasions. She continued to drink heavily and alcohol was her only source of calories. In July 2011 and October 2011 E signed advance directives saying that she did not want to be resuscitated or given any medical intervention to save her life. In September 2011, E had a hip-replacement operation and either required support or a wheelchair to mobilize. On 3 April 2012, a meeting with E, her family, and professionals agreed that all treatment options had been exhausted and she was admitted to a community hospital for palliative care and placed on an end-of-life care pathway with high-dose opiate medication, to which she was addicted. On 18 May 2012, the local authority issued an urgent application to the Court of Protection. They were concerned that E's position should be investigated and protected as E's death was imminent. She was refusing to eat and taking only sips of water.

The issues before the court were:[7]

1. Does E have the mental capacity to make decisions about her treatment?

2. If not, did she have mental capacity when she made an advance decision in October 2011, and is that decision valid and applicable?

3. If she lacks capacity and has not made a valid advance decision, is it in her best interests to receive force-feeding?

The Mental Capacity Act 2005 (MCA) is clear there is a presumption that a person has capacity to make a decision.[8] A person lacks capacity if at the material time she is unable to make the treatment decision for herself because of an impairment of, or disturbance in the functioning of the mind or brain.[9] The judge concluded that E had an impairment in the functioning of her mind due to anorexia, and although she was able to understand and retain information relevant to the decision and communicate her decision, she was incapable of weighing the advantages and disadvantages of eating in any 'meaningful way'[10] due to her obsessive fear of weight gain. Mr Justice Peter Jackson concluded that she lacked capacity to make decisions about her treatment.

On the question of the validity of the advance decision, the judge determined that a 'full, reasoned, and contemporaneous assessment evidencing mental capacity to make such a momentous decision'[11] was necessary, which had not been carried out. On the balance of probabilities, the judge concluded that the evidence as a whole indicated that E did not have capacity at the time of signing the advance decision in October 2011.

The court then turned to the question as to whether it was in E's best interests to receive further force-feeding. The assessment of best interests is governed by section 4 MCA which states that the court must consider all relevant circumstances including encouraging E to participate in the decision, consider E's values and beliefs, and take into account the views of E's parents and carers as to her best interests. On this point, Mr Justice Peter Jackson noted:[12]

> The beliefs and values that would be likely to influence E's decision if she had capacity are not easy to articulate. It depends upon an assessment of her true identity. Has she been ill for so long that her illness would remain part of who she is, even if she had capacity? Or is she still the person she was before anorexia took her in its grip?

E's parents stated:[13] 'We love her dearly but feel that our role should now be to fight for her best interests, which, at this time, we strongly feel should be the right to choose her own pathway, free of restraint and fear of enforced re-feed.'

The Body Mass Index (BMI) is a key marker in cases of anorexia. A BMI below 17.5 is one of the diagnostic criteria for anorexia nervosa. A healthy BMI is between 20 and 25. Dr Tyrone Glover, the court appointed expert in eating disorders, wrote: 'my long and detailed analysis of her care record indicates that E has remained at a BMI of less than 15 for at least six years. It is widely understood within Eating Disorder Psychiatry that many patients will not recover from the effects of malnutrition unless they have had their BMI increased to 17 or above. The only time that E's BMI was 'forcibly' restored to normal was during her treatment at the age of 15. It is of note that she went on to complete her A levels and gain a place at medical school in the ensuing years'.

Dr Glover concluded: 'E's BMI has not been raised to 17 or above for over seven years. Without this having been achieved it would be unsafe to deem the withholding of nutrition to be in her best interests.'

A specialist hospital placement had been identified, where the aim of the care plan would be to re-feed E and increase her BMI. Mr Justice Peter Jackson concluded that it would be in E's best interests for her to be fed, forcibly if necessary, and stated that 'I would not overrule her wishes if further treatment was futile, but it is not. Although extremely burdensome to E, there is a possibility that it will succeed.'[14] Four years later, E was still being treated at the specialist hospital.

Four other cases of patients with anorexia nervosa have been heard before the Court of Protection.[15] In all cases, a declaration was sought that it would be lawful and in the patient's best interests not to provide further force-feeding when the patient refused such treatment. In these four cases, the decision was made that it would be in the patient's best interests not to enforce further treatment. The key themes that emerged were that all treatments had been tried, and that they had not been successful. Further treatment was not thought to be in the patient's best interests as no benefit would be conferred by the intervention. However, the court emphasized that should the patient change her mind, then nothing should prevent treatment being given. The patients, carers, family, and treating team were all in agreement that further forced treatment would be of no benefit, and the court-appointed expert was Dr Glover, in all cases. Other key themes that emerged include the need for the patient to have control over her situation rather than having uncomfortable force-feeding enforced under the MHA, a situation often reminiscent of the abuse that many of these patients had experienced in childhood. As W stated of her treatment,[16] 'Currently I am struggling because I have no control over decisions in my life. I have no focus on things I would like in life that I am being denied.' When asked what the most important thing for W was, she replied: 'To make my own decisions and that treatment should not be enforced.'

W said that she did not wish to die and she had ambitions to return to education. However, her behaviour in restricting her food intake to such an extent that she threatened her own life was inconsistent with these stated aims. The treating clinicians, family, and close friends are thus left in an intolerable situation, perhaps reflecting the internal conflict within the sufferer of anorexia, that a need to control food intake outweighs every other consideration, including the usual goals in life. In each of the five anorexia cases that came before the court, treatment under the MHA including re-feeding had been tried for many years, with no noticeable improvement over time. These cases reflect the most severe end of the anorexia spectrum, and many other patients will be successfully treated. These cases only come before the court when recurrent treatment has failed, and the patient is clearly objecting to continued compulsory interventions.

Disputes Between Clinicians and Patients

In the cases discussed above there was generally a consensus amongst the patient, clinicians, family, and carers that further interventions were no longer of benefit to the patient. However, what happens when there is a dispute between the patient or their family, and the clinical team?

In the case of T,[17] Lord Donaldson of Lymington MR noted 'the more serious the decision, the greater the capacity required'. Thus, where a patient is refusing potentially life-saving treatment, clinicians will be more likely to bring a case to the Court of Protection if treatment decision-making capacity is in doubt.

C[18] led a life revolving around her looks, men, material possessions, and living the high life. She had been married four times, had numerous affairs, and moved on when the money ran out. She valued youth, beauty, and living a life that 'sparkles', above all else. In December 2014, at the age of 49, C was diagnosed with breast cancer. Her main concern was that treatment should not interfere with her ability to wear a bikini or make her fat. In August 2015, a long-term relationship ended and she lost her business and financial security. On 7 September 2015, C went to a beach, took 60 paracetamol tablets, and drank champagne in an attempt to commit suicide. When she woke up, she was worried about being in pain, and so called her general practitioner. She was admitted to a local hospital and subsequently to Kings College Hospital, having suffered liver and kidney damage, requiring kidney dialysis. By the date of the hearing at the Court of Protection on 13 November 2015, C was refusing further kidney dialysis. Without dialysis, she would die within three to seven days. With treatment it was possible, although not certain, that C's kidney function would recover and she would not need life-long dialysis. In order to administer dialysis to C against her will, she would require sedation rendering her unconscious for the duration of the dialysis. C could remove the dialysis tubes between treatments, risking further bleeding and infection each time a tube was replaced.

The issue before the court was whether C had the mental capacity to decide whether or not to consent to dialysis. Two psychiatrists within the treating Trust, Dr R and Professor P, were of the opinion that C lacked capacity to make this treatment decision as she was unable to use or weigh the relevant information as part of the process of making the decision. One of the psychiatrists, Dr R, was of the opinion that the black-and-white thinking expressed by C was preventing her reaching a 'balanced, nuanced, used and weighed' position. Professor P noted that C was unable to accept any future apart from the inaccurate view that the damage to her kidneys was irreversible and that she would require ongoing dialysis. However, the court-appointed psychiatrist, Dr Stevens, was of the opinion that C had capacity with respect to the decision to refuse further dialysis. C told him:[19] 'I know that I could get better; I know that I could live without a health problem, but I don't want it; I've lost my home; I've lost everything I'd worked for; I've had a good innings; it's what I've achieved.'

During her interview with the official solicitor on 10 November 2015, C stated: 'Everyone makes a choice. It would be nice if they could give me some choice. I am getting wheeled along. It's a bit unfair.'

C's daughter V stated: 'my mother would never have wanted to live at all costs. Her reasons for trying to kill herself in September and for refusing dialysis now are strongly in keeping with both her personality and her long held values.'

Having considered all the evidence available to him, Mr Justice Macdonald was of the view that C had the decision making capacity to refuse further dialysis. He acknowledged that his view differed from two of the psychiatric opinions:[20]

> Whilst I have some concern that Dr R in particular set the test for capacity too high in this case in looking for C to demonstrate significant using and weighing of information demonstratively ending with a balanced, nuanced, used and weighed position, the fact that I have differed from Dr R and Professor P is in large part a product of this being a finely balanced case in which a number of reasonable interpretations of the information available are possible.

Mr Justice Macdonald concluded: 'As a capacitous individual C is, in respect of her own body and mind, sovereign.'

C died a few days later.

It is important to distinguish these cases, where decisions have been reached following a significant period of treatment, from emergency situations. It is not uncommon for a patient who has been admitted following an overdose to refuse immediate life-saving interventions. In such a case, preservation of life is paramount. Legal protections are provided for patients in these situations by the MHA and the MCA. If treatment will alleviate the symptoms of a mental disorder, which can include self-harm, then it may be given under the MHA.[21] Section 5 of the MCA allows for medical treatment to be given in the best interests of a patient who lacks capacity to consent. Section 6 authorizes restraint of a patient who lacks capacity to consent to treatment if it is necessary to prevent harm and the restraint is proportionate to the likelihood and seriousness of that harm.

In the case of *Wye Valley NHS Trust v B* (2015),[22] the Court of Protection was asked to determine whether it would be in Mr B's best interest to undergo a leg amputation that Mr B was refusing. Mr B was a 73-year-old man with a longstanding history of mental illness and poorly controlled type 2 diabetes. He experienced persistent auditory hallucinations in which he heard the voices of angels and of the Virgin Mary. Mr B developed a chronic foot ulcer, a complication of diabetes, and was admitted to hospital in July 2014, alternating between general and psychiatric settings. Mr B refused medication for his diabetes and antibiotics for his foot. By August 2015 his mental health had improved but his foot was infected. Mr B allowed dressings to be changed but refused all other treatment. He was transferred from a psychiatric hospital to a general hospital on 12 September 2015.

The treating Trust applied to the Court of Protection for authority to carry out an amputation on Mr B's leg. They stated that Mr B would succumb to an overwhelming infection in a matter of days without this intervention, but his life expectancy with an amputation was around three years. Mr B lacked capacity to make treatment decisions because of a compromised ability to understand the information about his foot, and an inability to weigh the relevant medical evidence as part of the process of making the decision. The question before the court was whether it was in Mr B's best interests for the amputation to proceed. The court had to consider what weight to place upon Mr B's wishes and feelings as well as his religious beliefs. In his judgment, Mr Justice Peter Jackson stated:

> As the Act and the European Convention make clear, a conclusion that a person lacks decision-making capacity is not an 'off-switch' for his rights and freedoms.
>
> …
>
> the wishes and feelings, beliefs and values of a person with a mental illness can be of such long standing that they are an inextricable part of the person that he is.

Mr Justice Jackson went to meet Mr B. Mr B said:

> I don't want an operation. I'm not afraid of dying, I know where I'm going. The angels have told me I am going to heaven. I have no regrets. It would be a better life than this.
>
> …
>
> I don't want to go into a nursing home. I don't want my leg tampered with. I know the seriousness. I just want them to continue what they are doing … Even if I'm going to die, I don't want the operation.

I am ending this chapter with the words of Mr Justice Jackson, as they are salient thoughts for psychiatrists who, when approved by the Secretary of State under section 12, MHA, hold the unique position in British society of being able to detain a person against their will without a court order, for assessment and treatment of suspected mental illness.

He concluded:

> I am quite sure that it would not be in Mr B's best interests to take away his little remaining independence and dignity in order to replace it with a future for which he understandably has no appetite and which could only be achieved after a traumatic and uncertain struggle that he and no-one else would have to endure …There is a difference between fighting on someone's behalf and just fighting them. Enforcing treatment in this case would surely be the latter.

References

1. Mental Capacity Act 2005.
2. *Airedale NHS Trust v Bland* [1993] A.C. 789
3. *Airedale NHS Trust v Bland* [1993] A.C. at 863 and 864.
4. *Airedale NHS Trust v Bland* [1993] A.C. at 868.
5. *Airedale NHS Trust v Bland* [1993] A.C. per Lord Keith at 890.
6. Re E (Medical Treatment/Anorexia) [2012] EWCOP 1639.
7. Re E (Medical Treatment/Anorexia) [2012] EWCOP at para 46
8. Mental Capacity Act 2005 section 1(2).
9. Mental Capacity Act 2005 section 2(1).
10. Re E at para 49.
11. Re E at para 65.
12. Re E at para 78.
13. Re E at para 80.
14. Re E at para 138.
15. Re L [2012] EWHC 1639 (COP); *An NHS Foundation Trust v X* [2014] EWCOP 35; *Betsi Cadwaladr University Local Health Board v Miss W* [2016] EWOP 13; *Cheshire and Wirral Partnership NHS Foundation Trust v Z* [2016] EWCOP 35
16. *Betsi Cadwaladr University Local Health Board v Miss W* [2016] EWOP 13 at paras 29 and 30.
17. Re T (Adult: Refusal of Treatment) [1993] Fam 95, at para 113.
18. *Kings College Hospital v C* [2015] EWCOP 80.
19. *Kings College Hospital v C* [2015] EWCOP at para 54.
20. *Kings College Hospital v C* [2015] EWCOP at para 94.
21. Section. 63 Mental Health Act 1983; B v Croydon Health Authority [1995] CA Family 133.
22. *Wye Valley NHS Trust v Mr B* [2015] EWCOP 60.

Chapter 18

Women in Psychiatric Training

Georgina Fozard and Philippa Greenfield

Introduction

In common with other medical specialties there has been a gender shift in the composition of the psychiatric workforce. No longer is this a field dominated by men. In fact, in 2017 59 per cent of the trainees in psychiatry in the United Kingdom were women.[1] During our training we have discovered psychiatry can be a highly stimulating and rewarding career for a woman, but a path not without its challenges. We recognize that barriers to taking up and completing training are present. Some of these challenges are arguably shared with other high-pressure careers which were traditionally male-dominated, but others are unique to the nature of work in this field. During this chapter we will refer both to medical students and to psychiatry 'trainees'. By using this term we are generally referring to doctors who have completed medical school and (in the United Kingdom) their years as foundation doctors, and have begun training with psychiatry as their specialty.

Psychiatry: A Medical Specialty

Psychiatry training has been recognized as a career pathway that allows more time for work–life balance compared with other medical specialisms. However, following initiatives such as the introduction of the European Working Times Directive, which meant capped working hours across all training pathways, the numbers of junior doctors entering psychiatric training declined—an ongoing trend.[2] In recent years we have faced a recruitment crisis in psychiatry, across all subspecialties, with persistent difficulties in recruiting UK graduates.[3] With other challenges faced by trainees such as the recent Junior Doctor Contract changes in 2016/17 it is more important than ever that we proactively address recruitment to the specialty. With this in mind we will try to identify and address some of the barriers that may deter women in particular from embarking on or continuing this career pathway (many of which are more perceived or imagined than borne out in reality), but we also reflect from our first-hand experiences on the positive aspects of training in psychiatry for women and consider the valuable, arguably essential, contribution that women can make to the ongoing development of the profession.

There is no doubt that psychiatrists are needed now more than ever. One in four people in England will suffer with at least one psychiatric disorder,[4] and services have received less and less funding annually, accompanied by devastating cuts to in-patient beds. A longstanding culture of stigma about mental health issues seems to leach into the unconscious of politicians and even our colleagues in the National Health Service, meaning that as psychiatrists we have to fight harder for parity of funding in line with that allocated to other medical specialties. Mental health problems account for 23 per cent of the burden of disease in the United Kingdom, but spending on mental health services consumes only 11 per cent of the NHS budget.[5] Institutional bias against mental health remains a huge problem, but whatever the future structure of health service provision, more mental health professionals will be needed.

Barriers to Entering Psychiatric Training

Anecdotally, at medical school and during foundation training we found relatively more women medical students and junior doctors expressed an interest in psychiatry. We wonder whether a macho culture within the teaching hospital environment, or the way traditional medical schools favour those with maths, physics, and chemistry leanings rather than those with talents within the humanities or arts have contributed to medical school environments where the practice of psychiatry is at best misunderstood and at worst denigrated. We both suffered incidences of being patronized as students when we said we were interested in psychiatry: 'all you do is drink tea, it's not real medicine!' or (our favourite) 'do you want to do psychiatry because you suffer from mental health problems yourself?' If only we had found a witty retort to the urologist who asked this, such as 'did you want to be a urologist because you suffer from erectile dysfunction?' Unfortunately, these sorts of comments create a culture where any diligent student might worry that they will be shunned if they want to train in psychiatry. Perhaps this could be countered if there was more exposure to the specialty at an early stage (lack of exposure is a recognized problem).[6]

Fortunately, our experience was that the world of psychiatry was, by and large, a much brighter, thoughtful, and accepting place. Psychiatry is an incredibly rich, intellectually stimulating, and complex field. Much of the understanding gained during training is inaccessible to those taking a casual glance at the specialty, a great deal of what we do involves skill in weighing up nuanced risks and personality factors; most of our diagnoses cannot be made with a simple blood test. We found that as soon as we moved into training in psychiatry, never again did we have to deal with these sorts of comments, designed to undermine and plant self-doubt, and we embarked excitedly on learning a whole new area of medicine, the practice of which is so much more complex and varied than the diagnostic criteria and mental state examination we had touched on in medical school. Some junior doctors worry that they will lose their medical skills by becoming a psychiatrist, but this is not the case; we need to maintain our fundamental medical knowledge because people with the most severe mental illnesses die on average 15 to 20 years earlier than the general population.[7] Some of this risk may be accounted for by the side effects of psychiatric medication, thus there is no doubt that the physical health of our patients is our responsibility.

We have heard of junior doctors, perhaps hankering for the 'doctor as god' stereotypes of surgical wards and yesteryear, worrying that the bio-psycho-social model within psychiatry mean that as a psychiatrist one's skills will be undermined in a multidisciplinary team (MDT) of psychotherapists, social workers, nurses, and psychologists. This is backed up by research which shows one of the key barriers to medical students taking up training in psychiatry is a concern about lack of status and prestige.[6,8] On the other hand, we have found that the MDT made up of colleagues in other disciplines has afforded us a fantastic learning resource. Often psychiatrists take up leadership roles, and being literate in the myriad ways other disciplines approach and can help our patients, being open-minded, and able to consider the biological, social, and psychological factors that might need targeting at different times in a collaborative fashion, is crucial.

Empathic Ability

Are women more suited to a career in psychiatry than men? We wouldn't want to make such generalizations, but there is research showing women to have higher levels of emotional intelligence than men[9] which may manifest as an ability to empathize (Figure 18.1). With so much of our job being about helping people feel at ease and able to talk about difficult feelings and experiences, high verbal and empathic ability is crucial, and often a skilled psychiatrist can provide something therapeutic simply with gestures and words. To counter that, one of our patients said recently, 'I would prefer a man (as a doctor)—they are less emotional'. Still, we have often had feedback from service users, particularly women, stating that they have found it easier to open up to a woman. This is perhaps one area in which archetypes of the woman as somehow less threatening can be helpful. Even if we have not had the same lived experience as some of our patients, there are certain areas of female experience with which it might be easier to empathize as another woman; for example, about childbirth, miscarriage, or experiences of gender-based discrimination. Many perinatal psychiatrists who treat

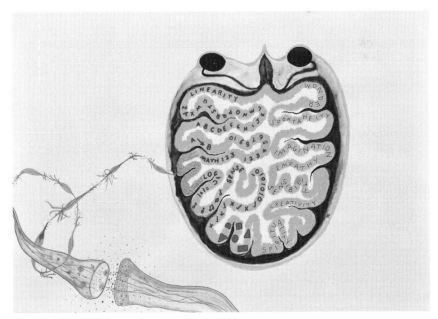

Figure 18.1 Artistic impression of brain hemisphere functions.
© Stephen Magrath, Wellcome Images. Reproduced under the Creative Commons CC-0

mental illnesses in women around pregnancy and birth are women themselves. Some women, when patients, request female doctors and nurses because this can help them feel more at ease, especially if they have suffered violence or abuse by men.

Challenges for Women Psychiatric Trainees

What are the particular challenges faced by women trainees?

Everyday Sexism

We have noticed certain challenges faced by ourselves and other women colleagues regarding age-old chestnuts about perceived age or physical appearance from patients. At the point of entering specialty training most trainees will have done at least two years as a foundation doctor, and most will still appear 'young' in the eyes of the public. Even as Senior House Officers (SHOs) and registrars we were on many occasions told we did not look old enough to be a doctor, and one of us has been told that we couldn't possibly make a decision regarding placing someone on a section 5(2) because 'you're not even 34' (see Figure 18.2).

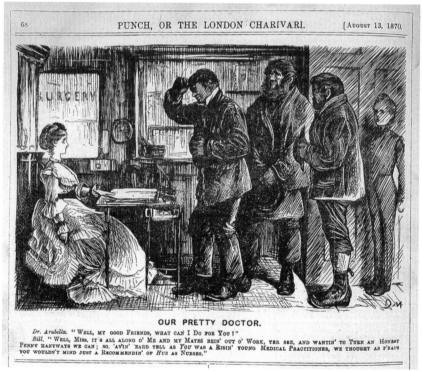

Figure 18.2 Our Pretty Doctor, 1870.

It is interesting to look back at the portrayals of psychiatrists in films and TV to see why the public perception of a psychiatrist favours the elderly, aloof male. It can be challenging to develop one's confidence as a clinician when, despite spending years in work and study, you are judged as trustworthy or not based on perceived age. We have discovered that with time and experience we have found ways to manage these sorts of comments and now find them less a reflection of our clinical ability or as criticisms that we ought to take to heart and more an echo of what might be the patients' anxieties, or what might be societal presumptions of what a professional 'looks' like. There is no doubt in our minds that wider everyday sexism also plays into this phenomenon.

This interplay between how competent we feel in ourselves as clinicians and what our patients might project onto us is complex and something we are always holding in mind during consultations. When starting out, psychiatry as a field can feel quite different to practise than mainstream medicine, which can further amplify the trainee's feelings of inadequacy and fear. Decision-making isn't always straightforward. The medications used are unfamiliar, there is complex interplay between risk factors, personality factors, the law, and the patient's own (sometimes negative) feelings about their illness and need for treatment. All these mean that decision-making is complicated.

Violence

Threats and a risk of violence from patients have been identified as some of the main barriers to medical graduates pursuing psychiatric training.[10] During our conversations with trainees from other medical training pathways, it is concern about personal safety that is cited as a key factor putting people off psychiatry. For some, this unfortunately stemmed from bad experiences as a student, feeling unsupported in medical student placement and perhaps having little space to discuss and put into context the behaviours and presentations of psychiatric pathology that they may have been exposed to for the first time. On first glance, and without adequate understanding, the presentations of those who are very unwell may appear unsettling or frightening. However, statistics clearly show that patients suffering with mental illness are not innately dangerous and in fact are much more frequently victims of abuse and violence themselves.[11] It appears that many of these concerns stem from the stigma that continues to plague the specialty, often not helped by negative media attention. The majority of patients and situations we face in psychiatry do not pose any danger to others. However, we cannot ignore the realities that are faced, particularly in certain settings such as acute admission wards, forensic units, and accident and emergency (A&E) departments, where staff find themselves working with patients with behaviour problems sometimes complicated by substance and alcohol issues. This is all compounded by cuts to staffing and budgets across the NHS that have been known to leave frontline professionals feeling more vulnerable and less well supported.

Dealing with violence at work is a reality across the NHS—just speak to colleagues in A&E. How do psychiatric trainees deal with this reality? One of us was chased through A&E by an angry patient awaiting assessment on one of our first night-shifts, which was a frightening but thankfully rare experience. We fully support policy taken on by NHS Trusts which have a low tolerance of aggression towards staff. However, we

note that within psychiatry we do sometimes end up having to be perhaps more tol-
erant of certain confrontational behaviours, or behaviours that might be perceived as
challenging or threatening if they are indeed manifestations of an underlying mental
disorder. We have found that with appropriate support and training in psychiatry we
are more mindful as a profession about our personal safety than those in other disciplines. In fact, we feel particularly equipped for managing risk and are called on
for support by colleagues encountering challenging patients in the 'general medical
population'. Why is this? We are more risk-aware. Our first day of induction covered
a lecture on keeping safe. Mental health trusts should all have lone-working policies
in place, personal and site alarm systems, and specific risk-management training such
as mandatory 'breakaway' training. More importantly, the skills we gain day to day
by working with patients experiencing a wide range of mental states, and an understanding of the Mental Health Act all provide us with skills in recognizing risk situations, verbally de-escalating these if we can, and the confidence and encouragement
to make the decision not to continue a consultation and to seek alternative support
when real risk is posed.

Stalking

It is not uncommon for psychiatrists to be stalked,[12] and we have at one time or another experienced unwanted intrusive comments and behaviours from people we have
treated. In a survey of psychiatric trainees across several NHS Trusts, 73 per cent reported some form of unwanted sexual behaviour directed towards them.[12] As various
social media platforms and email become more commonly used, it can be increasingly
challenging to maintain the boundaries within a therapeutic alliance. It is an increasingly common problem for trainees to find patients, or concerned friends and relatives
of patients, attempting to contact them via private social media and email accounts.
Doctors coming through core training now will be the first generation who will have
used Facebook to document their friendships, relationships, and private life since their
teens, making this relatively unknown territory for the profession. There is no doubt
that the experience of a clinician expressing concern and listening, can be misinter-
preted by some people, particularly if they are lonely and there is a disturbance of
mind. Although a problematic dynamic can emerge if not very carefully managed,
being aware of this possibility and frequent close supervision can mitigate negative
consequences.

Doctor, Heal Thyself

This phrase contains the essence of what we would suggest could be more explicitly addressed at the outset of psychiatric training, or even earlier in medical training. When
dealing with people inhabiting disordered mental states, the unconscious effects on
the mind of the trainee can be quite powerful. Although Balint groups, reflective
groups where doctors consider the emotional impact cases have had on them and
the possible reasons for this, and supervision afford great opportunities for trainees
to explore their countertransference reactions (the emotional reactions of the doctor
or therapist to being with the patient, which may at times be negative and hence must

be understood and mastered), for the most part the emotional path of a trainee is a private one, with different trainees experiencing different levels of stress and reflective learning at different times. Training in psychiatry can be thought of as a journey and a learning experience which is not just to do with acquiring knowledge and experience but also involves a constant process of reflection upon one's own personal emotional life as this is affected by the people we treat.

Rare but difficult experiences such as being stalked, being physically or verbally attacked, or of a patient committing suicide can all present assaults to the ego which can be extremely distressing. These are recognized as stressors faced by psychiatrists and psychiatric trainees.[13,14] Coupled with this, it is known that women psychiatric trainees report higher levels of work-related stress.[15] Sometimes it can be difficult for our usual support structures of friends, partners, and relatives, even other doctors, to understand these unique and at times traumatic events which are inevitable in the course of a psychiatrist's work. It is this emotional journey, and its rigour, that we feel could be more openly acknowledged at the outset of training in order to prepare trainees. While much of medical school and junior doctor training involves being literally 'thrown in' the deep end, we would argue that because psychiatry deals in emotions it is vital to inform trainees of the importance of an emotional journey during their training. This would serve to normalize some of the stresses of the job and help trainees to differentiate between their difficulties and the difficulties and projections of their patients. Equally, this would be helpful for junior doctors embarking on any career path, all of whom will deal with death and other traumatic human experiences at one point or another. We have found some of our most profound learning has been done in our own therapy, clinical supervision, and informally when debriefing from tough on-calls in the pub with our friends who are also psychiatrists.

With the notable exception of general practitioners (GPs), many doctors in medicine or surgery feel uncomfortable reflecting openly about the emotional impact of their work on them personally, and even less so to use this to inform their practice. At the beginning of psychiatric training it can feel strange to hear encouragement to have therapy, to reflect, and to become kind and compassionate to oneself following a medical education where emotional detachment was encouraged. It is as if having built up many layers of defences and a thick skin to get through the early years of doctoring, training in psychiatry is about stripping these defences away. Once one gets over any initial reluctance to open up, this is undoubtedly a privilege, and psychiatry leads the way in terms of caring for trainees' own emotional health compared to most other specialties.

We have noticed that having to take up the caring role an early age may be a factor that propels some women into a career in psychiatry. We note that the job affects how they later perceive taking up that caring role outside their work environment.

Is there such a thing as 'compassion fatigue'? It is an important step to recognize the roles we take on with others in our personal lives, and our reasons for doing so. It is also important to recognize how to look after ourselves and consider the balance between our personal and professional lives: this might involve putting down roots, establishing boundaries, or changing the sorts of social interactions we seek outside work.

Working in Liaison Psychiatry posts, embedded in general hospitals, can give trainees a real sense of what the specialty can offer in terms of helping other clinicians deal with traumatic cases and adverse events. Balint groups and reflections on psychosocial factors are fundamental facets of psychiatric training. Basic understanding about the dynamics of groups and the manifestations of splitting are parts of our training that mean we will always have a lot to add to MDTs. Indeed, a key competency requirement assessed in interviews for higher training is leadership, and we believe that psychiatric trainees have a particular head start in developing all the right skills to be effective leaders.

Women Leaders and the Importance of Mentoring

Unfortunately, there still is a lack of women in leadership roles within medicine.[16] It is recognized that having positive same-gender role models in medicine enhances recruitment to training.[17] We have found that it has been invaluable to have senior medical women's perspectives when navigating some of the challenges that emerge during psychiatric training.

Why and when have we needed this? For example, one of us found the tone of attack used by a lawyer in a tribunal was gender-focused, used apparently to undermine. Experiences such as this are difficult to endure, and harder still to combat. Another one of us found herself spoken down to and demeaned by a male medical consultant, displacing his frustration at having psychiatric patients on his ward. As bright and educated professional women, perhaps giving advice to senior men in other professions, we at times (and thankfully very rarely) have to deal with aggressive responses from men who feel the need to assert themselves and show who is boss. Sadly, sexism is still alive and kicking, and it can pull the rug out from under one's feet without the right support. In both these situations, it was the firm, wise, and supportive supervision and mentoring of strong women bosses which helped us make sense of our feelings after these unpleasant incidents and supported us in standing up to what was, essentially, male to female and senior to junior bullying.

Maternity Leave, the Gender Pay Gap, and the Junior Doctor Contract

The inevitable demands of juggling family life and maternity leave can cause difficulties for women psychiatric trainees[18] as they can across the board for working women. There are particular pressures within the health service today that mean that cover is often not found when women go on maternity leave. Budget cuts and pre-existing rota gaps mean that often Trusts are unwilling or unable to find cover (a problem confounded by the caps on pay to locum doctors). This can trigger significant anxiety in those who are about to leave their colleagues, and trigger resentment in those left to cover without extra resources. As junior trainees it can also be a struggle for those managing family demands and overnight on-call shifts and exams. Hopefully now there is more of an emphasis on equality but we urge Trusts to look into systemic issues that affect equality (funding cuts and 'efficiency savings', whereby staff on leave are not replaced) rather than simply paying the concept lip service. Even if individuals in the workplace take care to avoid behaving in a way that can make those in minorities feel unwelcome, it is the systems and structures around our employment and pay that send the real messages about how certain staff groups are valued.

Throughout 2016 junior doctors in the United Kingdom were in a stand-off with the Department of Health over a new junior doctor's contract, and trainees participated in strike action which was mandated by 98 per cent of the BMA's balloted trainee members. The new contract imposed by the government openly and unapologetically discriminates against women and care-givers, with an equality assessment stating this was 'necessary'. It also hit those who work non-resident on-calls particularly hard. One of the key sticking points in the contract which caused many people to agree to go on strike was the removal of yearly pay increments for those who train less than full-time or switch specialty. The effects of this element of the contract on the gender pay gap within medicine will be profound because it is usually women who take time out to have children and work part-time to care for them. Removing the increments will leave women stuck on the same pay for years as their male colleagues become consultants and thus move up the pay scales, and it will serve to reinforce a gender pay gap that is already present. In addition, with work up to 9 p.m. any day of the week now called 'plain time' (where previously weekends and all work after 7 p.m. would have attracted a higher rate), the cost of getting expensive childcare at weekends and evenings falls squarely on women doctors, and the contract does not offer to offset this.

As female psychiatric trainees of childbearing age, the contract fails to appreciate the way we work. Non-resident on-calls as a psychiatric registrar involve being up most of the night and driving to Mental Health Act assessments which may be at different sites; there is concern that those hours will prove difficult to log and claim. The government has made much of introducing 'flexible pay premia' for psychiatry trainees, because it is a specialty experiencing a recruitment crisis. Incentives are welcome but they are simply not adequate, given the cuts to overall pay found in other parts of the contract. It is disappointing that our NHS does not prioritize gender-pay equality, and it is hard to believe that this policy is not just a cynical way for the government to pay the workforce less, as greater proportions of women make up the junior doctor workforce.

Conclusions

Training in psychiatry involves embarking on a fascinating, stimulating, and at times emotionally demanding journey, which not only enables trainees to learn how to help their patients but also provides a privileged position at the interface of politics, sociology, science, psychology, and psychoanalysis, allowing us to gain particular perspectives on processes within organizations and events in the world at large. Women trainees face many challenges in pursuing their career in psychiatry, the most recent relating to contractual changes which discriminate against junior doctors who train less than full-time (LTFT), who are much more likely to be women with childcare responsibilities. Moreover, the deliberate underfunding of the NHS and social care by the current government and the lack of parity of funding for mental health services has led to an NHS in crisis, and a lack of resources for patients who are more vulnerable than ever. Women trainees have a crucial role to play in fighting for the right of equality for their patients and for themselves as professionals, and we have touched on the importance of women mentors and leaders to drive this forward. We have laid out what we think are some of the particular challenges for women trainees. Other people may have different perspectives but we can more than attest to how rewarding the gradual process of taking on these challenges can be. Psychiatry can be a wonderful career choice for women, and women's roles within the specialty are and should be promoted and encouraged. There is a great deal of collegiality, warmth, and encouragement already embedded within the culture of psychiatric training programmes and we hope that this strength will offer women psychiatric trainees the best chance to take on the significant challenges faced by our profession as it moves through stormy waters.

References

1. Royal College of Psychiatrists. Membership Data, Royal College of Psychiatrists. Available from: membership@rcpsych.ac.uk.

2. **Goldacre M, Fazel S, Smith F,** and **Lambert T** (2013). Choice and rejection of psychiatry as a career: surveys of UK medical graduates from 1974 to 2009. *British Journal of Psychiatry* **202**(3):228–34.

3. **Mukherjee K, Maier M,** and **Wessely S** (2013). UK crisis in recruitment into psychiatric training. *Psychiatrist* **37**:210–4.

4. **Bebbington P, Brugha T, Coid J, Crawford M, Deverill C, D'Souza J, Doyle M, Farrell M, Fuller E, Jenkins R, Jotangia D, Harris J, Hussey D, King M, McManus S, Meltzer H, Nicholson S, Palmer B, Pickup D, Purdon S, Sadler K, Scholes S, Smith J, Thompson J, Tyrer P, Wardle H, Weich S,** and **Wessely S** (2009). Adult psychiatric morbidity in England, Results of a household survey. Leeds: The NHS Information Centre.

5. **The Kings Fund** (2015). <http://www.kingsfund.org.uk/projects/verdict/has-government-put-mental-health-equal-footing-physical-health>.

6. **Eagles JM, Wilson S, Murdoch JM,** and **Brown T** (2007). What impact do undergraduate experiences have upon recruitment into psychiatry? *Psychiatry Bulletin* **31**:70–2.

7. **Thornicroft G** (2011). Physical health disparities and mental illness: the scandal of premature mortality *British Journal of Psychiatry* **199**(6):441–2.

8. **Malhi GS, Parker GB, Parker K, Kirkby KC, Boyce P, Yellowlees P, Hornabrook C,** and **Jones K** (2002). Shrinking away from psychiatry? A survey of Australian medical students' interest in psychiatry. *Australian and New Zealand Journal of Psychiatry* **36**:416–23.

9. **Salovey P** and **Mayer JD** (1990). Emotional intelligence. *Imagination, Cognition and Personality* **9**:185–211.

10. **Lambert TW, Turner G, Fazel S,** and **Goldacre M** (2006). Reasons why some UK medical graduates who initially choose psychiatry do not pursue it as a long-term career. *Psychological Medicine* **36**:679–84.

11. **Khalifeh H, Johnson S, Howard LM, Borschmann R, Osborn D, Dean K, Hart C, Hogg J,** and **Moran P** (2015). Violent and non-violent crime against adults with severe mental illness *British Journal of Psychiatry* **206**(4):275–82.

12. **McIvor RJ, Potter L,** and **Davies L** (2008). Stalking behaviour by patients towards psychiatrists in a large mental health organization. *International Journal of Social Psychiatry* **54**:350–7.

13. **Walter G**, **Rey J**, and **Giuffrida M** (2003). What is it currently like being a trainee psychiatrist in Australia? *Australian Psychiatrist* **11**(4):439–444.

14. **Holloway F**, **Szmukler G**, and **Carson J** (2000). Support systems 1. Introduction. *Advances in Psychiatric Treatment* **6**:226–37.

15. **Morgan JF** and **Porter S** (1999). Sexual harassment of psychiatric trainees: experiences and attitudes. *Postgraduate Medical Journal* **75**:410–13.

16. **Newman P** (2015). *NHS Women in Leadership: Plan for Action.* London: NHS Confederation (Employers) Company Ltd.

17. **Park J**, **Minor S**, **Taylor RA**, **Vikis E**, and **Poenaru D.** (2005). Why are women deterred from general surgery training? *American Journal of Surgery* **190**:141–6.

18. **Kohen D** and **Arnold E** (2002). The female psychiatrist: Professional, personal and social issues. *Advances in Psychiatric Treatment* **8**:81–8.

The Art of Listening

There's always one who's mastered the knack
of circular breathing, thereby becoming
uninterruptable. O marvellous man –

and sometimes woman – who can ex- and in-hale
this tautological excess without choking,
without even ruminating such delicious verbiage.

But what they are saying, amid the woosh and saliva
of variations, cadenzas, trills, is inevitably the small
but potentially interesting observation I made myself

five minutes earlier. Only now everyone agrees –
not in words, of course, for we're here to talk
about listening – but with *uh-huh nod mmm*

one by one stretching oblique across unpadded chairs,
elbows winged, hands clasping the backs of our necks,
shirt buttons gaping,

in what we'll learn next week is called *mirroring
the dominant pose*, which will not, on reflection,
shed much light on anything at all.

Emily Wills

Chapter 19

Women as Trainers in Psychiatry

Hannah Fosker and Ann Boyle

Women as Trainers and Leaders in Medicine

The world may seem to have progressed a long way regarding gender assumptions but often they appear to remain in stasis in the medical world. You will not meet many women in medicine who cannot recall a time they were assumed to have been the nurse. These assumptions have not abated, despite holding no statistical basis in our modern world where the majority of medical students are now female, and proportions of doctors from each gender are not far from 50/50.[21] The percentage of women making up the psychiatric workforce increased from 37 per cent to 67 per cent between 1974 and 1999.[3] Similarly, male nurses will most likely have been assumed to be the doctor at some point in their careers. Although nursing remains a predominantly female field, in mental health this majority is reducing, with almost a third of nurses in mental health now men.[9] Thus, in psychiatry we are perhaps striding more towards an unbiased work environment with regard to gender, more so than some other specialties.

However, the fact remains that women are under-represented in positions of leadership and senior academic roles. For example, only 26 per cent of Trust medical directors are women.[21] With 54 per cent of trainee doctors being women, this reduces to 32 per cent at consultant level. These percentages reduce even further when considering senior leadership roles; somewhere along the way, our junior female medics are stumbling before they make it to the top. Research has suggested barriers hindering a women's path to leadership positions include their personal expectations, the culture of medical organizations, and a desire for a better work–life balance.[21] The Medical Women's Federation Role Model report found that stereotypically masculine attributes continue to be perceived as necessary for success in leadership positions. This leads to a reduction in women applying for and reaching these positions. However, high-quality female role models can alter this and heighten women's confidence and expectations of themselves.[11] We need to prioritize encouraging our women colleagues up these ladders, with evidence that their presence at the top of an organization can lead to a change in the culture and improved organization-wide performance.[21]

How is This Being Challenged?

Diminishing numbers of women towards the top of the academic and professional pyramid in the medical world has not gone unnoticed. The Athena Swan Charter, established in 2005, aims to encourage advancement of women's academic careers in science, technology, engineering, maths, and medicine. It recognizes commitment to addressing gender inequality and tackling barriers to women's progression to senior academic and professional roles in those areas where attrition of women along the career ladder is recognized. Completion of a PhD and transitioning into a sustainable career in academia and higher education remains one of a variety of noted barriers to women's progression in academic medical careers. Breaking down this, and other walls, requires active engagement from senior roles throughout our organizations.[2]

Psychiatry has a commendable history of enabling women to navigate the career path and reach important positions as leaders and trainers. Women psychiatrists began working less than full-time in Oxford in 1966, two years before flexible training was formally introduced within the National Health Service (NHS). Increasing numbers of trainees have been taking up this opportunity in psychiatry, and there is a dedicated deanery lead for less than full-time training. For proof that such adaptation need not be a deterrent to great achievements consider Baroness Sheila Hollins (Professor of Psychiatry and former President of the Royal College of Psychiatrists and the British Medical Association) and Dame Fiona Caldicott (first woman Dean and President of the Royal College of Psychiatrists, Pro-Vice Chancellor of Oxford University, former chair of Oxford University Hospital NHS Trust, and former chair of the National Information Governance Board for Health and Social Care)[1](see Profile in this book). The deanery lead for less than full-time training provides links with various organizations, including the Medical Women's Federation, which works to actively encourage women to apply for leadership positions where thus far they remain under-represented.[8]

The Royal College of Psychiatrists also has a Special Interest Group dedicated to women (see Chapter 4). Originally named the 'Women in Psychiatry' special interest group at its inception in 1995, it is now called 'Women and Mental Health'. Although this new title may help to broaden its appeal and clarify its dedication to improving mental health in women, it continues to cite a key aim as supporting female psychiatrist's working lives, including career development in management and academic roles.[22]

The Pertinence of this to Psychiatry

The importance of senior figures in psychiatry lies not only with their aforementioned benefit to organizations but also in the importance of female role models to those developing their careers. Most women doctors are young (perhaps in part reflecting the sparsity of women entering the medical profession in the older generation of doctors), and over two-thirds of them have children.[12] Psychiatry's family-friendly reputation has been an ally in our well-documented recruitment battle, however the proportion of women entering psychiatry was reported to decline in Teifion Davies' 2013 study into recruitment. Here he postulated that our family-friendly appeal was diminishing as other medical specialties worked to improve their flexible training schemes.[15] He argued that the focus of recruitment should be on quality rather than quantity and cited women as the 'intellectual core of British psychiatry', in part due to their propensity to outperform their male counterparts in both written and clinical Member of the Royal College of Psychiatry (MRCPsych)examinations.

The Medical Women's Federation Role Models report described the impact and importance of good quality female role models, particularly for support in domains such as raising a family or maintaining work–life balance.[11] Research has shown the effects that positive role models can have on recruitment into psychiatry,[18] highlighting another advantage to women taking on trainer roles, with their reported benefit as role models in both personal and professional realms. This was supported in a 2009 study into recruitment into psychiatry from a Foundation Year Two post, in which two working mothers acted as trainers to junior medics undertaking an early placement in psychiatry, prior to applying for future training in a specialty of their choosing. Women trainees identified these trainers as positive role models, and positive support in this manner was found to be an influencing factor in future career intentions. With its higher proportion of women consultants, psychiatry is well placed to embrace, and benefit from, the feminization of medicine.[14]

Women trainers not only enhance our specialty's ability to entice, retain, and nurture high-quality junior doctors to pursue a psychiatric career but also provide high-quality senior clinicians with a proven aptitude for working with those with mental illness. Although undoubtedly great psychiatrists come in all shapes, sizes, and genders, there has been evidence to support the notion that women are predisposed by their attitudes and abilities to have a greater natural aptitude for psychiatry. This includes findings that women show higher levels of emotional intelligence (their ability to appraise, express, and regulate emotions).[18] Also, research has shown gender differences in rating psychopathology, hypothesized to suggest that women have an initial advantage in understanding mental state.[7] It would not be unreasonable to suggest that those skills making women naturals at psychiatry would also enhance their abilities to become effective trainers.

The advantages brought by women trainers to the junior psychiatric workforce, will reap benefits for all doctors passing through the speciality, including those who temporarily enter during their foundation training or along their pathway to a career as a general practitioner (GP) or indeed any other specialty. These junior doctors are expected to fulfil certain learning outcomes during this placement, developing within them transferable skills pertinent to a future career as a compassionate, empathic, holistic clinician, vital qualities as outlined in the Francis Report in 2013.[16,20] With female doctors' reported aptitude for these competencies, the benefits of good quality women trainers in psychiatry can have a far-reaching benefit to the future medical profession, nurturing compassion and empathy in doctors eventually entering all specialties.

Training in Psychiatry

Trainers in psychiatry are likely to have responsibilities for numerous types of junior doctors. This includes Foundation Year doctors or GP trainees, passing through the specialty for only a short time, and core and higher specialty trainees who are pursuing psychiatry as a long-term career. Although core values remain consistent throughout curricula, each cohort will have slightly differing aims in terms of the knowledge and skills they need to acquire.

Foundation-year doctors are expected to develop core communication skills, compassionate values, an ability to work within a multidisciplinary team to care for those with complex health problems, and hone their ability to perform an adequate mental state examination, knowing when to ask for help with further management of a patient with a psychiatric condition.[19] General practice trainees will also be expected to develop a level of knowledge about mental illness, both in terms of diagnosis and clinical management, as well as using the placement as an opportunity to hone communication skills. However, they will also be expected to develop a more in-depth understanding of local community resources and how to access these, and how to treat and assess psychiatric presentations in the context of their own community setting.[13]

During core psychiatric training, as well as developing knowledge of the diagnosis and treatment of psychiatric conditions through their placements within clinical teams trainees will be supported with taking their RCPsych Membership examinations (see Box 19.1). This currently consists of two written papers, each with multiple choice questions and extended matching items, and a practical exam (CASC— Clinical Assessment of Skills and Competencies). Through the written papers, knowledge across topics spanning the scientific and theoretical basis of psychiatry, clinical

---

Box 19.1 Examples of Multiple Choice Questions Found in MRCPsych Examinations

Clozapine is most likely to be associated with which of the following adverse reactions?

a) Cardiomyopathy*

b) Gingivitis

c) Lymphoedema

d) Retinitis pigmentosa

e) Sarcoidosis

A 25-year-old man tells you that whenever he turns the taps on in the bathroom he can hear his neighbour talking. Which of the following is he experiencing?

a) Extracampine hallucination

b) Functional hallucination*

c) Hypnopompic hallucination

d) Pareidolic illusion

e) Reflex hallucination

Source: data from MRCPsych Paper A—The Scientific and theoretical basis of Psychiatry, Sample Paper A Questions, © The Royal College of Psychiatrists. Available from: <http://www.rcpsych.ac.uk/pdf/Paper per cent20A per cent20sample per cent20questions.pdf>.

Box 19.2 Skills Required by Supervisors

Observer reflector
Information provider
Identifier of alternatives
Facilitator
Joint problem-solver
Process counsellor
Negotiator
Advocate

Reproduced from Advances in Psychiatric Treatment, 5(2), Cottrell D, Supervision, pp. 83–8, Copyright (1999), with permission from The Royal College of Psychiatrists

topics across a broad range of psychiatric sub-specialties, and critical review skills are tested. During CASC, clinical skills are assessed to ensure candidates are of competent standard to earn their RCPsych membership, and continue into higher levels of training within their chosen sub-specialty.[10,19]

Whichever category of trainee a trainer finds themselves teaching, the required skills are likely to be comparable. Training is likely to be delivered through interaction with patients and work on the ward, or in out-patient and on-call settings as well as through formal teaching sessions and relevant study days.

One aspect of training in which psychiatry leads the way in the medical world, is supervision. The Royal College of Psychiatrists and the European Federation of Psychiatric Trainees have both highlighted the importance of an hour of weekly protected supervision time between trainer and trainee.[4,6] Research has highlighted the uniqueness and value of this learning experience,[5] and it is something that is not replicated across other medical specialties. Cottrell looked further into what supervision time can and should entail, and highlighted the importance of ensuring this hour was high-quality, and that supervisors were adequately trained to fulfil this role (see Box 19.2). As well as discussion of day-to-day clinical work, this hour can be used to develop teaching skills, supervise research, and provide pastoral care through personal guidance and support.[17]

The Personal Perspective: From Trainer to Trainee

To gain a personal perspective of women as trainers in psychiatry, the following is a conversation between Dr Ann Boyle (Consultant Old Age Psychiatrist, Specialist Advisor for the Foundation Programme for the Royal College of Psychiatrists and Associate Postgraduate Dean at Health Education England) and Dr Hannah Fosker (a Specialist Registrar in General Psychiatry). They have known each other since Hannah's time as an undergraduate at Leicester Medical School. Ann has worked in numerous educational leadership roles, both within and beyond psychiatry training. She is also mother to a teenage daughter.

HF: Can You Tell Me About Your Career in Psychiatry, as a Trainee and then a Trainer?

AB: Well, I did the majority of my training in Leicester and progressed fairly quickly through the training scheme. There were not as many higher training places in the early 1990s so getting a senior registrar job was quite competitive. I remember six people being interviewed for one post when I was appointed. I did what would now be called dual training, even though I was already very clear that I wanted to be an Old Age Psychiatrist.

As a trainee, I do not think I appreciated how much being a medical teacher was part of every doctors' role. I was really involved with teaching when I was a senior registrar, mainly teaching medical students and Senior House Officers and I really enjoyed it. I suppose teaching was probably my 'Plan B' if I hadn't got into medical school. I helped my friends with maths and science at school—especially those who were struggling. I got into medical school in spite of, rather than because of, my school. So, I enjoyed teaching, or perhaps helping others in that way as not passing maths was even then a barrier to many career paths for school leavers. From being a senior registrar running tutorials, I then got involved with organizing the end of block medical student exams. I recall very clearly Professor Margaret Oates coming as external examiner from Nottingham and her getting right to the heart of a struggling student's problems during his viva. He had never shown up to tutorials and she managed to get him to start to talk about this, and get him the help he so clearly needed. He would now be called a student in difficultly. I was blown away by how sensitively she managed such a difficult conversation and understood for the first time that helping those learners who were struggling was one of the most challenging aspects of being a medical teacher. I became an organizer for the Membership exams in Leicester, which was a clinical exam centre at the time.

Then I became a consultant. Like now, your life changes and I recall that my training did not really prepare me for that transition. It was like falling off a cliff edge from a primrose path. A job came up to be a 'clinical tutor' and one of my mentors *told* me to apply. I was pregnant when I interviewed for the clinical tutor job, so becoming a lead trainer came hand in hand with becoming a parent. The role was largely a managerial one, but I remained an educational supervisor for trainees. It was around that time that the college began to mandate one-hour weekly supervision for each trainee, and working in a training role was beginning to be professionalized. I remember organizing a number of deanery and college visits; the whole quality-management agenda was in its infancy, and visits had a much lighter touch than they do now.

Around this time, the European Working Time Directive was introduced. I was responsible for leading the implementation in the Trust. Most colleagues were worried about the service implications, which were evident. I was more concerned about the effect on trainees, even though there would be shorter working hours which was great. I worried that they could become even more professionally isolated from the team and other trainee doctors, as well as having less ownership of evolving clinical problems, which affects experiential learning. These unintended consequences took some time to be apparent.

I was asked to become involved in developing psychiatry in the Foundation programme by the postgraduate dean locally and became an active and, I hope, valued member of the Foundation school faculty. I always saw our psychiatry trainees as isolated from the rest of medicine and from the acute hospitals, and observed the effects this had on stigma within the medical profession. Therefore, I viewed being part of the Foundation programme as a real opportunity for psychiatry. I have really welcomed Simon Wessely's work towards making us more medically relevant, and integrating us with the wider NHS, during his time as RCPsych President.

A few years later I was appointed as inaugural Head of School of Psychiatry, a job which was created out of the changes to training occurring at the time. There were other women (e.g. the current President Elect of the Royal College of Psychiatrists, Wendy Burn) who had also become heads of school at the same time. Many of them were from a similar background to me—in the middle of their career, with a background in education and training within their local trust. I then had to establish the educational governance structure, and navigate the changing relationships between the Royal College of Psychiatrists and what is now Health Education England, as well as the then regular Postgraduate Medical Education and Training board, to ensure collaborative working.

HF: As Someone who is Heavily Involved in Training, What Do You Think Led to You Wanting to Develop This Aspect of Your Career?

AB: I like developing people, and would have probably been be a teacher if I hadn't become a doctor. For me, developing a portfolio of skills and time for educational responsibilities, whilst remaining an active clinician, has sustained me both personally and professionally.

Some of my previous trainees have stayed in touch with me. I think it is because I have viewed the pastoral and mentoring components of the supervisory role as just as important as the clinical one. Plus, I am a psychiatrist so I am always interested in understanding people. I try to make the effort to show how grateful I have been for trainees' hard work, give them a present and a card, and say a proper goodbye. I think it's really important to do that. It is just a little touch of kindness. I don't think we value our trainees enough sometimes.

In a way, you have to treat the junior doctors as well as you treat your children. I find it rewarding, seeing them go and achieve something and become a success, a future leader. It is also rewarding to help those trainees who are in very difficult situations, which is harder, but in the end equally rewarding. I hope my former trainees will look after me too, when they are running the world and I am retired. I see you all as investment in the future NHS.

HF: What Specific Challenges Do You Think There are as a Trainer in Psychiatry, Perhaps when Compared to Other Specialties?

AB: The NHS is currently under enormous pressure, particularly in mental health services, and morale is low across every staff group. For me, all senior psychiatrists need to continue to 'big up, not talk down' a career in psychiatry to all trainees on each and every interaction. I try to be a visible and credible role model as a trainer, by demonstrating my professional values through my actions. We need to attract more UK medical school graduates to psychiatry, and we need to start thinking about tackling stigma earlier. For example, considering who is selected to medical school, and whether perhaps some of those four science A-level students may not be the best way to select doctors with an aptitude for psychiatry. I've got really into supporting sixth formers with their applications to medical school over the last five years. Supporting a future medical student to get into medical school is something they'll never forget. I am interested in social inclusion and very keen to support less advantaged students to become doctors.

Another challenge in psychiatry is maintaining our physical health knowledge and skills. We cannot leave physical healthcare to someone else. Junior doctors often come into psychiatry, and this hierarchical or segregated ideology is formed where the psychiatry trainees only want to learn about the mind, and the GP trainees and foundation doctors seem to me to be more involved in physical healthcare. Our patients with severe enduring mental illness are dying 15 years earlier than the general population, so we really need to upskill ourselves and fight for integrated healthcare. We cannot merely be proxy physicians but be alert to physical health problems and develop our initial clinical management skills. I am not sure that our current training structure or curricula are fit for this purpose. The foundation programme has provided us as a speciality to give many early doctors four months of postgraduate training in psychiatry, but we also need to think about what extra training psychiatrists need to look after our patients' physical healthcare now and in the future.

HF: What Specific Challenges do you Think are Presented as a Woman Trainer?

AB: My primary responsibility has to be to my family. Maintaining that balance between home and work is tough for anyone in a vocational career, any doctor, any nurse. Of course, men feel that too, it's not that mothers have the monopoly on that. But, particularly when I had a young child, at times my professional responsibilities weighed heavily on me. When there are clashes between important work commitments and events in my daughter's life, something has to give and I have had to make some difficult choices. My husband and daughter understand, I think, that I have tried to be a 'good enough' parent, and I have been blessed with a husband who has been very supportive.

I am glad to say I haven't been discriminated against because of my gender; I don't feel it has held me back at all. I have always sensed that, as a psychiatrist, the stigma surrounding my specialty was more of a disadvantage in medicine than being a woman. I have had some health problems in the past and I remember one medical doctor I saw asked 'what is it like being a psychiatrist?' I told him 'it's very busy, just like it's very busy for you'. Then he said, 'I think I would quite like being a psychiatrist, because I could take my dog to work and patients would just be brought to you.' People need to stop perpetuating these myths. I told him that actually most of my patients are detained in hospital and don't want to see me. He apologized. I was a patient at the time, lying on a bed, feeling very vulnerable.

Another time, I was having surgery, and there was a nice staff nurse looking after me post-operatively. At one point in my stay, he said, 'Ann, I feel like you could have been a good doctor, whatever specialty you did. Why did you decide to do psychiatry? Why did you waste yourself like that?' I think you don't realize the value of psychiatry until it touches you—be that personally, or through a patient, or through a trainee.

HF: I have certainly had similar experiences; my first clinical supervisor described my intended career choice as a 'waste of a good doctor'. It was really frustrating. I think he was trying to convince me to be an obstetrician, but it just made me more determined to become a good psychiatrist. What challenges do you think are faced by women trainers and trainees in our speciality?

AB: If you look at the recent industrial action, most of the issues are not gender-specific. Doctors want a different life now, more of a work–life balance. I used to work 100 hours as a house officer, but that isn't what people want now, nor is it right for our patients.

Balancing medicine and motherhood is becoming more challenging. I am not suggesting we should change our investment in training women less than full-time, but I do think that there are times in your career where you can't have it all. Take the Shape of Training report, which talks about being able to step out of training and have children, then come back; that's a really good idea, being able to do it more slowly. Rather than feeling you should progress straight to CCT (Certificate of Completed Training, i.e. consultant level) you can step in and step out. It is particularly hard for doctors who marry other doctors, which, let's face it, is a lot of people because you meet people at work. The pressure on those families now is greater than ever. With more females than males getting into medical school, and yet less women in leadership positions, I do worry about that. It is to be celebrated that in the Royal College of Psychiatrists we currently have a woman dean and a woman president—we are a more forward-thinking profession.

The burdens of annual assessment and appraisals, and revalidation, with all the hoops you need to jump though, are burdens to doctors of all levels and genders. The Pearson Report, which was recently commissioned by the General Medical Council (GMC) to look at consultant revalidation, spoke about how burdensome and exhausting it is. The NHS is in crisis and there is all this mandatory training. The results were published recently and Terence Stephenson, the current chair of the GMC, promised that he would look at the burden of mandatory training. He also acknowledged that there is a terrible amount of service pressure, but told us that we need to make sure we keep looking after the trainees. I suppose, as a trainer, I don't like it when some consultants complain about how terrible life is to the junior doctors. We need to support them. It is similar to how parents do not expose young children to the horrors of adulthood.

HF: There is evidence that female role models can be beneficial in terms of both professional and personal support to trainees. How do you feel about this? Do you feel any expectation to provide more of a personal support to women trainees? Perhaps, for example, in relation to balancing family and a career as a doctor. If so, does this present any challenges to maintaining your own personal boundaries in achieving this?

AB: I do think it is important to disclose things about your life, in a boundaried way. Everyone knows I have one child. I am sure if I had five I would not have as much time to invest in other people. My personal support isn't gender specific, though. I have invested time in supporting men trainees too, though I have supported many more women.

HF: What is the Most Important Lesson You Learnt from a Woman Trainer or Role Model in Your Medical Career?

AB: As an undergraduate in Ireland, and then as a newly qualified doctor before my psychiatric training, the only female role models I can remember are near peers—junior doctors who were really supportive. You worked a lot of hours, and looked after each other. I never worked with a woman consultant at that stage, and I can only remember a couple of women consultants who taught me at medical school. I didn't meet any women psychiatrists as an undergraduate.

The first woman consultant I worked for as a psychiatrist was Dr Sue Eason in Leicester. She was very inspiring, and glamorous. She was in the middle of her career, and was fantastically inspiring as a clinician, and she also had children. She ended up being the first medical director of the Trust, female or male. I only worked with her for six months but the most important pieces of advice she gave me were:

> It is no good being as good as the men, you need to be better than them. The only way to pass the exams is to read a lot of books, and work really hard. You have to dress properly at work to be respected (which she told me as I tended to wear jeans to work at the time). She also told me that your 40s are a great time of personal and professional development in medicine. I thought that was just middle-aged woman chat at the time, but actually, she was absolutely right. She was a powerful role model for me.

There were numerous inspiring women senior doctors around me at the time. I saw them ahead of me, having their children, then returning to work after three months off. Some went part-time, some did not. Less than full-time working did exist but fewer women seemed to avail of it. Working four days a week as a mother was normal in Leicester. There was no right or wrong way to combine medicine and motherhood. Psychiatry probably had more women doctors than other branches of hospital medicine.

HF: As a Woman Trainer, What Message Would You Most Like to Pass on to the Women Trainees of the Future?

AB:

◆ Look after yourself or you won't be able to look after anybody else.

◆ Aspire to be good enough. High-achieving perfectionists make excellent doctors but may fail to look after themselves to the same standard that they provide for their patients.

◆ Choose your husband or life partner wisely. Make sure they understand the demands and rewards of your career and can support you when you need.

◆ Be mindful that you can't have it all, all the time. Your career is a long one. At times, you will need to focus on your family and allow the professional stuff to simmer. I didn't do any work nationally until my daughter was in the later years of primary school.

◆ Also, your 40s really are a great period of development. You don't have to do it all as soon as you become a young consultant.

Ann left me with those wise words and then rushed off to take her daughter to a school trip.

References

1. **Psychiatrists' Support Service** (2013). 17 on LTFT training_final.pdf. London: Royal College of Psychiatrists. <http://www.rcpsych.ac.uk/pdf/17 per cent20on per cent20LTFT per cent20training_final.pdf>.

2. **Equality Challenge Unit** (2018). About ECU's Athena SWAN Charter. Equality Challenge Unit. <http://www.ecu.ac.uk/equality-charters/athena-swan/about-athena-swan/>.

3. **Goldacre MJ** (2005). Career choices for psychiatry: national surveys of graduates of 1974–2000 from UK medical schools. *British Journal of Psychiatry* 1 February;**186**(2):158–64.

4. Royal College of Psychiatrists (2013). <http://www.rcpsych.ac.uk/pdf/Core_Psychiatry_Curriculum_August_2016.pdf>.

5. **Rele K** and **Tarrant CJ** (2010). Educational supervision appropriate for psychiatry trainees' needs. *Academic Psychiatry* June; **34**(3):229–32.

6. **European Federation of Psychiatric Trainees** (2013). EFPT Recommendations on Standards of Psychiatric Training. <http://efpt.eu/wordpress/wp-content/uploads/2014/07/EFPT-STATEMENTS-2013-revision_2.pdf>.

7. **Fabrega H**, **Ulrich R**, and **Keshavan M** (1994). Gender differences in how medical students learn to rate psychopathology. *Journal of Nervous and Mental Disease* August;**182**(8):471–5.

8. **Medical Women's Federation**. <http://www.medicalwomensfederation.org.uk/about-us/campaigns/286-leadership-and-mentoring>.

9. **Health Careers NHS UK**. Mental health nursing infographic. <http://www.healthcareers.nhs.uk/sites/default/files/documents/Mental%20health%20nursing%20inforgraphic%20v2.pdf>.

10. **Royal College of Psychiatrists** (2018). MRCPsych Examinations. <http://www.rcpsych.ac.uk/traininpsychiatry/examinations/examinationstab.aspx>.

11. **Peters K, Ryan M, Toppin E, Leigh R**, and **Lucas A** (2014). The Role Models who Sustain Women's Career Engagement.<http://www.medicalwomensfederation.org.uk/images/ MWF_Role_Model_Report_May_2014_FINAL.pdf>.

12. **Sinden N** (2003). Patterns of child-bearing behaviour amongst female hospital doctors and GPs. *Family Practice* 1 August;**20**(4):486–8.

13. **Royal College of General Practitioners** (2018). <http://www.rcgp.org.uk/training-exams/ gp-curriculum-overview/document-version.aspx>.

14. **Boyle AM, Chaloner DA, Millward T, Rao V**, and **Messer C** (2009). Recruitment from foundation year 2 posts into specialty training: a potential success story? *Psychiatric Bulletin* 1 August; **33**(8):306–8.

15. **Davies T** (2013). Recruitment into psychiatry: quantitative myths and qualitative challenges. *British Journal of Psychiatry* 1 March;**202**(3):163–5.

16. **Francis R** (2013). Mid Staffordshire NHS Foundation Trust Public Inquiry, Francis R. Report of the Mid Staffordshire NHS Foundation Trust public inquiry: executive summary. London: The Stationery Office.

17. **Cottrell D** (1999). Supervision. *Advances in Psychiatric Treatment* **5**:83–8.

18. **Wilson S** (2006). The feminisation of psychiatry: changing gender balance in the psychiatric workforce. *Psychiatric Bulletin* 1 September;**30**(9):321–3.

19. **The Foundation Programme** (2016). The Foundation Programme Curriculum 2016 <http://www.foundationprogramme.nhs.uk/curriculum/Syllabus>.

20. **Boyle A, Davies S, Dogra N, Perry J**, and **Fosker H** (2016). The Foundation Programme in psychiatry: a qualitative study into the effects of a foundation placement. *British Journal of Psychiatry Bulletin* 1 October;**40**(5):281–4.

21. **The King's Fund**. Women and medical leadership. <https://www.kingsfund.org.uk/audio-video/women-and-medical-leadership-infographics>.

22. **Royal College of Psychiatrists**. Women and Mental Health Special Interest Group <http:// www.rcpsych.ac.uk/workinpsychiatry/specialinterestgroups/womenandmentalhealth. aspx>.

Chapter 20

How to Succeed in Psychiatry Without Really Trying: One Woman's Accidental Pathway to the Top of Her Profession

Wendy Burn

Introduction

I am writing this in late January 2017. The snowdrops are just beginning to open in the pale wintry sunshine, reminding me that soon it will be spring. A few days ago I heard that I had been elected as the next President of the Royal College of Psychiatrists. I will be the sixteenth holder of this office and the fourth woman President. It is still impossible to believe that this has happened, I am an ordinary 'jobbing' psychiatrist working in a busy old-age community post in Yorkshire. I am not an academic, I have never worked in London, and I have two children. How did this happen? This chapter gives me time to take stock and to reflect on how I got to where I am and a chance to share my progress with anyone who might want to follow a similar path.

Childhood 1958–76

I was born in Oxford. My father worked in a research post with the University; he was the son of Joshua Harold Burn, Professor of Pharmacology at Oxford University. My mother was a paediatrician who was advised to give up work when she encountered difficulty getting pregnant; this was the 1950s when it was still uncommon for women to work. Both my parents were doctors, my mother because she was passionate about medicine, my father because his father had insisted on it.

From as early as I can remember I wanted to become a doctor. I used to pore over my mother's copy of *Gray's Anatomy*, fascinated by the pictures illustrating the composition of the human body. I should have paid more attention to the words as later anatomy was nearly to be my undoing.

I started my education at the age of four at a small private school in Norham Gardens in Oxford called The Crescent. I liked the pupils and the teachers and would gladly have stayed there but when I was five I moved to my local state school, Botley County Primary School. My new school was completely different to The Crescent and I confess to feeling somewhat shocked by the change but I learnt some skills in physical combat which were helpful.

My academic progress at this school was limited. The class sizes were large. We sat in order of repeated test results and my best friend and I discovered that by copying each other's work we ended up sitting next to each other. This didn't inspire me to do my best and it looked as if I would fail my 'Eleven plus' examination which picked out the brightest pupils for the better secondary schools. I therefore moved schools again.

My next school was the private Manor in Abingdon, the preparatory school for St Helen and St Katharine. I joined at the age of nine for the last two years of primary school. It was difficult coming into a new school at that stage. Everyone had already established friends and I was behind in almost everything. I had to have extra hand-writing lessons in the lunch break; we were taught to write in beautiful italic script. Sadly, over the years, my writing has deteriorated but it is at least still legible. We were also taught to sew and I had to make a sampler of different stitches; I still use some them when forced to mend something.

The worst problem at the Manor was the food. We had no choice in this and had to finish everything on our plates. I have always detested root vegetables, especially carrots. These were served every Wednesday, together with mince with small bits of carrot in it. When we had finished eating we had to show our empty plates to the teacher in charge. The first time this happened I managed to force down the mince with the carrot pieces. Feeling this was a good compromise I took my plate to the teacher with the larger carrots still on it. She was furious when she saw it was not empty and told me I was impudent. I was sent with others who had not cleared their plates to the 'Stone Room', a small room with bare stone walls, and told to stay there until my plate was clear or lessons restarted. I resigned myself to spending Wednesday lunchtimes staring at a plate of carrots. The stakes were raised when the Headmistress told me that if I could not eat carrots I 'might be happier at another School'. I knew a threat when I heard one and decided something had to be done, but I also knew that I could not eat the carrots. After a lot of thought I decided I could hide the carrots down the thick green socks that we wore as part of our uniform. This worked brilliantly and I was able to leave the dining room with socks filled with carrots and remove them later. The problem was solved and I stayed at the school. We had regular practices for the Eleven plus exam at this school, including IQ tests. We then had to stand in a line in the order of our IQ scores. It is hard to imagine anything like that happening now. Thanks to the coaching I won a scholarship to St Helen and St Katharine and moved there at the age of 11.

St Helen had originally been started by nuns and there were still several on the teaching staff. There were strict rules around clothing, particularly skirt length, which was checked at the start of each term. Of course, we used to roll up our waistbands to make the skirts shorter. The teaching was good and I worked hard at the science as I already knew I needed this for medicine. The school was also strong on sport, not one of my strengths. I suffered frequent humiliation due to a system of the team captains picking their players. I was always amongst the last selected or sometimes not selected at all and had to run in circles around the pitches while others played. At least I never got my nose broken or a tooth knocked out by a lacrosse ball, which happened to several of the players. The horrible games lessons were followed by cold showers in an unheated pavilion. In summer, the pool was filled with cold water on the first day of term and we swam weekly whatever the weather. Not surprisingly, I hate sport, although to be fair many of my class mates seemed to enjoy it and still do.

I did reasonably well at school although never won a prize. I was not a prefect and had no other leadership roles, there was nothing to mark me out from the crowd. My A-Level results were ABC, in those days enough for medical school. I still have the postcard with these grades; we received our results by post the day after they were received by the school. The Headmistress has written 'well done' by the results.

In my spare time I joined the cadet branch of the St John Ambulance Brigade (Figure 20.1). We were trained in first aid and used to spend weekends at motorcycle rallies, car-racing and horse-riding events hoping for injuries that we could practice treating. We even had an ambulance for ferrying patients to hospital. I also joined Casualties Union. We used to simulate being ill or injured for first aiders or the emergency services to practice. I took part in several major disaster simulations.

In this part of my life I did stand out. I lead a successful team in various first aid competitions and won cups and trophies. It was where I learnt the huge advantage of teams and saw what a difference leadership and good joint working could make. I earned my Grand Prior award and had my picture in the local paper as a result.

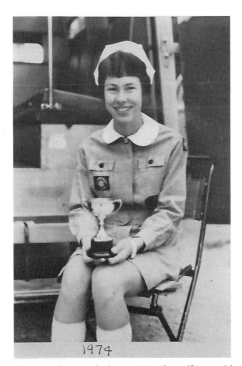

Figure 20.1 Wendy in her St Johns Ambulance Brigade uniform with a cup she had just won, 1974.

University 1976–82

I choose Southampton Medical School for my training. It was still a new medical school with a reputation for involving students with patients from the beginning, a system known as Early Medical Contact. The teaching took place in a rather bleak and modern building named Boldrewood. I was amazed to discover from a current Southampton medical student that it had to be demolished recently as it contained so much asbestos.

I loved medical school immediately but not for the right reasons. I shared my student accommodation with Arts students and joined the university theatre group. We put on productions in the university theatre; I acted as stage manager and remember the difficulty of making a seagull for the Chekhov play. There were parties every night and I developed an interest in punk rock and pogoed in the front row of many of the great bands; Siouxsie and the Banshees, Blondie, and the Ramones.

Sadly, medicine requires a huge amount of work and I failed the first year. I worked hard all summer but also failed the retakes and was told I would have to leave the medical school. This was one of the lowest points of my life and I had no idea what I was going to do. There was an appeals process which I entered into without much hope but to my huge relief and slight surprise, my appeal was successful and I was able to repeat the year and the exams. This time I was successful and progressed to the second year.

I had learnt my lesson and, apart from a spot of bother with orthopaedics, progressed smoothly through the rest of the course. I even managed to keep my interest in the theatre going. I was stage manager for the medical school Christmas revue and we took the show to the Edinburgh Fringe Festival where we got reasonably sized audiences and had a wonderful time.

My psychiatry placement was in Southampton with Dr Guy Edwards; I am still in touch with him. At the start of the attachment I had no thoughts of psychiatry as a career and spent the first week with my stethoscope round my neck so that people wouldn't think I was a psychiatrist. Guy Edwards was a strong advocate for the specialty and gave me more positive feedback than I had received in any other placement. He also gave me more responsibility. I was allowed to interview patients and present my findings in the ward meetings and even to write in the notes. I spent one day a week with the elderly in a different hospital. The psychiatrist there impressed me with his kindness to the patients. We were also given free cream cakes for some reason and I often wonder if that had more influence on my subconscious mind than I realized at the time.

House jobs 1982–83

After finishing medical school I had to do two six-month house jobs, one in medicine and one in surgery. My surgical placement came first: I spent three months at Lymington Hospital and three months in Southampton General. Lymington was a small cottage hospital which dealt with low risk surgery and had a small accident and emergency department where most of the injuries were from people falling off horses. This was a relatively easy posting and I learnt a surprising amount. The job in Southampton General was different. It was a really busy surgical unit and I was on a 'one-in-two' rota. This meant I worked from 9 a.m. one morning until 5 p.m. the next evening (32 hours), although we usually started before 9 a.m. and finished well after 5 p.m. I then had an evening and night off before starting again. Every other weekend I worked 9 a.m. on Friday morning to 5 p.m. on Monday with no guaranteed breaks. I worked in a team with a Senior House Officer (SHO), Senior Registrar, and Consultant, and we were kept going by team spirit and copious amounts of free beer on tap in the doctors' mess 24 hours a day. The massive advantage of this job was that no job that followed could ever be this bad. Even now when get I stressed at work I remind myself of what I survived in those three months.

My medical house job was with Professor (now Sir) Charles George in Southampton General Hospital. He was a clinical pharmacologist so I learnt a great amount about this area including the importance of understanding the mode of a drug's action and its half-life when prescribing. He wasn't a massive fan of psychiatry and I put off telling him of my career choice until the last possible minute when I was about to submit an application with his name as a referee. Unluckily that day, a psychiatry trainee reviewed a patient on our ward and prescribed an antidepressant. Professor George was very particular about how drug charts were written. They had to be done in capital letters and no mistakes were tolerated. The psychiatry trainee had prescribed amitriptyline but unfortunately had misspelt it. Coming across someone who could not spell what was then one of the most commonly used drugs in psychiatry did not improve Professor George's view of psychiatrists and when I told him what I wanted to do it he remarked that I was capable of better.

During my house year, two other important events occurred. At the end of my surgical job I had lived in hospital accommodation for six months and done nothing but work and sleep. As a result, I had saved enough to put down a deposit for a mortgage on a house. I bought a three-bedroomed Victorian semi for £22,700. I also met my husband William (Figure 20.2). It was not a *coup de foudre*; we barely noticed each other. He was a medical student doing a locum as a house officer and had to ask me

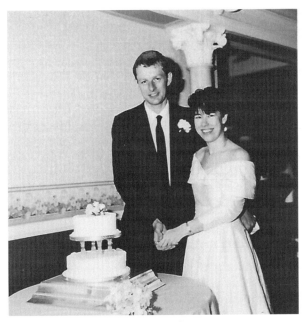

Figure 20.2 Wendy and William at their marriage in 1991.

or one of the other housemen to countersign his prescriptions. My main worry was that he would pester me for advice but he didn't and just got on with his work, much to my relief.

Psychiatric training in Southampton 1983–85

After my house jobs I thought I wanted to do psychiatry but I wasn't completely certain. In those days there was no pressure to rush straight into a training scheme. I contacted the local psychiatry tutor and was offered a locum SHO post. I started work at the Royal South Hampshire Hospital psychiatric department and loved it from the beginning. I moved on to Knowle Hospital, an old Victorian asylum that has now been converted to housing. While there I met William again; he was in the final year of his medical training and was placed with my team. This time we did notice each other and have been together ever since.

I decided psychiatry was the career for me and applied to join the Southampton training scheme. To my dismay, I was not given a post. In those days all jobs were competitive, including psychiatric ones, and I have never been good at interviews. However, of the two people who were appointed instead of me, one went into obstetrics and gynaecology and one left medicine completely, so it is reasonable for me to think that the interview committee made a mistake when they failed to give me a job.

At this point, Guy Edwards came to my rescue. He had received a research grant to look at how patients were assessed in medical wards following self-harm and whether the use of a structured questionnaire would improve things. I was appointed to carry out this research under his supervision. It went well and eventually led to a publication in the *British Journal of Psychiatry*.[1]

I would have happily stayed in Southampton and had never expected to live north of the Thames. William had different ideas and wanted to move to Aberdeen to give him more opportunities for the walking and climbing that he loves. We eventually compromised on Leeds, where he was successful in an interview for an anatomy demonstrator and I made an application for the psychiatry scheme.

As usual, I struggled in the interview. The heel of one of my shoes fell off and I completely forgot to mention that I'd heard that I had passed the first part of the Membership of the Royal College of Psychiatry (MRCPsych) examination that morning. There was a tricky moment when they asked why I wanted to train in Leeds. Now, a partner in the same region would be considered a good reason for choosing it and there might even be help available to ensure that we both got posts in the same deanery. In those days, following a boyfriend could be interpreted as a lack of commitment to a career. I therefore said that I was attracted to Leeds by the excellent reputation of the training scheme. To my huge relief I was offered a job.

Psychiatric training in Leeds 1985–90

My first post in Leeds was at High Royds Hospital, another Victorian asylum that has now been converted to private housing. It was a post working with the elderly and I loved it from the start; they have such interesting life stories and a degree of psychological robustness which I admire. There is also ample opportunity to keep medical skills going.

I went on to work in a day hospital, on a professorial unit, and in a general adult psychiatry post. One of my trainers was Professor Richard Mindham. He taught me psychiatry but I also learnt a fair amount about architecture from him. There was a second professor in Leeds, Andrew Sims, who wrote *Symptoms in the Mind: Textbook of Descriptive Psychopathology*. This has since been updated by Femi Oyebode.[2] If you only read one book on psychopathology, this is the one you should choose. I was also lucky enough to work for Dr Julian Roberts, one of the wisest people I have come across, who taught me a lot about how to influence people and systems.

I passed my MRCPsych examination and became a member of the College. I was considering an academic career and took up an old age academic post linked to Leeds University. My first placement was with Dr John Wattis; he was the Chairman of the Old Age Faculty of the Royal College of Psychiatrists and had to spend a lot of time in London. This allowed me free reign to manage the patients and I accumulated a large amount of clinical experience very quickly. I also learnt a huge amount from John who was one of the founders of old age psychiatry as a specialty. He wrote *Practical Psychiatry of Old Age*, a book I still use.[3]

After a year, I moved on to work for Dr Sasi Mahapatra in general adult psychiatry. This was an unpopular job with trainees as Sasi had at least twice as many patients as most consultants. He was considered unconventional by some of his colleagues but in many areas was ahead of his time. He dictated the letters to general practitioners (GPs) in front of patients and they always knew exactly what he considered their diagnosis to be. This was far from normal practice at the time and I was impressed by how well it worked.

I completed two years of what would now be considered 'higher training'; this had followed my year as a researcher and two years of what we would now call core training. At this point John Wattis obtained funding for a new old age consultant post. I was interested in this but thought I would not be eligible. Fortunately, John as Chairman of the Old Age Faculty had the power to deem me competent, which he duly did, and I was appointed.

Consultant career 1990–2017

My first consultant post had an interesting catchment area. It included the inner city with some of the poorest and most deprived people in Leeds, and the red-light district. The majority of assessments were done as home visits. This could be scary as I sometimes had to go after dark and there were no mobile phones in those days. The houses were often in an awful condition and I had to don a pair of Wellington boots for the worst visits. I also learnt to be very careful before sitting down and to check my notes for fleas after leaving the visit.

Soon after I started I was told by one of my colleagues that the youngest consultant should be the Royal College of Psychiatrists Tutor and I duly took up this post. I enjoyed my duties and made my first links with the College. The College ran an annual meeting for tutors; it was free and seemed to be designed to thank the Tutors who put a lot of work into their unpaid posts. Most were, like myself, relatively young, and the evening dinner was always a lively event. The meeting has evolved into the high-quality annual Medical Education Conference, complete with its own Twitter hashtag.

I was 31 when I became a consultant. Women consultants were still rare back then, and I was the first one at the hospital in Leeds. I was single when appointed but fairly soon I got married and became pregnant. I took a short amount of maternity leave and returned to work when my son was four-months old, in 1993. This was hard but he adapted well and we coped.

I had planned a fairly long gap before having another child but the person who ran the SHO training programme said that he would like me to take over when he finished and we established that to do this I would need to have my second baby fairly quickly and return from maternity leave. My daughter was born in December 1994. We already had a nanny in the house and I went back to work when she was three-months old.

I was rewarded with the Chair of the SHO training programme in 1995. I also became what was known as Clinical Tutor. This mirrored what is now Director of Postgraduate Medical Education and involved managing the study leave budget for Yorkshire. With the new roles came more responsibilities. One of the hardest tasks was allocating posts which we did every six months. Myself and the tutors would lock ourselves into a room with a cork board, labels with trainees' names, and coloured drawing pins and not emerge until we had finished. One terrible year when my daughter was about two I took the board home and left it in the hall. She found it and rearranged the labels and drawing pins by colour. Following this I learnt to write down the placements immediately.

I chaired the SHO training committee for five years. There were plenty of applicants for the training posts. Recruitment was all local to the Leeds training scheme. When we had a vacancy we placed an advert in the *British Medical Journal*, shortlisted those with the best applications, and offered the jobs to those who did the best interviews. This was an astonishingly simple but effective system.

I also began to be more involved with the College. I became an examiner for the old Part One clinical examination. This was fascinating as it involved travel all over the United Kingdom and we used real patients. When I first begun we would always stop for a proper cooked lunch and it wasn't unusual to be offered a glass of wine with the food. Following this, the examiners mellowed and I suspect that the examination was a little easier to pass in the afternoons.

Just as I finished chairing the training committee, a new post was created in Leeds; Associate Medical Director for Doctors in Training. I applied, was interviewed, and was appointed (I was the only applicant). I had managerial responsibility for all the trainees. The most important thing that I learnt was that if you are kind to the people you manage they will do their best for you. I also learnt how to spot depression in psychiatrists, who are generally not good at recognizing their own illnesses.

Around this time I joined my first College Committee as Regional Coordinator for Continuing Professional Development (CPD). The College was in Belgrave Square at that time and we met in the council room with a marble fireplace, ornate chandelier, and portraits of previous presidents on the wall. The meeting itself was interesting although I was too scared to speak. Regional CPD coordinators no longer exist but in the early days of CPD there was plenty for us to do including approving events for CPD.

I acquired another much more onerous role for the College, Senior Organizer for the clinical Part Two MRCPsych examinations. This consisted of hosting examinations in Leeds and finding patients for the candidates to interview. This was the most difficult and stressful event I have ever organized. The patients were naturally unwell and this could cause problems, but they were never as badly behaved as the examiners, who were completely unpredictable. I soon learnt to confine the examiners to one room with guards on the door or one would inevitably wander off and become lost.

I also took on a regional role as Programme Director of the Yorkshire Specialist Registrar Training Scheme in Old Age Psychiatry. I was responsible for recruitment, placements, and the annual Record of In-Training Assessment (RITA). This involved interviewing all the trainees annually and going through their training records and supervisor's reports.

In 2003, I took a big step up and became Chairman of the Yorkshire Psychiatry Speciality Training Committee. This meant I had oversight of all the psychiatric training in the part of Yorkshire covered by the then Yorkshire Deanery. There was more responsibility involved but at the time I took over things were relatively stable and initially it was not a time-consuming commitment.

All this changed when Modernising Medial Careers (MMC) was introduced in 2005. This was a radical overhaul of training which bought in centralized, computerized recruitment. The architects of MMC consulted widely but they totally ignored all the feedback they were given about the dangers and difficulties of the 'Big Bang' approach.

MMC turned into a disaster. In my view, the disengagement and unhappiness of the junior doctor workforce and the strikes of 2016 directly stemmed from this and we reaped the result of the problems sown at the time.

Somehow, the psychiatric training community managed to hold together and we rode out the storm. The one good thing to come out of MMC was the Schools of Psychiatry. The Yorkshire School was formed in 2007, I was appointed Head of School. In 2009, we combined with Sheffield to become the Yorkshire and the Humber School of Psychiatry with me as the Head.

I loved my time as Head of School. The post gave a real chance to influence training both nationally and locally but there was still plenty of opportunities for direct interaction with trainees and to help and support trainees who were struggling.

In 2011, the position of Dean at the Royal College of Psychiatrists became vacant. I decided to stand. There were five other excellent candidates and I did not expect to win. I can still vividly remember the phone call from Professor Dame Sue Bailey who was President at the time telling me that I had won the election and the feeling of disbelief that lasted for weeks.

Being Dean was fantastic. As College Officers posts are voluntary I continued in a full-time clinical post so there was lots of juggling of workload and time. Luckily, as a working mother I had learnt the skills needed and knew how to work efficiently and to time-shift.

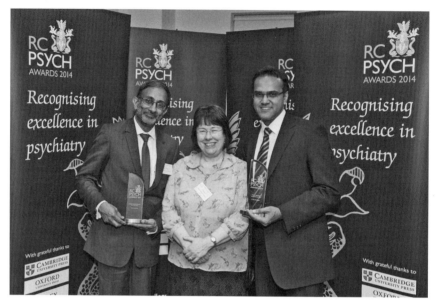

Figure 20.3 Wendy at the College award ceremony in 2014 with her friends, Manoj Kumar and Abu Abraham, who had won awards.

As Dean I had the chance to meet a huge number of psychiatrists from many different parts of the world (Figure 20.3). This reinforced my belief that the thing most psychiatrists have in common is their humanity and wish to help others. It never ceased to astonish me that if I wanted a piece of work done for the College we would advertise and then take our pick from more talented people than we could possibly use. Like me, they were all volunteers; the College runs entirely on the good will of its members.

Being Dean also gave me a chance to make a real difference at a national level. Changing things takes time, the smallest change being the result of huge amounts of work and negotiation, but it was possible. The MRCPsych examination stopped making a financial bonus and the number of papers was reduced from three to two. It became possible to get a liaison psychiatry endorsement if you were an old age trainee. It remained possible to be awarded a CCT even if you had needed some extra time to pass the MRCPsych. Work started on the introduction of awarding credentials. The College moved from a charming but unsuitable building that was rented to a much better one that we now own.

The five-year term of office flew past and all too soon I had handed over the role of Dean to the highly capable Kate Lovett. Half of all the previous Deans had gone on to become President of the College and I was frequently asked if this was my ambition. My answer was always no, but gradually things changed. I missed my involvement with the College and national decision-making. After much thought I decided to stand for election, encouraged by a woman past President who, when I consulted her, said 'If you don't stand you won't be elected'. I therefore collected the requisite signatures and threw my hat into the ring. The rest, as they say, is history.

Summary

What then have I learnt from reflecting on my career? What advice can I give to aspiring young psychiatrists? The title of this chapter is misleading when I consider it more carefully: I never planned a path to the top but I did always try my best. I worked as hard as I could, tried to be nice to people and to treat them as I would wish to be treated, and I never turned down an opportunity. I would advise anyone to do the same, even if this does not lead you to the top you will be left with great personal satisfaction and the world will be a better place for your presence.

References

1. **Burn WK**, **Edwards JG**, and **Machin D** (1990). Improving house physicians' assessments of self-poisoning. *British Journal of Psychiatry* July, 157;(1):95–100. DOI: 10.1192/bjp.157.1.95.
2. **Oyebode F** (ed.) (2014). *Sims' Symptoms in the Mind: Textbook of Descriptive Psychopathology*, 5th edn. Philadelphia, PA, Saunders..
3. **Wattis J** and **Curran S** (2013). *Practical Psychiatry of Old Age*, 5th edn. Boca Raton, FL: CRC Press.

Chapter 21

The Road Less Travelled

Sue Bailey

Why psychiatry?

Fifty years on it has all fallen into place. Why would anyone want to look after the body when one can experience the unique privilege of supporting those with troubled minds?

I come from a long line of far more intelligent and articulate women than myself, women who through social class and circumstances literally were never afforded the opportunity to go to university. They gained scholarships to attend local grammar schools but by then had 'carer' responsibilities and a family which could not afford uniforms or travel costs. One could ask why a scholarship grammar school girl, given that opportunity, choose medicine, when the delights of English history and politics awaited? Simple; the serendipity of life.

Having a neighbour who was the 'medical superintendent' of the local 'asylum' and being allowed as a sixth former to watch and learn as he 'mended' broken minds, I learned to respect the fact that every mind is unique. So, discovering that in order to practice psychiatry you had to train as a doctor, I applied to medical school.

Why child and adolescent forensic psychiatry?

I was in the first wave of problem-based learning medical students at Manchester University and fortunate to study medicine at a time when psychiatry was flourishing as a specialty under the leadership of Professor David Goldberg who, with colleagues, was pioneering community mental health across the city. Forensic psychiatry had just arrived in the north-west with two medium-secure units in Manchester and Liverpool, led by inspirational innovating forensic psychiatrists.

As a higher trainee in forensic psychiatry, I found myself sitting in sombre reflection in the confines of Her Majesty's Prison Manchester (Strangeways). Every man I had seen in clinic that afternoon had been subjected to all forms of unimaginable child adversity and abuse. I thought that perhaps if we could intervene earlier, outcome could be better, and so I undertook dual training in child and adolescent and forensic psychiatry.

What is forensic psychiatry?

Forensic psychiatry can be regarded as the study and management of behaviours which stop the individual from reaching his or her full potential while posing risks of harm to others. Such behaviours usually begin early, and we probably have a better chance of changing them in their early stages than we do when they are well established in adult life.

Future generations of professionals may give more emphasis to behaviour problems and less to the strange so-called diagnostic system to which we seem currently wedded.[1] If you enjoy critical careful analysis of complex sets of information, risk assessment, and management, forensic psychiatry is for you. It certainly gives you the opportunity to defend your opinion and views in the arena of Crown courts.

Why child psychiatry?

Why? Because working for child mental health matters.

Throughout my clinical life I have always worked in close partnership with patients and the voluntary sector because together our voice is stronger.

As current Chair of the Children and Young Peoples Mental Health Coalition,[2] there are some good reasons to become a children's mental health doctor.

Across the whole of psychiatry, we have good evidence-based treatments set in a bio-psycho-social understanding of diseases. Making a diagnosis is important but understanding how an illness affects a person's daily life is just as vital. Nowhere is this truer than for child mental health. It is hard for any government or society to focus on prevention when in reality we are living with a health system that remains reactive rather than proactive. Advocating good child mental health gives you the opportunity to be at the vanguard of change. Here are some hard facts:[3]

– 1 in 10, or about 850,000 5- to 16-year olds have a mental disorder, but only about 25 per cent receive any help (would this be accepted in childhood cancers?)

– Of these children, 3.7 per cent will have an emotional disorder such as anxiety or depression, 5.8 per cent will have conduct disorder, and 1.5 percent will have Attention Deficit Hyperactivity Disorder (ADHD). Child mental health has been so neglected that we have to rely on prevalence data going back to 2004. This is a prime example of lack of expenditure parity for mental health. Thankfully new prevalence data will be available in 2018 but before these findings become available, we know there is evidence that mental health problems are increasing in teenage girls.

– 28 per cent of pre-school children face problems that impact on their psychological development.[3]

– 32 per cent of girls aged 15, and 11 per cent of boys. Self-harm and approximately half of children with early onset conduct disorder have serious problems that continue into later life. These are the majority of the children I have seen assessed and treated through my clinical career.

Why prevention? Because 75 per cent of adult mental health problems begin before the age of 18, and 50 per cent by the age of 14. Why would you not want to be a child psychiatrist when we know young people with mental health problems are far more likely to drop out of full-time education by the age of 15, not be in education, employment, or training, have lower earnings, be in contact with the criminal justice, and have higher rates of relationship problems.

As a child mental health specialist you have a unique opportunity to alleviate suffering in the individual and to reduce the disease burden on society as a whole.

The practice of child and adolescent forensic psychiatry

Thirty years of experience in developing and working in adolescent forensic services gave me a rich clinical career, working in fantastic teams and across multi-agency systems, both nationally and internationally.

Opening the first medium-secure mental health unit for adolescents with mental illness who had harmed others whilst experiencing hallucinations and holding delusional beliefs was a team effort. The same was true in developing forensic community services for high-risk adolescents, working with local child psychiatry teams, juvenile prisons, residential special education units, juvenile justice services, social services, and the Magistrates and Crown Court Services. Locking up children presents the team with both treatment and ethical dilemmas. The 'forensic physician's dilemma' is playing one's part in keeping society safe while taking a human rights approach to young patients, remembering the imperative to protect, provide, and help young people to act as full participants in their own treatment and recovery whilst living behind high fences and in a 'home' with locked internal doors.

The great joy of this work is that of being part of a team: nurses, social workers, art, music, speech and language therapists, psychologists, psychiatrists, and a fully fledged school on site. Together, our jobs involved:

– the acute delivery of evidence-based interventions to treat psychosis, to discover a young person with underlying learning disability and/or features of autism or post-traumatic stress disorder (PTSD)

– helping children to come to terms with what they have done: perhaps a murder, a sexual offence, or destruction through arson

– helping support their families, often troubled, now themselves the victims of 'hatred' in local communities because of what their children have done

– helping young people deal with the 'fear and loathing' that comes with insight into the reality of their bloody acts

– saying sorry to victims or their families, getting a risk assessment right, meeting a child's multiple needs in mental health, physical health, education, relationships, helping them make a safe and fulfilling return to the community

– in high-profile cases, returning to the community on life-long parole with changed identities, helping the team to come to terms with a small number of cases where the illness is intractable, the risk to others high, and the move to adult high-secure mental health care when they reach age 18

I was persuaded by the late Professor Richard (Dick) Harrington that I could become a researcher, and I still continue to work with a team of researchers, all originally supported and nurtured by him.

What sort of research?

Over the years, the team has developed screening and assessment tools used by all sectors involved with young offenders, most recently the Comprehensive Health Assessment Tool (CHAT),[4,5] which covers screening and assessment of the mental and physical health, substance misuse, neurodevelopmental disorders such as autism, and acquired brain injury in young offenders. This is a tool used across secure and community settings for all young people in the youth justice system. I was Vice Chair of a national research and development programme in forensic psychiatry where, as well as screening and assessment tools, we developed and delivered research projects on cognitive behavioural therapy (CBT) interventions for young offenders and also seed-funded some of the early neuroscience studies on emerging personally disorder and juvenile psychopathy. Being involved in these initiatives prompts reflections on societal attitudes towards children, and young offenders in particular.

These include understanding human beings from a developmental perspective while being able to analyse the paths to antisocial behaviour, the links with mental illness, and learning how the unmet needs of troubled and troublesome youth, existing in troubled families and communities, could be met with better outcomes for them and reduced risk to others.

Every mental health worker knows that the 'child is the father of the man' and that adult behaviour has its roots in the developmental mix of genetics, intrauterine climate, and parenting and other environmental factors throughout childhood. There is a long and painful history regarding children as the architects of their own failings and thus neglecting to care for them appropriately.[6]

Few dilemmas have challenged the ideas of society about the nature of human development and the nature of justice more than that of children and young people in the juvenile justice system, especially those who have mental health problems, neurodevelopmental disorders, and learning disabilities. In the eighteenth and nineteenth centuries, children were seldom distinguished from adults and were placed with adults in prison. In the England of 1824, boys as young as nine years of age were held in solitary confinement for their own protection in ships retired from the Battle of Trafalgar. In the nineteenth century, legislation regarding children's rights was tied to the need for labour.

There have been periodic reactions against convicting, imprisoning, and punishing young people. The pioneers who sought to rescue both young offenders and those children offended against provided the beginnings of youth justice, care, and child protection. Both community and secure residential innovations in youth justice have been characterized by patterns of reforming zeal followed by the gradual embedding of the scientific evidence base from the dual fields of juvenile justice and the assessment and treatment of mental health problems in children and young people.

The overhaul of the youth justice system in England and Wales in 1998 with the introduction of multi-agency youth justice teams proved a turning point for progress in youth justice, paralleled across the United Kingdom, many parts of Europe, Australia, and New Zealand. Ten years earlier the development of Forensic Child and Adolescent Mental Health Services (FCAMHS) started to emerge alongside specialist secure in-patient services. A now vibrant European Association for Forensic Child and Adolescent Psychiatry Psychology and other involved professions (EFCAP) exists.[1]

Why work with and for the Royal College of Psychiatrists?

Early in my career I was an active member of the then College Psychiatric Trainees Committee. Inevitably, as an early years consultant, one becomes preoccupied with 'business back at base'. I reconnected with the College when I needed help and support dealing with the noise, distress, and response to the killing of the toddler James Bulger, and more particularly to the response to the children who killed him.

Mike Shooter, the President of the College was, with the public education team, very supportive of me and that is how, as a member, I become drawn into public education, became Chair of the Child and Adolescent Faculty, Registrar and eventually was elected President.

In parallel, working in a 'rare' field of medicine drew me into diverse committees across government departments and the world of civil servants and policy makers.

What struck me was that one family is very much like another; it is vital to listen, learn, and try and be helpful, however high-risk and difficult the circumstances. This is the art of intelligent kindness. This approach, grounded in the skills of child and adolescent and forensic practice, enabled me to seize the opportunity in the adverse circumstances of the introduction of a toxic Health and Social Care Bill (opposed by many across the profession), to fight for parity of esteem between mental and physical health, now enshrined in the Health and Social Act 2012.[7,8]

We can and all have to be leaders

As Elected Chair of the Academy of Medical Royal Colleges I found it somewhat strange when people started asking me 'what's it like being a leader in medicine?' I never did or do regard myself as a leader. The question caused me to reflect.

Psychiatrists led the way across medicine in sustainability, the benefits of exercise for improved mental and physical health outcomes, and in choosing wisely and shared decision-making across health.

Sustainability in medicine is about far more than carbon footprint. At its heart it is about patient empowerment and disease prevention, about being safe and calm in a stressed environment, and how, again, the practice of training that comes from psychiatry can be helpful.

What are the key ingredients in healthcare systems that work well both for good patient outcomes but also healthy workforce? For me this is about values-based, sustainable services,[9] where the workforce work in partnership with patients to make wise decisions (Choosing Wisely, Shared Decision-Making).[10] It is about individuals having emotional intelligence and relating to and with all parts of the system; above all, relating to fellow human beings with intelligent kindness.[11]

Good health is central to the lives of children, adults, and families wherever they live. Good health is also crucial for the realization of flourishing communities and the economic health of any nation.[12]

Successful health care organizations have the ability to collapse hierarchies, flatten organizational structures, to encourage clinicians to fulfil leadership roles, and to be valued and to value others. Good health organizations are collegiate rather than hierarchical. In collegiate systems everyone leads and everyone is a follower. Just watch a skein of geese as they fly across a sunset skyline. They alternate as leaders. If one goose is in distress and goes to the ground, two geese go with her for support and to ensure no single goose is ever left alone.

Clinical leaders need to have the ability and personal attributes that enable them to steer the activities of a group towards a shared goal while coping with change. This is no easy task. It requires the alignment of an organization with its values vision and objectives, and leaders to work with teams to create visions; management is about implementing these.

Emotional intelligence is a basic prerequisite, whether leading health teams or helping a violent troubled young person to gain safe autonomy. Important also are self-awareness (knowing how we feel), self-regulation (control of our emotions), empathy (knowing how others feel), and good social skills (for leaders to influence and inspire others, for troubled youth to be able to function in what they perceive as a hostile world that envelops them and seeks to destroy them). In reality, these are core skills any psychiatrist possesses and exercises in clinical practice every day.

What is the socio-political context for psychiatrists?

Austerity. Brexit. Lack of resources. It is time to stop bemoaning the problems with today's National Health Service (NHS) and act to solve them. Of course resources matter, so how can we help social care receive more resources which will, in turn, support our patient to live a good, healthy life? It is time to act and psychiatrists have a key role to play. The combination of facts and figures with emotional and intelligent kindness sits at the heart of the fundamental right to health for all, free at the point of access, the touchstone of our NHS. Health for all is indivisible from politics.

How can the organized efforts of society deliver public health for the whole population? What we lack in the current approach to healthcare delivery comes down to political will and strategic choice. The current postcode lottery when it comes to public health is simply not a good enough approach.[13]

Would moving to a system of place-based health work? This is our aspiration in 'DevoManc' where I enjoy the challenge of being a non-executive director of an acute Trust, where I see how more psychologically minded professionals could deal with pressures and retain a safe and positive sense of self.

How do we make the shift from treatment towards prevention? At present, we ask the wrong question of the public; we ask what health services do you want? What if we asked the individual 'what would help you enjoy life? The answer would reflect their lived experience at home, community, and at work, and also their hopes for their future.

This approach, which is truly values-based, would help build stronger, safer bridges for health and people. The shift is from institutions to people and places, from service silos to system outcomes, enabling a change of focus from the national to the local.[14]

Psychiatry took the lead in this over 40 years ago in setting up community mental health services, the recovery movement, person-centred care, and peer support, and sits at the heart of the Centre for Mental Health[15] of which I am privileged to be Vice Chair.

Encountering bumpy roads while moving forwards: Repair and healing.

As Chair of the Academy of Medical Royal Colleges, my life in 2015–16 was taken over by the junior doctors dispute. Why did this happen?

My personal view is that as we became preoccupied with the latest crisis or innovation in health we failed to recognize the rapidly changing world in which junior doctors learnt at work. We forgot the huge importance of generational differences and we forgot a basic tenet of the human condition:[20] we are social animals. Junior doctors were working in situations of increasing adversity, increasingly without any sense of meaning, purpose, or control, just like the men who sat in Manchester Prison 40 years ago. The inevitable drift was towards a toxic social identity, loss of well-being, anger, frustration, despair, helplessness. We forgot the basic importance of how we exist within and across social groups, and across and within communities of professional practice. I am now working to understand and meet the needs and aspirations of medical students, foundation doctors, and specialist trainees. I do not deceive myself that this will be a challenge and that healing takes time. Delivering flexibility in training, opportunities to learn and work abroad as part of training, as part of a global health community, need not mean an exit from UK medicine.

Psychiatry faces lots of challenges here in the United Kingdom but it also holds many of the answers to a future sustainable health and social care system in this country. Whatever our system of healthcare, there will always be jobs for psychiatrists.

Marching forward together

Psychiatry has come of age; all medical students would be better doctors in their chosen specialties if they had been given a real chance to learn about the best part of medical practice: supporting mental health of individuals in their real-life worlds.

2018 sees the centenary of the women's rights movement. Living as I do in Manchester, this has special meaning to me. My daughters were educated at the same school as the Pankhursts. Throughout my clinical life I have seen the growing influence of women in medicine and in particular in psychiatry as we celebrate the election of our fourth woman president.

Neither of my daughters chose medicine but instead work in social enterprises as artists, empowering vulnerable children, men, and women to have good mental health and well-being. The message from them is join the family of psychiatry because they see and experience every day the inequalities across society that impact on the mental health of those with whom they work. Whether this is children in gangs, children out of school, victims of child sexual exploitation, those with undiagnosed and untreated mental disorders, elders living well with and in spite of their dementia, veterans left with unresolved impact of trauma languishing on the streets and in prison, young men

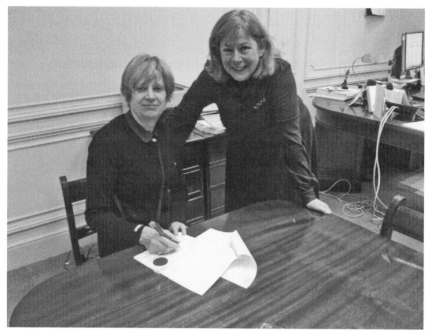

Figure 21.1 Dame Sue Bailey, President, and Vanessa Cameron, Chief Executive of the Royal College of Psychiatrists taking keys to new premises for the College at 21 Prescott Street, London, in 2013.
© Royal College of Psychiatrists

with autism misunderstood, troubled, and in trouble, there are roles for psychiatrists and other mental health professionals.

Our message, as a family, is march, women, march[16] into psychiatry; join the best family in medicine. Come and join the road less travelled (see Figure 21.1).

References

1. **Gunn J** (2017). Foreword. In: Bailey S, Chitsabesan P, and Tarbuck P (eds). *Meeting the Mental Health Needs of Young Offenders*. Cambridge: Cambridge University Press pp. xiii–xiv.
2. <http://www.cypmhc.org.uk>.
3. <https://www.centreformentalhealth.org.uk/missed-opportunities>.
4. **Chitsabesan P, Lennox C, Theodosiou L, Law H,** and **Bailey S** (2017). Assessment of young offenders' mental health, physical, educational and ??? needs. In: Bailey S, Chitsabesan P, Tarbuck P (eds). *Meeting the Mental Health Needs of Young Offenders*. Cambridge: Cambridge University Press, pp. 41–54.
5. **Shaw J** (2014). The development of the comprehensive health assessment tool for young offenders within the secure estate. *Journal of Forensic Psychiatry and Psychology* **25**(I):1–25.

6. **Maughan B** (2017). Origins of offending in young people. In: Bailey S, Chitsabesan P, and Tarbuck P (eds). *Meeting the Mental Health Needs of Young Offenders.* Cambridge: Cambridge University Press., pp. 11–237 <http://www.legislation.gov.uk/ukpga/2012/7/contents/enacted>.

8. **Bailey S** (2013). Whole-person care: From rhetoric to reality; achieving parity between mental and physical health. <http://www.rcpsych.ac.uk/usefulresources/publications/collegereports/op/op88.aspx>.

9. **Kemp V** and **Williams R** (2017). Psychosocial resilience, psychosocial care and forensic mental health. In: Bailey S, Chitsabesan P, and Tarbuck P (eds). *Meeting the Mental Health Needs of Young Offenders.* Cambridge: Cambridge University Press, pp. 24–38.

10. <http://www.choosingwisely.co.uk>.

11. **Ballatt J** and **Campling P** (2011). *Intelligent Kindness: Reforming the Culture of Healthcare.* London: Royal College of Psychiatry.

12. **Crisp N, Stuckler D, Horton R, Adebowale V, Bailey S, Baker M, Bell J, Bird J, Black C, Campbell J, Davies J, Henry H, Lechler R, Mawson A, Maxwell PH, McKee M,** and **Warwick C** (2016). Manifesto for a healthy and health-creating society. *Lancet* **388**: e24–27.

13. **Bambra C** (2016). Health Divides: Where You Live Can Kill You. Past, present, future p207. Bristol: Policy Press.

14. **Get well soon—re imagining place-based health** (2016) New Local Government Network Collaborate—thinking—culture—practice.

15. <https://www.centreformentalhealth.org.uk/making-recovery-a-reality>.

16. **Hawksley L** (2013). March Women March Andre Deutsch.

The Other Women in the Wardrobe

The thinner one.
The one who wears the trousers.

The one in beige and caramel, soft-centred,
seamless, goes with everything.

The one too good to wear.

The plain one, just about hanging together
thanks to the lost skill of invisible mending,
and her mother's needling –
it'll do and *fancy is as fancy does.*

The girl on the top shelf
with nothing underneath.

The non-iron, windproof, all-in-one reversible
that zips and folds obligingly to fit the smallest space.

The cast-off, in someone else's favourite shade.
The bargain one that's near enough her size.

The sister contrived from 25 lemonade bottles
who biodegrades to a good mulch.

The gadget-mum with non-slip shoulders,
hooks and clips for everything
they didn't know they'd need.

The mutton dressed as wolf.
The jackal in cashmere.
The kid in a tracksuit.

The woman who's left already, on the early train,
in a suit like his,
man-made, with synthetic trim.

Emily Wills
(Reproduced from *Unmapped*, published by The Rialto, 2014)

Index

Notes: Tables, figures and boxes are indicated by an italic *t, f* and *b* following the page number *vs.* indicates a comparison.

Abraham, Abu, 286*f*
academic careers, intellectual disability, 116
ACCORD-MIND trial, dementia risk, 239
admission, depression management, 82
Adverse Childhood Experiences Study, 164
AEGIS (Aid for the Elderly in Government Institutions), 209, 214
affective (mood) disorders, 77*b*
Age Discrimination Act (2010), 68
ageism, 65*t*
AGENDA (Alliance for Women and Girls at Risk), 57, 69
Aid for the Elderly in Government Institutions (AEGIS), 209, 214
ALA (alpha linoleic acid), 237–8
alcohol consumption, 140
  dementia risk, 240
Alder Hey Children's Hospital, 202
Alliance for Women and Girls at Risk (AGENDA), 57, 69
Allitt, Beverley, 135, 144
alpha linoleic acid (ALA), 237–8
Altschul, Annie, 231*f*
  career, 231–2
  life of, 230
  principles of, 231
  see also Hockey, Lisbeth
Alzheimer's disease (AD), 198–9, 233
Alzheimer's Disease International (ADI), 195–9
Alzheimer's Society, 189, 195–9
ambivalence, mothers in child sexual abuse, 168
anorexia, right to life *vs.* self-determination, 246–9
antidepressants, 83*b*, 83*t*
antioxidants, 237
antisocial personality disorder (ASPD), 69
APOE gene, 235
Appleby, Helen, 209
Arie, Tom, 190
Armstrong-Jones, Robert, 47, 50
Ashworth Hospital, single-sex wards, 129
ASPD (antisocial personality disorder), 69
The Assault on Truth (Masson), 162–3
Association for Contentious Trust and Probate Specialists, Graham, Nori, 190
Association of Medical Superintendents of Lunatic Asylums, 39
asylums, 125, 219–21
  closure of, 15
Athena Swan awards, 178
Athena Swan Charter (2005), 11, 61, 116, 268–9
attachment styles, old age, 184

Bailey, Sue, 289–97, 296*f*
  child and adolescent forensic psychiatry, 289
  research, 292
Balint, Enid, 8
Balint groups, 8, 258
Balint, Michael, 8
Barrie, J M, 166
Barry, James (Margaret Ann Buckley), 25
Barton, Russell, 209
Battle Hymn of the Tiger Mother, 94
BDNF (brain-derived neurotropic factor), 241
Beach, Fletcher, 45
Beard, Mary, 136–7
de Beauvoir, Simone, 178
behaviour, motherhood, 159–60
Berloff, Max, 212
Betrayal Trauma: The Logic of Forgetting Childhood Sexual Abuse (Freyd), 165
Bicknell, Joan, 113, 114*f*
Bion, Wilfred, 155
black and minority ethnic (BME) third sector, 226
Black, Carol, 34, 63–64
Black, Dora, 104–7, 104*f*, 106*f*
  career, 105–6
  life, 105
  posts held, 104–5
Black, John, 64
Blackwell, Elizabeth, 25
Bland, Anthony, 245–6
Bland case, 245–6
BMA *see* British Medical Association (BMA)
BME (black and minority ethnic) third sector, 226
body image, ageing effects, 181–2
Books Beyond Words (Hollins), 115, 115*f*
borderline personality disorder (BPD)
  gender bias in secondary services, 69
  historical child sexual abuse, 169
Bowlby, John, 93
Boyle, Ann, 269–75
Boyle, Helen, 47, 50–51, 50*f*
BPD *see* borderline personality disorder (BPD)
Brading, Alison, 4–5
brain-derived neurotropic factor (BDNF), 241
brick mother, 158–9
British Medical Association (BMA)
  advisory service for women (1980s), 34
  Caldicott, Fiona, 53
  Garret Anderson membership, 26
  women, admission of, 45
British Medical Journal (BMJ), Friern Hospital correspondence, 10
British Psychological Society, 57
Brockington, Ian, 99

Brodaty, Henry, 197
Buckley, Margaret Ann (James Barry), 25
bullying, 65*t*
Burn, Wendy, 277–87, 279*f*, 281*f*, 286*f*
    childhood, 277–9
    consultant as, 283–7
    house jobs, 280–2
    psychiatric training, 282–3
    university, 280

Caldicott, Fiona, 52–55, 52*f*, 53*f*, 54*f*, 55*f*, 59, 269
    career, 53–54
    roles of, 52
Caldicott Principles, 54, 54*b*
The Caldicott Report, 53–54
Cameron, Vanessa, 296*f*
CAMHS (Child and Adolescent Mental Health), 58
capacity
    right to life *vs.* self-determination, 247–8
    treatment refusal, 249–50
career breaks, 58
Care Programme Approach (CPA), 85, 225
Care Quality Commission (CQC), single-sex
    wards, 125
carers, 66
Care Services Improvement Partnership (CSIP),
    women carers, 66
'caring for babies,' dementia care, 16–17
CASC (Clinical Assessment of Skills and
    Competencies), 268–9
case studies
    caring for patient with intellectual
        disability, 117–18
    countertransference reactions, 156–9
    early trauma and containing mind, 153–5
    historical child sexual abuse, 170–1
    long-term care, 222
    motherhood, 158–9
    old age, 181, 185
    prison, 141–2
    Women's Mental Health Units, 127*b*
Castle, Barbara, 33, 202
CCT (Certificate of Completed Training), 273
CEMD (Confidential Enquires into Maternal
    Deaths), 98
Certificate in Psychological Medicine,
    Medico-Psychological Association, 44
Certificate of Completed Training (CCT), 273
Chalmers Watson, Alexandra, 30
CHAT (Comprehensive Health Assessment
    Tool), 292
Chekov, Anton, 223
Chicago Health and Aging study, dementia and
    antioxidants, 237
Child and Adolescent Mental Health (CAMHS), 58
childhood abuse
    mental illness and, 17
    see also historical child sexual abuse (HCSA)
children
    psychiatry, 290–1
    rejection, 155–6
children and adolescent forensic psychiatry, 289, 291
children, murder of, 143–4
Children's Commissioner Report on Childhood
    Sexual Abuse (2015), 165

Clayton, Harry, 196
Climbié, Victoria, 138
Clinical Assessment of Skills and Competencies
    (CASC), 268–9
clinical leadership roles, intellectual disability, 113
clinical trials, epidemiological studies *vs.*, 235
Clouston, Thomas S, 43–44
Clunis Report (1994), 226
Clytemnestra, 135–7
CMHTs (community mental health teams), 225
cognition, 233
    assumed decline in old age, 179
    training in dementia, 241
cognitive behavioural therapy (CBT), 82, 84*b*
cognitive reserve, 235
College Continuing Professional Development
    (CPD), 60
Collins Report (2012), 12
communication, maternal mental illness, 97–98
community care, 224–6
    deaths in, 15
community mental health teams (CMHTs), 225
Community Psychiatric Nurses (CPNs), 222
compassion fatigue, 259
compassion-focused therapy, 84*b*
Comprehensive Health Assessment Tool
    (CHAT), 292
Confidential Enquires into Maternal Deaths
    (CEMD), 98
Confidential Inquiry into Premature Death of
    People with Learning Disabilities, 111–12
Conolly, John, 39
consent, guidance from GMC, 18
*Considering the Predictive Value of the Risk
    Assessment Score* (Wills), 148
constructive dismissal, 65*t*
containing mind, 153–5
Continuing Professional Development
    (CPD), 284–5
CoP *see* Court of Protection (CoP)
coping, depression, 79–80, 81*b*
co-production, 86*b*
cosmetic surgery, old age, 183
countertransference reactions, 156
    case study, 156–9
Court of Protection (CoP), 245–52
    clinician–patient disputes, 249–52
    right to life *vs.* self-determination, 245–9
coworkers, psychiatry barriers, 254–5
CPA (Care Programme Approach), 85, 225
CPD (Continuing Professional
    Development), 284–5
CPNs (Community Psychiatric Nurses), 222
CQC (Care Quality Commission), single-sex
    wards, 125
Cremona, Anne, 58
Crews, Frederick, 165
criminology, gender bias, 138
Crossman, Richard, 205, 212
crystallized intelligence, 241
CSIP (Care Services Improvement Partnership),
    women carers, 66
culture
    old age, 183
    women's roles, 178

Cyriax, George, 196
Czech Republic, gender pay gap, 13

Dave, Rupal, 109–10
Davey, Francis Sophia, 91
Davies Committee, 213
Davies, Messler, 171
Davies, Sally, 34
Davies, Teifion, 266–7
DBMA Counselling and Doctor Advisor
    Service, 80*t*
death
    anticipation of, 180–1
    contemporaries of, 179–80
    spouse of, 184
defamation, 65*t*
dementia
    'caring for babies,' 16–17
    cognitive training, 241
    crystallized intelligence, 241
    definition, 233–4
    diagnosis, 18
    epidemiological studies vs, clinical trials, 235
    genetics of, 234–5
    multimodal prevention strategies, 242
    old age, assumption in, 179
    prevalence, 233
    risk factors, 236, 236*t*
    risk reduction, 233–44
    types of, 233
dementia with Lewy bodies (DLB), 233, 234
Department of Health (DoH)
    Improving Working Lives initiative, 60, 62
    women carers, 66
Department of Health and Social Security (DHSS),
    Alzheimer's Society, support for, 196
depression, 75–76
    coping, 79–80, 81*b*
    dementia risk, 236*t*, 240
    management, 81–84
Deprivation of Liberty Safeguarding (DOLS), 87
DevoManc, 294
Dewar, Margaret Cochran, 47
DGHs (district general hospitals), 3
DHA (docosahexanoic acid), 237–8
DHSS (Department of Health and Social Security),
    Alzheimer's Society, support for, 196
diabetes, dementia risk, 236*t*, 239
Diagnostic and Statistical Manual 5 (DSM-5)
    historical child sexual abuse, 164
    intellectual disability, 111
diet, dementia risk reduction, 237–9
The Disappeared (Wills), 229
disclosure, historical child sexual abuse, 167–8
discrimination in practice, Women's Mental Health
    Special Interest Group, 64–65, 65*t*
dismissal, constructive, 65*t*
district general hospitals (DGHs), 3
DLB (dementia with Lewy bodies), 233, 234
DNAR (do-not-attempt-resuscitation) orders,
    18, 245–52
DocHealth, 80*t*
docosahexanoic acid (DHA), 237–8
doctors
    mental health of, 78–79*b*

opportunities for, 194
perceived glut of, 31
special treatment of, 79, 80*t*
Doctors Support Network (DSN), 80*t*, 87–88
DoH *see* Department of Health (DoH)
DOLS (Deprivation of Liberty
    Safeguarding), 87
domestic violence, 10–11
    mental illness and, 17–18
Donaldson, Liam, 63
do-not-attempt-resuscitation (DNAR) orders,
    18, 245–52
Dovem, Emily Louise, 47
Drayton Park Crisis House, 226
DRCOG (Diploma of the Royal College of
    Obstetricians and Gynaecologists), 9
drug abuse, 140
    old age, 182
drug reps, 8
drugs *see* pharmaceuticals/medications
DSM-5 *see Diagnostic and Statistical Manual 5*
    (DSM-5)
DSN (Doctors Support Network), 80*t*, 87–88
Duties of a Doctor (GMC), 15, 16*b*

Eason, Sue, 274
ECT *see* electroconvulsive therapy (ECT)
Edinburgh Postnatal Depression Scale
    (EPDS), 96–97
Edwards, Guy, 280, 282
EFCAP (European Association for Forensic Child
    and Adolescent Psychiatry Pathology), 291
Effectiveness of Services for Mothers with Mental
    Illness (ESMI), 97–98
eicosopentaenoic acid (EPA), 237–8
elderly *see* old age
Electra, 136
electroconvulsive therapy (ECT), 75–76, 75*b*
    training in, 221
Elgar, Sybil, 122, 123
Eliot, T S, 180
Elliot, Patricia, 32
Ely Hospital (Cardiff), malpractice in, 213
emotional abuse, 168
emotional impact of psychiatry, 259
emotional intelligence, 293–4
empathic ability in psychiatry, 255–6
Emson, Daksha, 65, 98–99
Enoch, David, 209
EPDS (Edinburgh Postnatal Depression
    Scale), 96–97
epidemiology
    mental health, 140
    studies *vs.* clinical trials in dementia, 235
Equality Act (2010), 13
Equality Challenge Unit's Athena Swan charter *see*
    Athena Swan Charter (2005)
equality work, Women's Mental Health Special
    Interest Group, 62
equal pay, 34–35
    see also gender pay gap
Equal Pay Act (1970), 3, 13
Erikson, Erik, 95
ESMI (Effectiveness of Services for Mothers with
    Mental Illness), 97–98

Estonia, gender pay gap, 13
Etychegoyer, Alice, 60
European Association for Forensic Child
    and Adolescent Psychiatry Pathology
    (EFCAP), 291
European Working Time Directive, 253, 270
evil, illness *vs.*, 135–6
exercise lack, dementia risk, 236*t*, 240–1
expressive therapies, 84*b*

Facebook, motherhood, perception of, 95
False Memory Syndrome Foundation
    (FMSF), 165
family unit, isolation from, 95
Fawcett, Henry, 47
FCAMHS (Forensic Child and Adolescent Mental
    Health Services), 291
feminist themes, 16–18
femme fatales, 177
Ferenczi, Sandor, 163
financial aspects
    intellectual disability, 111
    maternal mental illness, 98
    motherhood, 95
    old age, 183
First World War, 28–30
fish oils, 237–8
Five Year Forward View for Mental Health, 219
Fleurey, Eleonora Lilian, 46–47, 46*f*
FMSF (False Memory Syndrome Foundation), 165
folate, 238
Fonda, Jane, 178
Forensic Child and Adolescent Mental Health
    Services (FCAMHS), 291
forensic psychiatry, 289–91
forensic service patients, 66–67
formal supervision, prison, 142–3
formulation, psychiatrists, 74, 74*t*
Fosker, Hannah, 269–75
Foundation Year doctors, training in
    psychiatry, 267–8
France, gender pay gap, 13
Francis Inquiry, 21
Freud, Sigmund
    historical child sexual abuse, views on, 162,
        163, 168–9
    mother–infant relationship, 152–3
    Oedipus complex, 162, 166–7
Freyd, Jennifer, 165
Freyd, Pamela, 165
Freyd, Peter, 165
Friern Barnet Hospital
    closure of, 219–20
    Murdoch, Claire, 219–22, 222–3
    non-consensual sex as part of culture, 9–10
    Rands, Gianetta, 9–11
    ward name changes, 222–3
frontotemporal dementia (FTD), 233, 234
Fry, Elizabeth, 215
FTD (frontotemporal dementia), 233, 234

GABA (gamma amino-butyric acid) neurons, 5
Garrett Anderson, Elizabeth, 26, 27*f*, 39, 40, 45
Garrett Anderson, Louisa, 29
gender awareness, prison staff, 143

gender bias/imbalance
    Medical Schools Council (2012) report, 11
    mental health wards, 69
    secondary services, 69
gender binary, 178–9
Gender Differences in Prescribing conference, 66
Gender Discrimination Act (2005), 68
gender pay gap, 13, 65*t*
    challenges to, 13–15
    psychiatry, 260–1
    see also equal pay
gender-sensitive facilities, 66
gender-specific therapists, historical child sexual
    abuse, 169–70, 171
General Medical Council (GMC)
    Duties of a Doctor, 15, 16*b*
    establishment of, 25
    women, acceptance of, 43
George, Charles, 281
Gerada, Claire, 68, 78*b*
Germany, gender pay gap, 13
Gibbs, Amy, 208
Gilligan, Carol, 14
Glaugeaud-Freudenthal, Nine, 99
Glover, Tyrone, 248
GMC *see* General Medical Council (GMC)
Godlee, Fiona, 34
Goldberg, David, 289
Goodmayes Hospital, 189
Graham, Nori, 189–201, 191*f*, 198*f*, 226
    career, 190–5
    challenges, 199
    elderly mentally ill care home provisions, 199–200
    family issues, 194
    key figures, 190–2
    old age psychiatry, 192
    opportunities for women doctors, 194
    recruitment issues, 193
    retirement, 200
    skills for change, 198
    voluntary organizations, 199
Graham, Philip, 190
Great Ormond Street Hospital, 105, 106
Greeks, wickedness, 136–7
Green Allison, Helen, 122–4, 122*f*, 123*f*
    career, 122–3
Greenfields, Marilyn, 195*f*
Grogan, Amelia, 47
Gurland, Archie, 190
Gurney, Russell, 27

Hamilton, James, 99
Harrington, Richard, 291
Haslam, Michael, 10
HCSA *see* historical child sexual abuse (HCSA)
Health and Social Act (2012), 293
Health for Wealth, 80*t*
health problems, psychiatry, 258–60
Helen Allison School, 123, 123*f*
Henderson, Jane B, 47
Henry-Gutt, Rita, 33
Her Majesty Prison Holloway, 134
    closure of, 143
Her Majesty's Prison Manchester
    (Strangeways), 289

Herman, Judith, 164
hidden learning, 21–22
Hidden Learning (McKay Knight), 21*f*
High Roads Hospital, Leeds, 282–3
Hindley, Myra, 144
historical aspects, 25–37
    First World War, 28–30
    parity, fight for, 30–31
    post-Second World War, 32–35
    qualifications, 25–28
    Second World War, 32
    between wars, 31–32
historical child sexual abuse (HCSA), 161–75
    acknowledgement of, 165
    case study, 170–1
    development, course of, 162
    effects of, 161–2
    gender-specific therapists, 169–70, 171
    historical perspectives, 161–6
    large scale population studies, 164
    mothers' role in, 166–9
    psychiatric illness and, 165–6
    publications, 163–4
    traumatic memory, 163
    see also childhood abuse
Hockey, Lisbeth, 230*f*
    career, 231
    life of, 230
    principles of, 231
    see also Altschul, Annie
Hodgeson, Helen, 209
Hollins, Sheila, 114–15, 114*f*, 269
Hollyman, Julie, 58
Hood, Alexander, 32
Horder, John, 190
hormonal changes, barriers to work as, 42
hospital admission, intellectual disability, 112
hospital closures, 223–4
humanistic therapies, 84*b*
human rights, intellectual disability, 116
hyperglycaemia, 239
hypertension, 236*t*, 237
hypothyroidism, 182

ID *see* intellectual disability (ID)
illness, evil *vs.*, 135–6
IMHAs (Independent Mental Health Advocates), 10
Improving Working Lives initiative, Department of
    Health, 60, 62
Independent Mental Health Advocates (IMHAs), 10
Inglis, Elsie, 29–30, 29*f*
insight oriented therapy, 84*b*
Institute of Psychiatry, Psychology and
    Neuroscience (IoPPN), 67
intellectual disability (ID), 109–21
    academic careers in, 116
    care for, 117–18
    clinical leadership roles, 113
    definition, 111
    diagnosis and assessment, 109–10
    future work, 116–17
    hospital admission, 112
    human rights, 116
    mental health, 111–12
    motherhood in, 118–19

pharmacological treatments, 112
physical health, 111–12
psychiatrist's role, 112
psychiatry in as career, 119
research, 113–15
teaching and training, 116
treatment options, 112
International Classification of Diseases (ICD-10)
    (1992), 77*b*
International Classification of Diseases (ICD-11), 166
interpersonal therapy (IPT), 84*b*
intimacy, old age, 183–4
IoPPN (Institute of Psychiatry, Psychology and
    Neuroscience), 67
IPT (interpersonal therapy), 84*b*
Irish College of Physicians, 27
Irish orphanages, 17
isolation from family unit in motherhood, 95

Jagannadhan, Annie B, 47
Jex-Blake, Sophia, 25–26, 26*f*, 27–28, 43
job-share
    refusal of, 58
    see also part-time working
Job Share Register, 59
Jones, Mabel, 50
Julius Caesar (Shakespere), 178
Jung, Carl, 182
Junior Doctors
    contract in psychiatry, 260–1
    Rands, Gianetta, 7–8

Kemp, Norah, 47
Keogh, Alfred, 30
Kerr–Haslam Inquiry (2005), 10
Kerr, William, 10
King's and Queen's College of Physicians of Ireland
    (KQCPI), 43
King's College, London, Institute of Psychiatry,
    Psychology and Neuroscience, 67
Kinsey, Alfred, 164
Klein, Melanie, 153, 154
Knowle Hospital, 282
Kohen, Dora, 61, 65
Kouao, Marie-Therese, 138
KQCPI (King's and Queen's College of Physicians
    of Ireland), 43
Kumar, Channi, 99
Kumar, Manoj, 286*f*

Lady Chichester Hospital, 50–51, 50*f*, 51*f*
Lady Margaret Hall (Oxford)
    Green Allison, Helen, 122
    Rands, Gianetta, 4
large scale population studies, historical child
    sexual abuse, 164
Lawrie, Jean, 32
Laycock, Thomas, 43
leadership
    qualities of, 293–4
    underrepresentation of women, 268
LEA (Local Education Authority) Grants, 7
learning disability *see* intellectual disability (ID)
Less Than Full-Time Training (LTFT), 64
Levin, Enid, 193

Licentiate of the Society of Apothecaries, 26
life line, 80–81
life-sustaining treatment, stopping of, 245–6
   see also do-not-attempt-resuscitation
      (DNAR) orders
Lindsay, James Murray, 46
literature review, Women's Mental Health Unit
   provision, 130–1
Little House on the Prairie, 94
Little Women, 94
Local Education Authority (LEA) Grants, 7
London School of Medicine for Women, 27
   see also Royal Free Hospital (RFH)
long-stay wards, 207–8
   staff practices, 211
Lovett, Kate, 286
low educational achievement, 236*t*
LSD (lysergic acid diethylamide) therapy, 222–3
LTFT (Less Than Full-Time Training), 64
lysergic acid diethylamide (LSD) therapy, 222–3

Magistrates and Crown Court Services, children
   and adolescent forensic psychiatry, 291
Mahapatra, Sasi, 283
Making Part-time Work, Medical Women's
   Federation, 62
management, prisons, 142
Mann, Anthony, 190, 193
Manning, Carl, 138
MAOI (monoamine oxidase inhibitors), 83*t*
Marcé, Louis Victor, 91
Marcé Society, 99
marriage, perception as barrier to career, 33
Marshall, Jane, 60, 64
Mason, Fiona, 62, 66–67
Masson, Jeffrey, 162–3
maternal function *see* motherhood
Maternal Mental Health Alliance (MMHA), 101
maternal mental illness, 91–103
   detection of, 96–97
   historical cases, 91, 92*f*
   impact of, 98–99
   medication, 97
   modern perinatal psychiatry, 99–101
   psychiatric mother and baby units, 93
   risk of violence, 98–99
   social services, fear of, 97
   specialist services need, 97–98
maternity leave, psychiatry, 260–1
Maudsley–Garrett Anderson debate, 39–49
Maudsley, Henry, 39, 40*f*, 48
   women, attitudes to, 42–43
MBU (Mother and Baby Inpatient Unit)
   (Nottingham), 93
McDonald, Liz, 100
McKay Knight, Sophie, 21*f*
McKim Thompson, Ian, 34
media coverage, historical child sexual abuse, 164
Medical Act (1878), 26
Medical Act (1978), 33
Medical Act (Qualifications) Bill (1876), 27
medical model, depression management, 81–82
medical psychotherapists
   diagnostic function, 152
   Mental Health Trust, 151–2

Medical Schools Council (2012) report, 11
Medical Training Application Service (MTAS), 11
Medical Women's Federation (MWF), 30*b*, 64
   foundation (1917), 28
   Making Part-time Work, 62
   Role Model Report, 268
   Role Models, 267
   Second World War, 32
   between the wars, 31
medications *see* pharmaceuticals/medications
Medico-Psychological Association (MPA)
   Boyle, Helen, 50–51
   Certificate in Psychological Medicine, 44
   woman president, 47
   women, attitudes to, 39, 42–43, 43–44
   women membership, 46–47
Mediterranean diet, 238–9
melatonergic antidepressants, 83*t*
Mellanby, Jane, 5
Member of the Royal College of General
   Practitioners (MRCGP), 9
Member of the Royal College of Psychiatrists
   (MRCPsych), 119
   Burn, Wendy, 282
Mencap, 118
Mental Capacity Act (2005), 18, 112
   right to life *vs.* self-determination, 247–8, 251
mental health
   disorder prevalence, 253
   doctors of, 78–79*b*
   epidemiology, 140
   gender discrimination in wards, 69
Mental Health Act (1983)
   capacity and right to life, 245
   right to life *vs.* self-determination, 251
   training in, 221
Mental Health Assessors, 87
Mental Health Foundation Trusts, Women's Mental
   Health Unit provision, 131
Mental Health Trust (MHT), 149
   medical psychotherapists, 151–2
mentoring, psychiatry, 260
MHT *see* Mental Health Trust (MHT)
mild cognitive impairment, 234
Miller, Jonathan, 195, 195*f*, 197
Miller, Noreen, 196
MIND diet study, 238–9
MMC (Modernising Medial Careers), 285
MMHA (Maternal Mental Health Alliance), 101
modern ageing, 181–3
Modernising Medial Careers (MMC), 285
Modernising Medical Careers initiative, 64
Moffett, Elizabeth Jane, 47
monoamine oxidase inhibitors (MAOI), 83*t*
mood charts, 80–81
mood (affective) disorders, 77*b*
Moodscope, 80–81
Moral Welfare, 164
Morris, Jerry, 190–1
Mother and Baby Inpatient Unit (MBU)
   (Nottingham), 93
motherhood, 149–60, 150*f*
   absence in historical child sexual abuse, 167
   behaviour, symptoms, meanings, 159–60
   case study, 153–5, 158–9

challenges of, 95
child rejection, 155–6
cultural perceptions, 93–95, 94f
identity development, 149–50
intellectual disability in, 118–19
mental illness *see* maternal mental illness
perception as barrier, 33
psychiatric services, 158–9
psychoanalytic theory, 152–3
risk-management panel, 156–8
transference, 150, 158–9
Mothers and Babies: Reducing Risk through
    Audits and Confidential Enquiries
    (MBRRACE-UK), 98
Mott, Frederick, 50
Mounty, Jane, 58
MPA *see* Medico-Psychological Association (MPA)
MRCGP (Member of the Royal College of General
    Practitioners), 9
MRCPsych *see* Member of the Royal College of
    Psychiatrists (MRCPsych)
MTAS (Medical Training Application Service), 11
multi-professional teams, maternal mental
    illness, 97–98
Murdoch, Claire, 219–28
    21st century, 227–8
    changing principles of care and, 221
    Harry case study, 222
    training, 221
Murphy, Elaine, v, 191f
Murray, Flora, 29
Murray, Robin, 73
Murrell, Christine, 31–32
MWF *see* Medical Women's Federation (MWF)
My Small but Significant Body of Work (Wills), 56
myxoedema madness, 182

Napsbury Hospital, 105
NaSSA (noradrenergic and specific
    serotonergic antidepressants), 83t
National approval Scheme PM79 (Part III), 58–59
National Audit on Violence, 130
National Health Service (NHS)
    equal pay study (1947), 32
    ombudsman establishment, 213
    part-time working, 59
    Practitioner Health Programme, 80t
    primary care service, 3
    single-sex wards in 1990s, 125
National Institute for Health and Care
    Excellence (NICE)
    intellectual disability guidelines, 116–17
    medication for maternal mental illness, 97
    start of (1999), 18
National Institute for Mental Health in England
    (NIMHE), 66
National Programme Board for Gender Equality on
    Women's Mental Health, 67
Newhouse, Muriel, 32
NHS *see* National Health Service (NHS)
NICE *see* National Institute for Health and Care
    Excellence (NICE)
Nielsen, Dennis, 144
Nightingale, Florence, 215
Nightingale House, 190

NIMHE (National Institute for Mental Health in
    England), 66
Noman, Conolly, 46
non-consensual sex, 6–7, 7–8
    Friern Hospital, as part of culture, 9–10
noradrenergic and specific serotonergic
    antidepressants (NaSSA), 83t
normal functions, pathologizing of, 16–17

Oates, Margaret, 93, 98
obesity, 236t, 239
obsessive compulsive disorder (OCD), 98
occupational therapists (OTs), 82
OCD (obsessive compulsive disorder), 98
Oedipus complex, 162, 166–7
Olbtich, Oscar, 202
old age, 177–88
    care by relatives, 183
    case study, 181, 185
    cosmetic surgery, 183
    cultural differences, 183
    drug addiction, 182
    fables about, 179
    financial constraints, 183
    intimacy, 183–4
    mental illness care home provision, 199–200
    modern ageing, 181–3
    psychological changes, 179–81
    sexuality, 183–4
    terminology change, 182
old age psychiatry, 192
One Flew Over the Cuckoo's Nest, 75b
OOPE (out-of-programme experience), 119
Oppenheimer, Catherine, 59
Orange, Margaret, 47
Orestes, 136
The Other Woman in the Wardrobe (Wills), 298
OTs (occupational therapists), 82
out-of-programme experience (OOPE), 119

Paedophile Information Exchange (PIE), 16
PALS (Patient Advice and Liaison Service), 10
PAR (population attributable risk),
    dementia, 236
part-time working, 59
    Advisory Service (1962), 32
    need reduction, 68b
    see also job-share
The Pathology of Mind (Maudsley), 48
Patient Advice and Liaison Service (PALS), 10
patient-led decision making, intellectual
    disability, 112
Patient Management Problems (PMPs), 60–61
patients
    current issues, 69
    gender ratio, 66
    notes, 221
    resuscitation, 18
Pearson Report, 273
Pechey, Edith, 27, 43
Pemberton, Max, 73
Pendleton's rules, 8
perinatal services
    losses of, 65t
    provision of, 99

personality disorders, historical child sexual abuse, 169
person-centred therapy, 84*b*
PFIs (Private Finance Initiatives), 12–13
pharmaceuticals/medications
  access to, 78–79*b*
  depression management, 82, 83*b*, 83*t*
  maternal mental illness, 97
PHP (Practitioner Health Programme), 65
phrenological bust, 110*f*
physical inactivity, dementia risk, 236*t*, 240–1
physical perfection, ageing effects, 181–2
PICUs (psychiatric intensive care units), 60
PIE (Paedophile Information Exchange), 16
plagiarism, Maudsley, 41–42
PMPs (Patient Management Problems), 60–61
Polson, George, 211
population attributable risk (PAR), dementia, 236
Postnatal Special Interest Group, 66
post-traumatic stress disorder (PTSD), 166
Powick Hospital, malpractice in, 213
Practical Psychiatry of Old Age (Wattis), 283
Practitioner Health Programme (PHP), 65
Prince, Martin, 198
prison, 135–47
  case study, 141–2
  challenge of, 141–2
  child murder, 143–4
  numbers and problems, 139–40
  psychiatry/psychology limitations, 144
  risks and opportunities, 142–3
  self-harm rates, 140
  social backgrounds, 140
Private Finance Initiatives (PFIs), 12–13
protection, Women's Mental Health Units, 129
PSS (Psychiatrists' Support Service), 65, 80*t*
psychiatric intensive care units (PICUs), 60
psychiatric mother and baby units, 93, 97
psychiatric services, motherhood, 158–9
psychiatrists
  academic development of, 60–61
  definition, 74
  formulation, 74, 74*t*
  media images, 257
  socio-political context, 294–5
  training and development, 73–74
Psychiatrists' Support Service (PSS), 65, 80*t*
psychiatry, 253–4, 253–63
  barriers to entry, 254–5
  emotional impact, 259
  empathic ability, 255–6
  gender pay gap, 260–1
  health problems, 258–60
  Junior Doctor contract, 260–1
  maternity leave, 260–1
  mentoring, 260
  sexism, 256–7, 256*f*
  stalking, 258
  training, 11–13
  see also training
  violence, 257–8
psychoanalytic theory, motherhood, 152–3
psychodynamic therapy, 84*b*
psychological changes, old age, 179–81

psychotherapy
  depression management, 82, 84*b*
  myths around, 180–1
PTSD (post-traumatic stress disorder), 166

qualifications, historical aspects, 25–28
Queens' University of Ireland, 27

Ramsay, Rosalind, 58
Ramsey, Mabel, 31
randomized controlled trial (RCT), 235
Rands, Gianetta, 3–24
Rape Prosecution Working Party, 67
RCPsych *see* Royal College of Psychiatrists (RCPsych)
RCT (randomized controlled trial), 235
recovery
  definitions of, 86–87*b*
  dimensions of, 87*b*
Recovery Colleges, 219
recruitment issues, 193
recurrent unipolar depression, 76, 77*b*
reflective space, prison, 142
Regional Health Boards (RHBs), 209
Registered Mental Nurse (RMN)
  opportunities for, 222–3
  training, 221
Remembering, repeating and working through (Freud), 163
research
  Bailey, Sue, 292
  intellectual disability, 113, 115
  under-recognised women's role, 178
retirement, 87–88
  life changes, 179
  Rands, Gianetta, 20–22
reversible monoamine oxidase inhibitors (RIMA), 83*t*
RFH *see* Royal Free Hospital (RFH)
RFHSM (Royal Free Hospital School of Medicine), 5–7
RHBs (Regional Health Boards), 209
Rhodes Farm Clinic, 106
right to life, self-determination *vs.* in anorexia, 246–9
RIMA (reversible monoamine oxidase inhibitors), 83*t*
Rimmer, Elizabeth, 197
The Rising Tide, 192
risk-management panel, motherhood, 156–8
RMBF (Royal Medical Benevolent Fund), 80*t*
RMN *see* Registered Mental Nurse (RMN)
Robb, Barbara, 205–18, 206*f*, 207*f*
  AEGIS (Aid for the Elderly in Government Institutions), 209
  family, 206–7
  long-stay wards, work against, 207–9
  malpractice in other areas, 213
Roberts, Julian, 283
Robertson, Mary, 60
Robinson, Kenneth, 32, 208, 212
Robinson, W M, 31
Role Model Report, Medical Women's Federation, 268
Rolph, C H, 209, 212
Rowe, Phyllis, 209

Roxan, David, 213
Royal Army Medical Corps, 29
Royal College of Nursing, 57
Royal College of Psychiatrists (RCPsych), 11
    Bailey, Sue, 293
    Caldicott, Fiona, 53
    Clinical Assessment of Skills and
        Competencies, 268–9
    membership examination, 268–9, 268b
    membership of see Member of the Royal College
        of Psychiatrists (MRCPsych)
    recovery definitions, 86b
    supervisors, 269, 269b
    see also Women's Mental Health Special Interest
        Group (WMHSIG)
Royal Free Hospital (RFH)
    admittance of women, 7, 43
    Black, Dora, 105
    Murdoch, Claire, 222, 225
    see also London School of Medicine for Women
Royal Free Hospital School of Medicine
    (RFHSM), 5–7
Royal Free Psychiatry Senior Houser Officer (SHO), 9
Royal Medical Benevolent Fund (RMBF), 80t
Royal South Hampshire Hospital, 282
Russell, Gerald, 190, 193

SAC (Society for Autistic Children), 122
Safeguarding Vulnerable Groups Act (2006), 16
safety, Women's Mental Health Unit provision, 130
Salem witch trials, 137–8
Sans Everything: A Case to Answer (Robb),
    205, 209–10
Scott Calder, Jane, 32
Scottish Women's Hospitals (SWH), 30, 31
secondary services, gender bias, 69
Second World War, 32
selective serotonin reuptake inhibitors (SSRIs), 83t
self-determination, right to life vs. in
    anorexia, 246–9
self-harm rates, prison, 140
senior academic roles, underrepresentation of
    women, 268
Senior House Officers (SHOs), 74
serotonin and noradrenalin reuptake inhibitors
    (SNRIs), 83t
Sewall. Lucy, 25
Sex Discrimination Act (1975), 3
Sex in Mind and Education (Maudsley), 40–41
sexism
    psychiatry in, 254, 256–7, 256f
    Royal Free Hospital School of Medicine, 5–7
sexual harassment, 65t
sexuality, old age, 183–4
sexually transmitted diseases, old age, 183
sexual molestation claims, psychosis as, 9–10
Shared Parental Leave (SPL) scheme, 95
shared socializing, prison, 142–3
Sheffield Women in Medicine Group, 11
Shooter, Mike, 293
SHOs (Senior House Officers), 74
Shove, Edith, 27
Sick Doctors Trust, 80t
Silverston, Rosalie, 33
Sims, Andrew, 283

single mothers, 95
Slattery, Zoe, 191f
Slaughter, Anne-Marie, 14–15
SNRIs (serotonin and noradrenalin reuptake
    inhibitors), 83t
social backgrounds, prison, 140
social media
    motherhood, perception of, 94–95
    old age, 183
social services, removal of children, 97
Society for Autistic Children (SAC), 122
socio-political context, psychiatrists, 294–5
Somerville College (Oxford), 189
Southampton General Hospital, 280–1
Southampton Medical School, 280
South Ockendon Hospital (Essex), malpractice
    in, 213
SPL (Shared Parental Leave) scheme, 95
Spotlight, 226
SSRIs (selective serotonin reuptake inhibitors), 83t
staff, community- vs. hospital-Women's Mental
    Health Units, 128–9, 128b
stalking, psychiatry, 258
Stephenson, Terence, 273
St George's Hospital (London), 113
St. John Ambulance Brigade, 279
Stobart, Mabel St Clair, 28–29, 28f
Strangeways (Her Majesty's Prison
    Manchester), 289
Strangham. Lucia, 47
suffragettes, 4, 4f
supervisors, Royal College of Psychiatrists,
    269, 269b
support groups, depression management, 84
Survey of Adult Carers in England
    (NHS Digital 2012–13), 117–18
Sutcliffe, Peter, 144
Swanson, Catherine, 32
SWH (Scottish Women's Hospitals), 30, 31
symptoms, motherhood in, 159–60
Symptoms in the Mind: Textbook of Descriptive
    Psychopathology (Sims), 283
syndrome, 233
systemic therapies, 84b
systolic hypertension, 237

Taws, Elizabeth, 191f
Taylor, Joanne, 135
TCAs (tricyclic antidepressants), 83t
teaching, intellectual disability, 116
team working, 254–5
terminology change, old age, 182
Thatcher, Margaret, 12–13, 220–1
The Memory Wars (Crews), 165
Time Unveiling Truth (Detroy), 6–7, 6f
tobacco smoking, 236t, 240
Tormes, Yvonne, 168
TPD (Training Programme Director), 11–12
trainers, 268–76
    advantages for women, 267
    challenges to, 271–3
    development of, 271
    female role models, 274
    future work, 275
    personal perspective, 269–75

training
  flexibility in, 58
  intellectual disability, 116
  national changes, 64
  nineteenth century, 43
Training Programme Director (TPD), 11–12
transference, motherhood, 150, 158–9
trans people, 125–6
trauma, case study, 153–5
traumatic memory, historical child sexual
  abuse, 163
treatment issues, Women's Mental Health Unit
  provision, 130
Treves, Frederick, 28–29
tricyclic antidepressants (TCAs), 83*t*
Tuke, Batty, 43
Tuke, Harrington, 43

Understanding Alzheimer's Disease and Other
  Dementias (Graham & Warner), 190
Underwager, Ralph, 165
unequal pay *see* gender pay gap
United States (US), women, attitudes to, 45
University College Hospital (London)
  Graham, Nori, 189
  Woodford-Williams, Eluned, 202
University of Birmingham, 105
University of Utah Medical School, 105–6

vagina dentata, 177
vascular dementia, 233, 234
violence
  criminal acts, 140
  psychiatry, 257–8
VITACOG study, 238
vitamin B12, 238
vitamin C, 237
vitamin E, 237
Voisin, Maria, 99
Voluntary Aid Detachment, 206*f*
voting rights, 31

WAAC (Women's Army Auxilliary Corps), 30–31
Wakefield, Hollinda, 165
Walker, Joan, 32
Walter, Harriet, 178
Warner, James, 190
Waters, Eric, 60
Waterstone, Jane, 44–45, 44*f*, 47
Wattis, John, 283
West, Rosemary, 144
WHC (Women's Hospital Corps), 29
When Father Kills Mother (Black), 106*f*
Whitehead, Tony, 209
Whittingham Hospital (Lancashire), 213
WHO *see* World Health Organization (WHO)
wickedness, 136–8, 177
Wilcock, Gordon, 195
Wills, Emily, 2, 56, 148, 229, 264, 298
WIM (Women in Medicine), 64

Wisner, Katherine, 99
WIST (Women in Surgical Training), 64
witches, 14, 14*f*, 137–8, 177–8
WMHSIG *see* Women's Mental Health Special
  Interest Group (WMHSIG)
WMHUs *see* Women's Mental Health Units
  (WMHUs)
Women Doctors: Making a Difference (2009), 34
Women in Medicine (WIM), 64
Women in Mind networking, 68
Women in Psychiatry Special Interest Group
  (WIPSIG) *see* Women's Mental Health Special
  Interest Group (WMHSIG)
Women in Surgical Training (WIST), 64
Women in the Criminal Justice System Reference
  Group, 67
Women's Army Auxilliary Corps (WAAC), 30–31
Women's Hospital Corps (WHC), 29
Women's Mental Health: Into the Mainstream
  (2002), 66
Women's Mental Health Special Interest Group
  (WMHSIG), 57–72, 266
  academic development of women, 60–61
  beginning of, 58–59
  data, 61
  discrimination in practice, 64–65, 65*t*
  early years, 59–60
  future work, 67
  gender equality work, 62
  international view, 69
  mental health of women service users, 65–66
  mission statement, 62, 63*b*
  national changes to training, 64
  national interest in careers, 62–64
  research topics/publications, 60*t*, 61
  support for psychiatrists, 65
  tenth anniversary (July 2005), 61, 62*b*
Women's Mental Health Units (WMHUs), 125–33
  case history, 127*b*, 128*b*
  community *vs.* hospital wards, 126–9
  evidence for, 129
  provision challenges, 130–1
Women's National Service League, 28
Woodford-Williams, Eluned, 202–3, 202*f*
working hours, 58–59
work–life balance, 68–69
  psychiatry, 253
World Health Organization (WHO)
  maternal mental illness, 93
  mood (affective) disorders, 77*b*
  Women's Mental Health Special Interest Group,
    support for, 69
World in Action, malpractice in hospitals, 213
Wye Valley NHS Trust v B (2015), 251–2

Yorkshire Specialist Registrar Training Scheme in
  Old Age Psychiatry, 285
youth justice system, 291

Zito, Johnathan, 226